The mind and
its discontents

International Perspectives in Philosophy and Psychiatry

Series editors: Bill (K.W.M.) Fulford, Katherine Morris, John Z Sadler, and Giovanni Stanghellini

Volumes in the series:

Mind, Meaning, and Mental Disorder
Bolton and Hill

What is Mental Disorder?
Bolton

Postpsychiatry
Bracken and Thomas

Philosophy, Psychoanalysis and the A-rational Mind
Brakel

The Philosophical Understanding of Schizophrenia
Chung, Fulford, and Graham (ed.)

Nature and Narrative: An Introduction to the New Philosophy of Psychiatry
Fulford, Morris, Sadler, and Stanghellini

The Oxford Textbook of Philosophy and Psychiatry
Fulford, Thornton, and Graham

The Mind and its Discontents
Gillett

Dementia: Mind, Meaning and the Person
Hughes, Louw, and Sabat

Talking Cures and Placebo Effects
Jopling

Schizophrenia and the Fate of the Self
Lysaker and Lysaker

Body-subjects and Disordered Minds
Matthews

Rationality and Compulsion: Applying Action Theory to Psychiatry
Nordenfelt

Philosophical Perspectives on Psychiatry and Technology
Phillips (ed)

The Metaphor of Mental Illness
Pickering

Trauma, Truth, and Reconciliation: Healing Damaged Relationships
Potter (ed)

The Philosophy of Psychiatry: A Companion
Radden

Feelings of Being
Ratcliffe

Values and Psychiatric Diagnosis
Sadler

Disembodied Spirits and Deanimated Bodies: The Psychopathology of Common Sense
Stanghellini

Essential Philosophy of Psychiatry
Thornton

Empirical Ethics in Psychiatry
Widdershoven, McMillan, Hope and Van der Scheer (eds)

Forthcoming volumes in the series:

Psychiatry of Cognitive Neuroscience
Broome and Bortolotti (eds)

Mapping the Edges and the In-between
Potter

The mind and its discontents

SECOND EDITION

Grant Gillett
Professor of Medical Ethics,
Dunedin Hospital and Otago Bioethics Centre,
University of Otago Medical School,
Dunedin,
New Zealand

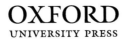

OXFORD
UNIVERSITY PRESS

OXFORD

UNIVERSITY PRESS

Great Clarendon Street, Oxford OX2 6DP

Oxford University Press is a department of the University of Oxford.
It furthers the University's objective of excellence in research, scholarship,
and education by publishing worldwide in

Oxford New York

Auckland Cape Town Dar es Salaam Hong Kong Karachi
Kuala Lumpur Madrid Melbourne Mexico City Nairobi
New Delhi Shanghai Taipei Toronto

With offices in

Argentina Austria Brazil Chile Czech Republic France Greece
Guatemala Hungary Italy Japan Poland Portugal Singapore
South Korea Switzerland Thailand Turkey Ukraine Vietnam

Oxford is a registered trade mark of Oxford University Press
in the UK and in certain other countries

Published in the United States
by Oxford University Press Inc., New York

© Oxford University Press, 2009

British Library Cataloguing in Publication Data

Data available

Library of Congress Cataloging in Publication Data

Data available

Typeset in Minion by Cepha Imaging Private Ltd., Bangalore, India
Printed in Great Britain
on acid-free paper by
CPI Anthony Rowe, Chippenham, Wiltshire

ISBN 978-0-19-923-7548 (Pbk.)

10 9 8 7 6 5 4 3 2 1

Contents

Acknowledgements

First edition

As I review the tortuous path that has led to the present work, the late Kathy Wilkes stands out as the most formative philosophical force in my life. She is responsible for beginning me on the voyage of discovery that has, over the last 12 years, culminated in my writing this, and throughout that journey, things that she said to me have been gradually understood and incorporated into my own work. In many ways, the memory of Oxford broods over the work as it has always treated me well with an abundance of keen and penetrating minds and an overall charity of academic companionship highly stimulating to restless and impatient souls such as myself. Figures who stand out from that period include John and Hilary Spanos, two dear friends and very sharp minds, and Michael Lockwood, a constant source of curly questions and sound intuitions.

Bill Fulford has always pushed me along and been accommodating and encouraging to fledgling efforts in the philosophy of psychiatry, but I am not alone in owing him a great deal for my development in this area. Other thinkers who have stimulated, indulged, discussed their own work, and lavished time on me include Eric Matthews from Aberdeen, Stuart Youngner from Cleveland, Paul Mullen from Melbourne, and Alastair Hannay from Oslo, who played a very important role in my development as a thinker by working with some fairly unformed material and seeing potential in it, which must, in retrospect, have been fairly well hidden.

Tom and Cynthia Murray are very special friends: their house was a site where much of this was written, and Tom's Bioethics Center at CWRU was a place where many of the ideas were 'noised abroad' and benefited from input and discussion by his gifted students particularly Nancy Johnson, Felix Pesa, Carol Donley, Melissa Cappeart, and Jason Schroeder. They have my special thanks for contributing so much to the polishing of the ideas so that they were fit to appear in the book. Warren and Glen Brookbanks are stalwart friends and an inspiration to me for years, and it was Glen who contributed the delightful Vicar story in Chapter 13.

Carl Elliot was a colleague at a crucial time in developing these ideas and we remain good friends, much to my benefit, ever since. In the last few years, John MacMillan has pulled me through the philosophical hoops required to iron out difficult points in the analysis and himself thrashed out many of the Husserlian and phenomenological analyses in the book. Rachel Gillett, my daughter, has helped me with both bibliographical research and intelligent discussion of many themes. Shirley Gillett, my partner, has been a constant source of new ideas, which I have always shamelessly appropriated; she is one of the most honest and insightful academics that I have ever worked with. Cathy Mason and Mark, her partner, were good for penetrating discussions of many of the key ideas and providing encouragement to carry on. A further special friend who I get to see far less often than I would like but whose clarity of thought is a model for me is Olaf Gjeldsvik in Oslo.

Other groups and friends have heard and responded to chapters and excerpts, including The Psychiatry and Philosophy Group at Otago, in particular Chris Wiseley, Sarah Romans, Trevor Siverstone, Richard Mullen, David Clarke (Monash University), Neil Pickering, and John Dawson. The Philosophy Department at Otago has always been an interested group, despite their almost unanimous disdain for continental philosophy, and some of my sharpest critics and most demanding interrogators are there. Special thanks must go to Paul Griffiths, Colin Cheyne, Alan Musgrove, Andrew Moore, Charles Pigden, and David Ward. The Philosophy Departments at Canterbury University, Massey University, Newcastle University, Brown University, and Auckland University have also heard and improved various bits. Others have all made some contribution including Dewey DuCharme and Priscilla Szekeles (special thanks for Aristotle on dreaming) of Akron University, Michael Schwarz of Cleveland University Hospitals, Jack Copeland and Derek Brown both of Canterbury University (Christchurch, NZ), Lyn Stevenson of the Professional Ethics Program at Harvard and a fellow student from graduate days in Oxford, and Denise Russell of Sydney University.

Friends and colleagues at Otago University are too generous to overlook and have all been a great source of commentary and development of my ideas: they include Mark Olssen, John Morss, Judith MacFarlane, Barbara Nicholas, Lynley Anderson, Robin Hankey, and Paul Smith.

The book is dedicated to my, superficially, most crazy daughter Lizzie, because of her quickness of wit, insight into human nature, and fascination with all things psychological (inherited from her mother). She is disarmingly open in her affection to her friends and those who know her, highly organized in her personal life, great fun to be with, and a very shrewd commentator on all my foibles and failings.

This one's for you Lizzie.

Acknowledgements

Second edition

The main contributions to this edition have been made by my excellent students in Roots of Postmodernism and Contemporary Continental Philosophy at the University of Otago. Those who have helped me develop my thinking for that course, including Gilbert May, Catherine Dale, Tim Mehigan, and several members of our English Department, have all contributed to the new emphases and moments of scholarship to be found in the second edition. In addition, a small and supportive group of enthusiasts including John McMillan, Carl Elliot, Neil Pickering, Maren Marijke Frerichs, Kati Taghavi, Sheila Bloomer, Kristen Steslow, Joshua Ben, and Flora Huang have participated in a discussion group of key passages of *The Mind and Its Discontents* to help me improve it. Bits of the new edition have benefited greatly from discussions at The University of Toronto, University of British Columbia, University of Hull Department of Philosophy and of course, the international network of philosophy and psychiatry conferences and meetings. This one is still for you Lizzie!

Introduction

The liberty of the individual is no gift of civilization. It was greatest before there was any civilization, though then, it is true, it had for the most part no value, since the individual was scarcely in a position to defend it. The development of civilization imposes restrictions on it, and justice demands that no one shall escape those restrictions. What makes itself felt in a human community as a desire for freedom may be their revolt against some existing injustice, and so may prove favourable to a further development of civilization; it may remain compatible with civilization. But it may also spring from the remains of their original personality, which is still untamed by civilization and may thus become the basis in them of hostility to civilization. The urge for freedom, therefore, is directed against particular forms and demands of civilization or against civilization altogether. It does not seem as though any influence could induce a man to change his nature into a termite's. No doubt he will always defend his claim to individual liberty against the will of the group. A good part of the struggles of mankind centre round the single task of finding an expedient accommodation—one, that is, that will bring happiness—between this claim of the individual and the cultural claims of the group; and one of the problems that touches the fate of humanity is whether such an accommodation can be reached by means of some particular form of civilization or whether this conflict is irreconcilable.

Sigmund Freud (1930/1985)

Freud believed in a version of the romantic myth of the noble savage. Man (the gender is important) was the master of nature with elemental drives and desires intrinsic to his nature and largely a heritage of his biological or evolutionary genesis. In this guise, he is transformed at one level by civilization but at a deeper level he retains the primitive dispositions barely held in check by a veneer of culture. As an elemental, romantic man, he is constrained by the straitjacket (or rather 'corsets') of civilization and attempts to assert his freedom and express his essential nature.

This is an appealing and popular picture. It informs many works of pop culture and psychology, but more importantly, it informs much of contemporary psychology as is evident in the fact that psychologists often try to study behaviour in human beings by using animal models and assuming that basic mental mechanisms are preserved fundamentally intact and only modified in their function by the imposition of social and cultural variables.

I believe this picture to be seriously flawed and will develop an alternative drawing on clinical psychiatry but also contemporary philosophy of mind and post-structural thought that sees a human being as a problematic being who straddles the worlds of meaning and actuality. As such he or she brings meaning to bear on a contingent and situated life that requires one to adapt to a life-world into which one is thrown at a certain point and which provides resources for the skills and equipment that one needs to get by and construct a livable life story.

This book discusses themes and controversies in psychiatry and draws out their philosophical significance for our conception of the human psyche (or soul). There is an increasing body of writing on philosophy and psychiatry and a journal (*Philosophy, Psychiatry, and Psychology*) aimed at the growing international community of scholars writing and thinking in this area. In the present work, I develop and extend my own approach to the philosophy of mind and psychiatry to elucidate the nature of phenomena involving disorders of thought and action. The approach is derived from Wittgenstein in that it focuses on rules and meaning as the essence of mental content but goes further to engage with phenomenology and post-structuralist discussions of human subjectivity. Its philosophical ancestry is my *Representation, Meaning, and Thought* (1992) and the underlying thesis that thought and meaning are embedded in and emerge from interpersonal activity, a milieu that is the ground for developing our normal psychological techniques of adaptation to being-in-the-world-with-others but also a source of tensions and strange anomalies. There are probably biological underpinnings for many disorders of thought but these interact in a complex way with features of context and discourse to shape the human psyche.

I will therefore develop a social and interactive account of the psyche and use it to explore a variety of clinical problems ranging from the overtly psychotic to the borderline normal. The thought that each human individual is a unique product of meaning and contingency, discourse, and biology who uses techniques developed in social and cultural settings to deal with the challenges that life throws up helps us understand not only psychiatry but also the normal workings of the psyche as observed in psychology and explored in philosophy.

Mind and personality are dynamic productions sensitive to human beliefs and attitudes, and mental explanation is a complex culturally produced phenomenon as discussed in post-structuralist approaches to the human condition. The major areas of clinical psychiatry raise interesting philosophical issues clustering around our conception of the human individual and provide a phenomenologically rich understanding of human subjectivity as an understanding of the way that the body is inscribed by a cumulative life of encounters with others.

The approach remains broadly Wittgensteinian in that it focuses on rules and meaning as the essence of mental content and intersubjectivity as a distinctive feature of human forms of life but engages more extensively with philosophers such as Heidegger, Foucault, and Lacan to explore a more nuanced approach to the development of mental life and mental disorders in response to lived experience. I will extend the idea that a human individual, even if we treat him or her as an individual who is subject to biological forces and causal influences, is a social production, and health is integrity in one's adaptation to the human life-world, not merely the absence of biological imbalance. As in the first edition, we are left with the conviction that being fully human is a mode of being existentially and ethically haunted by the spectres of mental illness.

The chapters are as follows:

(1) **Mind, brain, and psychiatry**: This chapter explicitly examines the philosophical problem of mind and brain in relation to the theoretical and diagnostic issues that arise in psychiatry and the types of explanation employed by different approaches to psychiatric disorder. The psyche is conceived to be much as Aristotle thought it to be, a mode of functioning in which meaning becomes incarnate in lived human life.

That position finesses dualism and critical scientific realism and moves us directly to an exploration of the mirror world of language and thought and the way it reflects on human beings and shapes their lives. The chapter touches on the diversity of problems encountered in clinical psychiatry with specific reference to personality disorder and psychosis and discusses Jaspers' distinction between causal and meaningful approaches to explanation but then reconceptualizes that distinction to take account of the complex entanglement of the psyche in situated, embodied human subjectivity. The chapter concludes by exposing the arguments commonly used to justify a biological approach to psychiatry.

(2) **Psychiatric categorization**: Psychiatric diagnosis is related to judgements (both descriptive and evaluative) from various social perspectives. The particular problems arising from psychiatric diagnosis including determinations of efficacy of treatment and political abuse of psychiatry reflect the complexity of those judgements and the responses of the individual to them. The chapter examines Szasz's claims concerning the myth of mental illness and Laing's focus on the interpersonal and social dimension of existential unease, arriving at a discursive naturalism that is messy in terms of traditional categories of biological or scientific realism about psychiatric disease. Structures of signification and their genealogies, expressed in the medicalization of social problems, are deconstructed in post-modern critiques of the idea of psychiatric categories and mental illness in general. A more modest scrutiny argues for a narrative conception of human identity and personality that is an enactment of metaphors and formative self-understandings of lived engagement with the world and that can be deeply maladaptive for a variety of reasons.

(3) **The treatment of aliens**: Aliens are neither people nor things, they are abject. The idea that human beings could be alienated and thus drift outside the normal bounds of moral discourse shapes the metaphysics of mental disorder in terms of abjection in relation to 'the normal human condition' and informs psychiatric classification and treatment. The contrast between objective (thing-related) and reactive (person-related) attitudes to human beings is developed by Strawson in his discussion of freedom, but is highly pertinent to psychiatric classification and treatment. I will explore the links between this idea, abjection or alienation, and Fulford's contrast between factual and evaluative aspects of clinical judgement. I will also explore the ways in which the tension between these attitudes pervades psychiatric practice and the puzzles surrounding our relations with those who are other 'by reason of insanity'.

(4) **The depths of the self**: This chapter is the key to the book in that it lays out a theory of the psyche that is critical of traditional ideas about the unconscious. Human beings are storytellers running a narrative of their own experience on the basis of their ongoing engagement with the world. The unconscious is invoked to explain gaps in that narrative, but Freud's Victorian psychic hydraulics is altogether too reifying of that which is by nature not determinate in form. Lacanian problematizations of the psyche as an imago enunciated under the name of the father are explored and linked to inscriptions on the body made by complex

historical events befalling individuals and human groups. The meaning for one's self-understanding of 'outing' the unconscious into a world of discursive engagement with others is both difficult and emancipatory and forces us to look at the selves we do not like to portray ourselves as being (and can be bound up in knots by).

These first four chapters form the foundational orientation of the book and allow the more focused clinical material to be explored and discussed with slightly different highlights from those appearing in the first edition.

(5) **Thought in disarray**: The psychotic disorders pose the problem of rationality and normality in thought and the way in which we should understand them. The norms governing thought are determined in the intersubjective context in which mental content is defined, and they create cognitive skills in an individual that are used in attunement to the world and judgements about oneself. That analysis informs an interpretation of insight, delusion, and hallucination as phenomena of importance in understanding the fundamental biological mechanisms affecting conjoint attention and social perception and their relation to phenomenological approaches to the psychoses. Correctly knowing one's place in the world is a complex cognitive attainment, not merely an immediate product of introspection, and psychotic thinkers lack the integrity of self and cognition needed for that achievement so that they display *a fortiori* many things we tend to overlook in philosophical thinking about the psyche.

(6) **The black dog and the muse**: Churchill often referred to his recurring mood problem as his 'black dog', and he is one of many gifted individuals (such as Shelley, Cowper, and Schumann) considered to have a bipolar mood disorder. The understanding of mood disorder has now shifted its focus onto biology and the genetics justifying a philosophical exploration of emotion, imagination, creative thought, and their relation to biology and meaning. That exploration is enlivened by attention to Foucault's understanding of the relations between creativity and insanity and becomes deeply relevant to the moral problems of treatment and the alleged dampening of personality, well-being, and creativity by lithium. It is also instructive in considering problems associated with genetic selection and the choices between dual selves that therapy can force on us.

(7) **Fidgets**: Attention Deficit Hyperactivity Disorder (ADHD) and the use of drugs to treat it raise significant questions about the nature of psychiatric disorder and what we do to ourselves when we medicalize life (particularly the irregularities of childhood). We therefore need to question the integrity of the diagnostic category involved and examine accusations that child psychiatry and the pharmaceutical industry together are causing an expanding and threatening medicalization of the normal problems or immaturities and experimentations or freedom of children who are exploring what it is to be new (unformed) human beings looking for information. This provokes an interesting discussion of our sociopolitical use of psychiatry and therapeutic interventions to regulate our dealings with those we are making in a situated, or our own, human image.

(8) **I and the other robots**: Childhood autism is a curious disorder in which children find it difficult to accommodate themselves to the normal social world and tend

to be unresponsive, indeed almost robotic in their interpersonal behaviour. The problems of thought and development that follow this disorder are pervasive and affect all of the child's activity. The nature of this disorder and its obvious relevance to the growing body of work on developmental epistemology make the condition and its phenomenology very interesting to philosophers. Unfortunately, philosophers often lose sight of the basicness of intersubjectivity and our dealings with others in the development of the psyche and so produce individualistic theories of psychological development and epistemology. A discussion of autism and other defects in which children are isolated from the shared human life-world for other reasons helps to illuminate the real nature of our human being-with-others.

(9) **Moral insanity and evil**: The psychiatric problems surrounding society and the psychopath bear directly on our notions of responsibility and moral judgement. The philosophical analysis of intentional action is directly relevant to the understanding of psychopathy and the impulsiveness that characterizes it. It is greatly enhanced by a neo-Aristotelian account of action, continence, and practical wisdom. I shall examine the neuropsychological and other features of psychopaths that help us understand their problem and try to relate these to notions of criminal responsibility and desert and also to radical evil and culpability as it arises in extremes of violent and criminal behaviour.

(10) **'My name is Legion for we are many'**: Whereas schizophrenia is popularly thought of as split personality, the actual problem of mental 'splitting' is most dramatically seen in multiple personality disorder, which is in the family of dissociative disorders. The problems of identity raised by this disorder can only be assessed against an adequate theory of personal identity and that requires a more nuanced view than any of those on view in the standard body identity versus psychological state essentialism debate. I shall outline a discursive and existential view that also helps explore the vexed issues around nosology, the reality of the disorder, and social constructionism. Hacking's conception of the looping effect of human kinds and a view of the psyche as a quasi-stable discursive construction, which allows one to tell one's own story, offer a rich hunting ground for a philosophical discussion of memory and identity.

(11) **I eat therefore I am not**: Anorexia is a quest for lightness of being, the meaning of which shapes the performative identity of its sufferers. The shaping of the soul and/or body in anorexia and the eating disorders is a reaction to the strains of living in a world of nature according to impossible discursive demands. The elements of the psyche are both the demons driving our behaviour so that our biological nature is sustained but also signals with significance. Anorexia is a quintessentially postmodern disorder because it can only be understood as a reaction of an embodied subject to the construction of a woman according to the valorizations and legitimations of post-classical modernism.

(12) **The meaning of hysteria**: Hysterical patients do not evaluate their symptomatology in the same way as others and are therefore labelled as deceptive. In fact, a number of patients with this disorder are revealed to have underlying neurological disorders and they all tend to show a style of cognition not well suited

to self-knowledge. This again raises the question of right judgement and the discursive (psychosomatic) skills involved in the complex interaction between underlying neurocognitive abnormalities and the social factors that play an obvious role in the disorder. The resulting insights refocus our attention on self-reflective judgement and the skills involved in the narrative achievement that is a coherent and meaningful life in which one takes one's place among others as their equal.

(13) **The good that I would do**: We all show lack of judgment, weakness of the will, self-deception, and irresponsibility of varying degrees. The more dramatic versions of these found in overt psychopathology and the philosophical analysis of character, thought, and action that have been used to examine them will elucidate these common problems in such a way as to inform and challenge some theories of mind and meaning. When we move from the more dramatic disruptions of personality to the more common problems arising in everyday psychiatry outpatients, we find the relation between autobiography and meaning are essential in our understanding of the persons involved. It emerges that the care of the self, centered on the link between the subject and the truth is a key aspect of personal integrity and self-knowledge.

(14) **Concluding autobiographical postscript**: This will draw together the content and analysis undertaken throughout the book.

Throughout the book, I have tried to sequester discussions mainly for those with a professional interest in philosophy in the appendices concerning the following:

(A) Metaphysics and the mind

(B) Natural kinds and causality

(C) Consciousness, thought, and intentionality

(D) Varieties of alienation

(E) The problem of other minds, theory-theory, and simulation theory

(F) Actions, reasons, causes, and the will

(G) Sructuralism and post-structuralism

(H) The philosophy of personal identity

Chapter 1

Mind, brain, and psychiatry

Sherrington recalls that as a student in Germany the Professor put one of the Betz cells from the cerebral cortex and labelled it 'the organ of thought'. A few days later a tumour of the brain was being demonstrated in the pathology department and one of the students asked: 'And are these cells also engaged in thinking, Herr Professor?'

(Drury, p. 60)

Aristotle, along with the Hippocratics, realized that the brain was the seat of those diseases which affected human powers of sensibility, movement, and intellect, a position that has become the philosophical view that the mind (or better, *psyche*) is a complex of cognitive techniques structured by meaning that, if deployed adequately, adapt the individual to the human life-world. Neuroscience is often regarded as the 'base science' as we try to understand the physical and social or interpersonal influences on psychological disorders, and the physicalist assumption (that the mind is a way of describing brain function) carries with it a theoretical framework of mechanism and antecedent causes following Pavlov, Hebb, and Watson. The alternative seems to be that there is 'mind stuff' or 'a soul', an entity with attributes not realized in the brain, inside a human being.

There is, however, a kind of naturalism that locates human beings in a world of meaning (structured by culture, rituals, and symbols) so that the psyche is a set of functions engaging that world of meaning with the trajectory of the situated embodied being in the actual world. That is not dualism—the belief that there are two different kinds of stuff in the world (mind stuff and physical stuff)—but neither is it physicalism because it eschews the philosophical view that the basic stuff of reality can adequately be described by the language of core natural sciences such as physics, chemistry, and physiology. It regards patterns discerned in the biological, social, and moral sciences as equally valid ways of describing and explaining what goes on in the world (particularly in relation to human thought and action).

In fact, Cartesianism (of any kind) is problematic in that a domain of events uniquely accessible to an 'inner self' is a dubious idea whether in *mentalist* or *materialist* drag. The notion that there are special 'mental' events and states with an 'other', ineffable kind of being or existence—a *Cartesian mentalist* position—or that the inner states and events comprising the mind are actually physical or brain states and events (even if described in other words)—the *Cartesian materialist* belief—both posit an 'inner' and an 'outer' that displaces the (embodied) human subject from its life-world. Wittgenstein argues that such inner 'goings-on' understood as mental states are a fiction and that mind-talk reveals the way we use the meanings available in our culture to organize and direct our activity in the world. Therefore, the debate as to whether our beliefs, attitudes, and desires (*inter alia*) are best construed as mental or physical and/or neurophysiological is misconceived because *the mind* comprises relational and discursive properties intrinsic to human agency and subjectivity in a world structured by meaning, myth, symbolism, intersubjectivity, and interpersonal relationships.

These disclaimers are *metaphysical*—they concern what things really are, or 'the existence and character of the known' (Weinberg & Yandell, 1971, p. iv)—and therefore inseparable from *ontology*—a study of the sorts of things that really exist. A metaphysical belief (e.g. minds and thoughts are in reality nothing but brain processes) is part of physicalist ontology—the claim that *all that really exists* are physical events and objects (including states of the brain). But this should all be taken a bit more slowly and the implications for theories of mind and meaning must be laid out quite carefully to understand psychiatry and the phenomena associated with mental disorders.

1.1 **Philosophical preliminaries[1]**

Questions such as 'Is the mind real?' or 'Are there really such things as mental states?' aim at a realistic understanding of the world. But commonsensical realism—the idea that there really is 'a world out there'—is not the same as philosophical realism—the claim that the world out there is independent of our ways of thinking about it, an idea that is problematic when we notice that the world is changed and we ourselves are affected by our ways of thinking (Hacking, 1995; Lacan, 1979).

Kant observed that any characterization of the world and its contents is created by rational thinkers, and therefore, he problematized the claim that we can get to know things as they are in themselves. Some thinkers follow Hegel and use Kant to ground a collective definition of truth (prominent in certain strands of postmodern thought). Hundert (1989) remarks, 'it is our experience with objects that enables us to objectify them' (p. 57) and focuses on 'modes of living experience which characterize our uniquely human way of being in the world' (p. 83), thereby underlining the importance of lived experience in understanding ourselves in general and suggesting that first-person experience (suitably illuminated and deepened both by psychological theory and philosophical analysis, especially of mental disorders) may be vital to our understanding.

The human mind is a joint product of physiological states and events and sociocultural or interpersonal reality, and an adequate science of the mind therefore begins by recognizing that we are beings-in-the-process-of-becoming shaped by discursive contexts. Therefore, talk of electrons, calcium channels, serotonin reuptake, neurones, action potentials, brain circuits, information, thought, attitudes, and so on embodies ways of categorizing things, none of which have a claim to be absolutely basic in understanding the human mind. Neuroscience, for instance, is constructed from human concepts contributing to certain kinds of explanation (complexes of theoretical, observational, and conceptual terms serving certain ends). Thus, the apparent

---

[1] The brief account in the text is developed more fully in Appendix A.

basicness of even a term such as *neurone* is deceptive; one ought to ask, 'Basic, in terms of what kind of explanation?[2] The present work accepts the following twofold claim:

(A) There can be interesting metaphysical explanations.

(B) The nature of the objects, properties, and facts to which our concepts correspond is not fixed independently of the concepts that correspond to them. (Morris, 1992, p. 15–16)

The first implies that we can learn things from talk about electrons, synapses, and bipolar disorder but that those truths are couched in terms dictated by our beliefs about those things. Therefore, whereas it is an objective fact whether something is or is not, for instance, *the sum of 2 and 2* or *an act of violence*, our thoughts about 'sums' or 'acts of violence' rely on concepts such as <addition>, <violence>, and <action>, the concepts concerned being subjectively generated (by thinkers of a certain sort with certain interests). The subjectivity here is also present in the judgment that '5' really is (objectively) a prime number, a truth that is made available by the concepts <5> and <prime>, and that reflects the fact that cognition adapts us, as subjects, to the world by organizing our experience in ways that order and unlock the possibilities of what is around us.

The view is neither philosophical realism nor idealism: to be discovered, in a realist view, is to be stumbled across (perhaps after an active search), whereas an idealist posits that all the things 'out there' are a function of our mental impressions and ideas (or representations) and that we can know no more about them than what those ideas reveal. In this view, it seems possible for the world of experience to be a notional or representational 'illusion' (perhaps shared). But we exist as thinking beings interacting within a domain of objects and events in ways that are ordered by the use of concepts to divide things into categories that enable us to do actual things in our world (such as constructing a simple light source from a battery, a bulb, and wire connections) so that when we discover something we find a new point of attachment for our concept system in the world around us, an attachment that then articulates our dealings with the world. (We find, for instance, that wire is a conductor, an objective fact accessible once we have concepts about electricity, giving us an entrée into one variety of energy use and storage, and an understanding of certain natural phenomena.)

Concepts therefore empower us by discerning and constructing regularities and connections between different situations (a shared process). When a person thinks of a thing in a certain way, for example, as a frog, both the cognitive role (frogs are little amphibious animals) and conditions grounding the judgment (one should only think <that is a frog> when the thing in front of one is a frog) organize that person's interactions with the world (perceptual and motor) according to rules governing that concept and the skills involved in following them. Our concepts and categorizations are tools or techniques identifying aspects of the world worth taking into account, an important (pragmatist) strand in Wittgenstein's account of rule following and truth that coheres with a (commonsensical) realistic view of knowledge (Gillett, 1995). Notice that the key idea is a set of classifications adequate to open up the relevant domain in

---

[2] Again, I deal with the problem of 'basicity' or reduction in Appendix A.

terms of our interests and projects, a consideration that is important in philosophical understandings of psychology and psychiatry.

1.2 **Psychiatry as a domain of knowledge**

Psychiatry is a biomedical science and therefore largely accepts that its suite of disorders reflects recognizable malfunctions in the human system. The basic sciences of pathology and physiology explain dysfunctions by correlating phenomenological descriptions with pathophysiology so that, for instance, the concept of goitre (an enlargement of the thyroid gland) is now thought to involve two different disease types, one caused by an autoimmune attack on the thyroid gland and the other by (neoplastic) tumours in the gland. Medical science thrives when pathology makes important distinctions in clinical phenomenology (clusters of symptoms, response to treatment, and natural history) by making use of pathophysiological explanations (such as the difference between inflammation and a neoplastic growth).

Another partner in the enterprise is therapeutics. A pragmatist of any stripe recognizes the close, indeed, conceptual relation between our concepts and what we do, so that conceptions of dysfunction (or illnesses) and their underlying causes (diseases) are negotiated in the light of effective treatments. For instance, neuropharmacology studies the actions of drugs in different illnesses so as to disclose the organization and biochemistry of the dysfunctional physiological pathways. The efficacy of a drug such as carbamazepine in two apparently disparate conditions—Temporal Lobe Epilepsy and non-diagnosable aggression—is taken to indicate common features that would otherwise never have been noticed. Or, the fact that a stimulant ameliorates Attention Deficit Hyperactivity Disorder (ADHD) where, prima facie, we might expect sedative or tranquilizing drugs to have the desired effect (in fact, they can worsen behaviour in genuine cases) suggests hypotheses about the 'real nature' of that disorder (in terms of brain function)[3].

The role of pathophysiology and pharmacology in explaining and modifying conceptions of disease affects our fundamental categorizations in medicine so that we think of the underlying reality of human illness in terms of biophysical descriptions. This tendency has eclipsed more tolerant, because less well-defined, phenomenological descriptions, particularly where biology (and neurobiology) is the focus of psychiatric research. But problems arise when we notice that significance or meaningfulness (and therefore, sociocultural context) pervades and influences psychiatric phenomenology. These problems cast doubt on biomedical conceptions of psychiatric phenomena (despite the orthodoxy that the mind comprises causal mechanisms realized in the brain), an approach somewhat at odds with the thought that 'the reality we represent cannot be determined in advance, and is, in its foundations, interpersonal' (Bolton & Hill, 1996, p. 162).

The appeal to interpersonal and discursive psychology directs us towards an examination of practices, institutions, and situated individuals as the foci of psychiatric

---

[3] The present work suggests that the brain and the situated context of the human being whose brain it is are holistically connected in their function and interaction.

attention and suggests a rapprochement between the ontology of the natural sciences (causes and physical objects) and those of the moral sciences or humanities (meanings and the structure of thought).

1.3 Causes, meanings, and the relation between mind and the world

Karl Jaspers has distinguished between *explaining* a psychological disorder and *understanding* its meaning to the patient. 'It is not absurd to think that it might one day be possible to have some rules which could causally explain the sequence of meaningfully connected thought processes without paying heed to the meaningful connections between them' (Jaspers, 1913/1974, p. 86). Jaspers' speculation prompts a philosophical inquiry into mind, meaning, causality, and psychological explanation that begins by distinguishing between tracing the causal origins of various psychic events and states and appreciating their meaning to the patient. Causal explanations (as in the natural sciences) consider individuals 'objectively' as complex biological organisms. By contrast, the meaning of an event to a human being emerges 'while we gather experience in our contact with human personalities' (Jaspers, 1913/1974, p. 84). A further distinction, between 'rational' and 'empathic' understanding, reveals that some of our thinking is governed by the 'rules of logic', whereas other elements reflect a person's individual psychology (or subjectivity). Empathic contact is not as concerned with explanation as it is with addressing a person as a person so that it reflects the way that the person understands what is happening to him and our 'reactive attitudes' are kept in play (Strawson, 1974, p. 1ff). We can then attend to and be guided by a (careful) negotiated synthesis of our objective appraisal of *both* the psychological forces *and* the meanings that are operating[4].

Jaspers sees clinical psychiatry as, in part, a process of helping the patient begin to understand the 'gaps' in his or her story (Freud, Lacan). The resulting clarification of psychic life increases the patient's ability to articulate his or her 'malady of the soul' (Kristeva, 1995). Consider a young man, Albert, who beats his wife whenever he fails in some way, for instance in his job, as a husband, or as a father. An empathic view may reveal that (a) he has never learned to cope with his own failures, (b) he resorts to aggression when he feels inadequate, (c) mastering relevant life skills will allow him to grow in character and maturity, and (d) the result will be less harm to himself and others.

Jaspers' (1923/1997) further claim that 'extraconscious' phenomena can cause psychological disorders (although traces of meaning may 'haunt' them) does not, however, imply that the causes of psychiatric disease can be understood 'without paying heed to meaningful connexions' (as in a reductive view of psychiatry quite different from that endorsed by Jaspers).

In the potentially reductive view, we accept not only a distinction between causal and meaningful connections but also the view that psychiatric disorders are caused (and mainly affected) by events such as changes in neurotransmitters or other

---

[4] I shall discuss reactive and objective accounts of persons in Chapter 3.

biological variables. Combined with the thesis that such non-meaningful causes encompass the only 'objective' way to understand psychiatric disease, we are then led to think that the meaning of the disease to the patient is an epiphenomenon with no role in explaining the mismatch between the patient and the world[5].

Causal processes identified by Jaspers (1913) include the normal mechanisms underlying everyday phenomena such as 'habituation, memory, after effect, fatigue, etc.' (p. 365) and also abnormal reactions such as dissociation, paralysis, fixations, and precipitation of psychosis. Each reactive 'alteration in the extraconscious foundations is a theoretical construct; we have to conceive of it as causally conditioned and analogous in some way with the manifest somatic sequelae of an emotional upset' (p. 384). The theoretical construct is invoked to explain certain manifestations in terms of a change in posited psychic mechanisms. They are thought of as physiologically moderated in the same way as the bodily reaction to emotion so that (when normal) they are compatible with the integrity of personality and 'a possibility of full illumination through self-reflection' (p. 366). An abnormal process represents 'an exaggerated or entirely new kind of transformation', taking us from symbols and meanings that inform life experiences (even when they are very stressful) to an absurd and incomprehensible fracture or splitting affecting one's conscious adjustment to life events. Jaspers accepts that, in relation to 'psychic commotion', there is no sharp divide between 'psychologically incomprehensible' events and processes (such as those triggering a psychosis) and the lesser disturbances we can reconstruct the effects of and make meaningful in terms of their effects on our lives (being put in prison, for instance). This 'fuzzy boundary' implies that an adequate understanding of psychic responses to life events cannot completely disregard meaningfulness (and therefore, the life story of the patient) in trying to comprehend the maladies of the soul because traces of meaning are inextricably interwoven with physiological disturbances.

Breaking down the sharp divide between causal and meaningful connexions allows us to make use of neurophysiology and neuropsychology in a truly scientific spirit (as Freud [1986] tried to do).

> It is probable that the chain of physiological events in the nervous system does not stand in a causal connection with the psychical events. The physiological events do not cease as soon as the psychical ones begin; on the contrary, the physiological chain continues. What happens is simply that, at a certain point of time, each (or some) of its links has a psychical phenomenon corresponding to it. Accordingly, the psychical is a process parallel to the physiological, 'a dependent concomitant'. (pp. 176–177)

Freud is a realist about the physiological and psychic events making up the subconscious mind, believing that they determine the psychic life of the patient in a way that is unattractive to a holistic (or humanistic) view that embraces the meaningful and discursive influences and regards subjective realities as part of what the brain deals with. Consider, for instance, the person who sees a young couple arm in arm in the park and is wistfully reflecting on the delights of young love until he recognizes the woman concerned as his fiancée.

---

[5] Causality and psychological explanation are discussed in Appendix B.

The idea that real explanations are and must be biological is hard to shake. One route to it is through factor analysis-based dispositional theses about human personality functioning such as those of Eysenck and his followers. Eysenck (1965) himself, deeply influenced by psychometry, behaviourism, and statistical analysis, looked for clusters of responses on personality questionnaires, analysing these to see if any (statistical) effects explain some of the variance seen . Inspired by faculty psychology, Eysenck took human character types such as '*sanguine* (cheerful and active), *melancholic* (gloomy), *choleric* (angry and violent), and *phlegmatic* (calm and passive)' (Gleitman, 1991, p. 690) to indicate quantifiable influences on behaviour, positing neural mechanisms that correspond to underlying dimensions of personality (considered as underpinning individuality).

> [W]e have determined the existence, at a descriptive level, of two important dimensions of personality, extraversion/introversion and neuroticism/stability . . . dimensions . . . powerfully determined by heredity and likely, therefore, to have [a] physiological, neurological, or biochemical basis in the nervous system of the individual.
>
> (Eysenck, 1965, p. 66)

Eysenck subsequently introduced a third dimension called *psychoticism* (actually related to attributes more characteristic of the psychopath than of patients with any of the psychoses).

Eysenck's (1987) basis in learning theory lead him to speculate about the kinds of brain structures involved in terms of approach, avoidance, and arousal by drawing on information from both conditioning studies and experiments with psychotropic drugs. He noted that highly articulated patterns of behaviour implicate cortical inhibition of lower centres in such a way that excess cortical activity 'produces inhibited (introverted) behaviour . . . Alcohol, a depressant drug which lowers the arousal of the cortical centres, produces extraverted, uninhibited behaviour; it frees the lower centres from cortical control' (p. 246), a key to current understandings of ADHD, psychopathy, and schizophrenia.

Eysenck's (1965) work concerns, on the one hand, patterns of association between questionnaire and inventory responses and, on the other, measures of excitability and non-specific arousal in the brain and their responses to broad categories of drugs such as the benzodiazepines, amphetamines, and alcohol. It seems to show dimensions of organization in responses to psychometric instruments measuring 'personality', and two basic dimensions in measurements of arousal, one indicating inhibition and the other facilitation of perceptual, learning, and motor activity (p. 70). He used his observations to account for individual differences in psychology and psychiatric phenomenology.

But we should ask, for instance, 'What is it, in the history of an individual, that makes certain (extraconscious) patterns of reactions adaptive or maladaptive in certain situations?' The most plausible answer may invoke certain biological predispositions but is likely also to implicate the individual's learning history, whether remembered or not (Raine, 2002). When the individual understands the influences and tendencies manifest in his or her behaviour, we can talk about conscious mental life and meaningful connections within it, but where there is a 'gap' (in cognitive penetrability), we invoke unconscious and subconscious mechanisms.

Imagine, for instance, a young woman Carrie who thinks she has seen a ghost in her basement. Now, she may be slightly suggestible and have relatively high scores on the neuroticism scale, but why should she think of ghosts unless there is a set of meanings in her history and the discourses that have affected her that make available the idea that a person can, in some sense, be present after their death. She may then be influenced by the cognitive connections and associations of the concept <ghost> in ways that she may not fully understand when she applies it to her basement 'encounter'. The thesis that psychology and psychiatry should be responsive to a person's lived experience implies that 'the meaningful' is central not only to the content but also to some extent to the form of psychiatric disorders[6]. For the minute, we need to examine the relation between meaningful connections and causal or biological connections in understanding the life-world of a human being (Husserl, 1970).

1.4 Causal claims in psychology and psychiatry

Bolton and Hill (1996) premise their study of the mind and mental disorder on the idea that meaningful connections are, in reality, causal and biological. Their position rests on a metaphysics (similar to that of Davidson) in which causal transactions in the brain underpin connections between mental phenomena such as thoughts and attitudes. On their view mental explanation is a subtype of causal explanation in virtue of the realization of mental states by brain states subserving organism–environment interactions that we conceptualize in terms of intentionality and thought[7].

Many accounts of the mind hold that to explain a thought, intention, or action is to specify what caused it. The relevant causes, one might think, are most plausibly found in the underlying microprocessing architecture of the brain and obey the laws of neurophysiology. But can we explain the microprocessing structure of the brain entirely in neurophysiological terms? When we ask that question, the cultural and discursive embedding of the development of human cognitive and neural function immediately invokes the historical, cultural, and social contexts that shape human cognition. But can the complex events, fashions, contingencies, and historical movements affecting a person be captured by neuroscience or has the explanatory task now exceeded the bounds of any natural science, as is claimed by some thinkers (Bhaskar, 1979; Harre, 1983; Taylor, 1964). In this vein, Wittgenstein (1980) remarks, 'I am not aiming at the same target as the scientists and my way of thinking is different from theirs' (p. 7e). Nevertheless, at the end of the day (or when the real push comes to real–causal–shove), for those of a scientific bent, the 'real events' in the mind are described and explained in neurobiological terms.

The argument showing why that view is wrong begins by examining the nature of mind, thought, and neurobiology. It rapidly emerges that mechanistic causation of one material state of affairs by one appropriately related in space and time is not what

---

[6] I will pick up this discussion in relation to Anorexia in Chapter 11.

[7] The arguments are developed more fully in Appendices A and B.

we are aiming at when we relate a subject's behaviour to his or her situation; rather, we are mapping the individual's behaviour onto a structure of rules and meanings and the skills involved in negotiating them[8]. We are, in psychological explanation, *either* tracing the meanings of events as the subject sees them and making sense of that subject's interaction with the world in the same terms *or* positing extraconscious mechanisms that are distorting the application of cognitive skills. The resulting brain–world exchange may or may not be comprehensible in neuroscientific terms but embodies a rationale for a more situated and holistic account. Such a conception of mental explanation alters our view of psychological disorders in a way that has profound implications for theoretical psychiatry[9].

1.5 Thinking and the human mind

Thoughts and the concepts articulating them are aspects of the mind, the cognitive aspect of the (Aristotelian) form of a human being. For Aristotelians, as distinct from substance dualists, this aspect of the human form depends in a special way on the operations of the (embodied and situated) brain but does not imply that, at the most fundamental level, we can only explain human mental life in terms of brain processes so that we are committed to a biological conception of psychiatry. In understanding a person as a thinking subject, we notice that (i) she or he is able to follow rules shared with others, and (ii) she or he is embedded in dynamic human interactions where the relevant rules have been imparted as the basis of the meanings instantiated in life and experience (around here).

Wittgenstein, as did Aristotle, derives his view of the acquisition, refinement, and communication of concepts (the building blocks of thought) from our natural history. An ecological view of that sort implies that salient cultural and social patterns configure neural networks to realize regularities arising in human life in a natural (and radically restructured or domesticated) environment. Human ecology is ecology in a human life-world, itself humanized by human activities and signifiers (themselves promiscuous artefacts or tools for use in it). With this in mind, we can consider the explanatory patterns found in psychology.

1.6 Shaping the human cognitive engine: meaning and the brain

The human brain is a repository of meanings and, throughout life, it stores experience in terms of the meanings available 'around here' and the responses that exploit them. Those meanings are governed by rules arising within the language of a community and the classifications used in that community to group stimulus patterns in terms of their significance (Gillett, 1991). The rules embed and produce patterns of association or articulation in human behaviour and the role of speech in thought is increasingly

---

[8] All of which, under the guise of causality, are important in Bolton and Hill's account; so, my quibble with them is metaphysical but also affects our respective explanatory frameworks.

[9] It is discussed more fully in Appendix B.

recognized in theoretical, clinical, and experimental work on cognition (Dennett, 1991; Karmiloff-Smith, 1986, 1992; Luria, 1973; Vygotsky, 1929/1962). Words structure brain function in ways illuminated by certain features of neural network theory and practice (Gillett, 1989; Harre & Gillett, 1994). In brief, a neural network registers certain configurations of activity associated with significant objects by creating preferred excitation patterns so that arbitrary sound patterns, combined with inputs from the environment, are used to form 'semantic complexes' (as in the writings of Vygotsky, Luria, and Freud, in different ways).

Freud (1986) discusses 'object presentations'—comprising two complex patterns of association, one verbal and the other situational—formed in the mind by experience: 'A word is thus a complex presentation . . . There corresponds to the word a complicated associative process into which the elements of visual, acoustic, and kinaesthetic origin . . . enter together' (p. 182).

Meanings (or significations, the semantic types associated with signs) are marked by arbitrary or conventional symbols used in human discourse as part of different activities and they facilitate connections within and between stimulus patterns. Luria (1973) characterizes a word as a 'complex multidimensional matrix of different cues and connections' (p. 306), a conception that is useful in understanding Lacan's (structuralist) doctrine of the signifier and the signified as key terms in psychology and particularly the psychology of the unconscious. The neural network theory suggests that meanings, construed in this way, shape or influence the microprocessing structure of the brain by setting up nodes of preferential excitation linked to patterns of information and then forming connections between those functional nodes (in a way that is tailor-made for structuralism).

Informal, Parallel Distributed Processing (PDP), or network-type systems have another intriguing feature. They generate selective processing patterns best where clearly differentiated stimulus groupings repeatedly arise but, even where the significant groupings of stimuli do not fall into readily apparent discrete, detectable patterns, we can 'piggyback' the extraction of significance on 'teaching stimuli', marking what is worth noting. In the real world, such correlative marking stimuli could arise in two ways:

(i) Feedback from motivational circuits to information-detecting systems; and

(ii) Symbolic markers associated with objects and events in the environment.

Humans (and other animals) modify their behaviour as a result of motivational information such as the availability of food or other affordances (Gibson, 1966). They also have innate propensities to detect certain kinds of information, but more important than these, in the human case, is that the infant or child imitates and learns from the responses of other human beings so that 'any view which . . . construes the child as a solitary inquirer attempting to discover the truth about the world must be rejected' (Hamlyn, 1973, p. 184). The responses of other people cue the learner as to what is worth attending to (Gillett, 1987). Therefore, a connectionist approach to causality and explanation can dovetail beautifully with discursive theories of mind (Gillett, 1993c).

In the discursive view, we begin with words and their meanings (or passages of discourse and their formative effect on mental life) as a starting point common to a diverse range of theories about the mind and mental content. We must thread our way through these various approaches (including the view of mind and meaning that informs Bolton and Hill's [1996] work) to arrive at a view that is adequate to relate psychiatric phenomena to human discourse and its interactive structures.

Bolton and Hill (1996) argue that the information mediating the organism's interactions with the world is encoded in functional states in the brain. They are agnostic about the structure implementing the model but insist that it causally generates mental life. Their summary claim is as follows:

> The brain can be said to encode meaning or information, though not because there is a one–one correspondence between meaningful states and neural states . . . Encoded meaning is based in organism–environment interactions, and can be applied to the brain only insofar as the brain serves in the regulation of those interactions. (p. 116)

Their causal claim about mental explanation rests largely on its predictive power:

> This theory-driven predictive power apparently makes unavoidable the conclusion that explanations that involve meaningful mental states are in some sense causal, and it lies at the basis of replies to all arguments to the contrary. (p. 118)

The argument is vulnerable to an alternative not relying on causality (such as Wittgenstein's philosophy of mind). Wittgenstein often used the analogy of chess to point out the difference between mental (or rule-governed) and physical (or causal) explanation, a difference that turns on the differing conceptions of rule following, only one of which equates rule following with natural regularities such as cardioregulatory responses (Bolton & Hill, 1996, p. 221ff). The rules of chess do not cause me (reflexively or automatically as a matter of biological fact) to move the pieces in a certain way; they provide constraints that delineate valid moves in the game and provide a framework for the development of certain skills (unlike a cardiorespiratory reflex that causes my body to react in a certain way that I do not control).

The discursive view of mental explanation is tied to rule following because it locates a person in a sphere of discourse where she or he must develop skills relevant to the relationship between the self and world. These skills structure what-it-is-like-to-be that person (seeing an aspect—'the substratum of this experience is the mastery of a technique'), and render his or her responses understandable (Wittgenstein, 1953, p. 208e), so as to build competence into his or her life. It is as if one were to successfully locate a person on a map of human activity and associated points of attachment to the world and then say, 'Ah, now I see where I am or you are!' This is not a causal explanation despite its explanatory and predictive power about what the individual experiences and how they respond to that experience (Gillett, 1993a, 1993b).

Bolton and Hill (1996) distance themselves from the physicalist view of explanation—'that ultimately all causing goes on at a physical level' (p. 175)—in that they believe that some causal (or functional) laws are specific to information processing and they argue that, in a sense affected by subjective features of experience, mental explanations depend on physical properties that may be specific to the agent (p. 213). To that extent, they agree with the claim that mental causation must somehow emerge from the supervenience of the mental upon 'fundamental physical processes' (Kim, 1993 , p. 138), a position assuming that 'the only alternative to biological design, in our sense of "design", is sheer coincidence, freak accident' (Millikan, 1995, p. 262). However, the discursive view offers an alternative to this stark choice.

Millikan (1993) is surely right that successful creatures are likely to have cognitive mechanisms allowing them to use external or environmental cues rather than internal ones. But, if that is so, then their action structures are intentional (in the phemomenological sense: they are essentially directed upon objects in the environment outside the mind). Tyler Burge (1995) puts it thus:

> [A]n illuminating philosophy of psychology must do justice . . . to psychology's attempt to account for tasks that we succeed and fail at, *where these tasks are set by the environment and represented by the subject him- or herself.* The most salient and important of these tasks are those that arise through relations to the natural and social worlds. (p. 201)

The evidence of neuroscience is that brain function is shaped to lock on to environmental targets and track them (Luria, 1973) and, for human beings, the significant targets may be culturally determined. We need to add one further ingredient to the picture in order to derive a view of psychological explanation adequate to current thinking in cognitive neuroscience.

Many of the most basic and primitively appreciated elements of our mental world are socially or interpersonally mediated, things such as a sense of belonging, discerning the fact that others like me, guilt, rejection, and so on. Other significant features reflect complex discourses: the baroque qualities of Handel's music, the tension in the air, or the Impressionism of a Turner painting.

It seems that signification and situated sociocultural reality combine to shape the microprocessing structure of the brain that 'encodes' the recognition routines for these features. We may be able, at one level, to understand the shifting patterns of excitation in the brain as a result of the confluence of conditions, the parsed utterance, and the intentions of the speaker, and so on, but at another level, the processing patterns reflect the complexities of discourse. Therefore, psychological explanations incorporate the holistic interaction of law-like (physical nature) and non-law-like domains (the intentional world of speakers and hearers)[10]. What is more, there are rules governing the use of terms in a language, conventions governing the communication of speakers intentions, internal or individual influences on a discursive interaction (involving 'immense scope for creativity and change' [Bolton & Hill, 1996, p. 263]), and massive causal particularity in ecologically real situations. At any given moment, the network state of the brain may be unique so that its activity is not predictable on the basis of quasi-scientific generalizations and our best indicator of what is going on might be empathic—trying to 'get on the same wavelength' as the individual concerned. We are helped by two aspects of human interaction:

(i) We tend to use terms to signify regularities salient to human beings; and

(ii) Human thinking is built from these, often shared, ways of understanding what is going on.

---

[10] I will discuss natural kinds and laws of nature in Appendix B.

These orienting clues, along with an intuitive understanding of how people relate to each other as we learn skills (and response strategies) from others, generate an understanding of human psychology grounded in subjective experience and intersubjectively validated.

Therefore, even if we inhabit a shared human world massively transformed from its natural state so that the resources of biology are not likely to cope well with our modes of activity, we have skills that are adapted to the human life-world and the intersections of subjectivity within it. The skills are, however, realized in brain function and therefore vulnerable to anything that disrupts brain function (such as physical or pharmacological insults).

1.7 **The uniqueness of the cognitive individual**

The focus on discourse or speech as an interpersonal activity reminds us of Lacan's (1977) dictum: 'the function of language is not to inform but to evoke' (p. 86). In language, we use discursive skills to do things to each other and we modify ourselves as a result. Thus, the words shaping the brain are not pure causal codes linked to objects in 'the world out there' but are tools that evoke, arrest, penetrate, signify, and subject us to interpersonal effects that need to be dealt with in a way that affects a person's life story. A liveable story transcends the natural world and incorporates quasi-stable answers to the implicit question 'How should a person live?' (Taylor, 1989) In that way, norms (or values) inform the mind in ways that are interpersonal, reflecting cultural mores and not mere natural regularities. Thus, if the shape of human brain microprocessing is significantly shaped by words (as used in actual interpersonal situations), then (human) psychological explanation and the functions of the (human) cognitive engine are neither biologically individualistic nor likely to involve 'bottom-up' determination of behaviour (as Dennett and others have noticed).

The richness of our language reflects our practices, our interpersonal dealings with one another, and the many different projects and purposes individuals bring to the diverse contexts in which layers of meaning are added to the skeleton function of a word (as it may be grasped by a child or someone with the pedantic approach to word meaning typically found in certain types of autism or in the notion of an ideal [logical] language)[11]. Therefore, a normal human being, shaped by participation in discourse, evinces in his or her psyche the complexity, nuances, informality, and located individuality of human relationships and interactions that make up a life. The microprocessing structure of the brain is therefore an accumulation of 'complex multidimensional matri[ces] of different cues and connections' (Luria, 1973) realizing in an individual situated human life trajectory the 'imperative of the word as law that has formed [us] in its image' (Lacan, 1977, p. 106).

Word meanings, as they function in human cognition, embody a cluster of connections widely articulated within our record of cumulative experience even though they also have a core and normative set of connections. For instance, the term *trumpet* has core connections to ideas about music, a particular type of instrument, and a characteristic

---

[11] As (seemingly) valorized by Frege and certain neo-Fregean kinds of logical realism.

sound but a looser set of connections (perhaps varying from person to person) important in psychological explanation (for instance, to ideas about pageantry, judgement, courage, and so on). Ideal theories connecting words to (physical or natural) things are unlikely to capture the dynamic interconnectedness of psychological phenomena because they (necessarily) neglect the highly varied formative contexts that shape these associative meanings. The norms of rationality reflect accepted and shared ways of thinking found in discursive groups (Stich, 1990). Thus, in sorting reason from unreason, we need to be sensitive to the human context giving rise to the thinking concerned. A general calculus (based on universal word meanings and canons of rationality) that neglects the holistic nature of such human contexts is unlikely to help us in understanding the psyche, but an understanding of the repertoire of cognitive skills human beings use in their adaptation may be very informative. What is more, the basic human features common to the lives of different human groups enable some intertranslation between different discourses such that individuals and groups who have different sociocultural origins can explore and clarify their points of agreement and disagreement. Davidson (1984) points out that the framework of mutual comprehension is rich enough to sustain quite diverse interpretations of the world and allow fruitful discussion of them.

It should now be clear that the present approach to philosophy of psychology is highly congenial to a certain kind of psychiatric practice and therapeutic discourse focusing on the individual patient and his or her story and situating that person in a human context.

1.8 **The discursive turn in psychology**

Discourses, exchanges with other human beings, shape human cognition so that the domain of the interpersonal is the basis of understanding and meaning. We constantly adapt, refine, and rearticulate our thoughts about what is around us, in part, on the basis of the responses of others who share the concepts we use and participate in the normativity that surrounds us (a domain of 'reactive attitudes' [Strawson, 1974]). A human being is exquisitely sensitive to the uses of signs (and thereby, the associated concepts) by others so that any human being's relationships with the world are 'traced by language and dissolved by ideas' (Foucault, 1984, p. 83), a process of inscription that invokes both linguistic interactions and their cultural context in our formation as subjective beings. This is true both of my conception of what is *out there* and of what is *in here* so that my conception of who and what I am is also responsive to my interactions with others both through their actions towards me and their speech about me (Hacking, 1995; Lacan, 1977).

The discursive production of the mind has significant implications for psychological explanation:

(i) Discursive explanations locate the subject in relation to the discourse she or he inhabits.

(ii) Therefore, they reveal the individual's position vis-à-vis the power relations obtained in the discourse.

(iii) It allows us to understand subjectivity as dynamic, reactive, and structured by the significations available to organize patterns of thought and action.

But we ought to notice that these explanations (in terms of meanings) are not internal causes of the subject's mental life, a highly significant proviso in conceptualizing the unconscious, traditionally conceived as the locus of internal processes causing behaviour but not consciously accessible to the thinking subject. The discursive approach analyses the experience of the subject and the significations informing that experience as always already situated so that subjectivity is structured by linguistically informed situations, an emphasis consistent with the idea that physical or non-intentional causes and conditions, intentional configurations escaping reason or reflection, and cultural realities all deeply affect a person. The style of explanation is genealogical in that it trades in power relations and discursive positions of the person, acknowledging (with Freud) that many of the most important influences on subjectivity have their origins in early childhood when intentionality is being constructed[12].

Human beings cue their offspring in terms of their own responses to things around them and also greatly extend the range and productivity of the child's information gathering by actively imparting to the child a set of shared concepts. Although nobody (at least since a Tsar of Russia who wanted to discover the language of the Garden of Eden) has been cruel enough to raise human infants in isolation from normal social contact, we can guess the result. The Tsar's experimental children (who survived) were said to be imbeciles, and when we study perception and infant learning, we find that the child gleans vital orienting cues from others (Butterworth, 1991). Indeed, contemporary children raised without the normal level of 'parenting' and social contact with adults are poor not only in social but also in cognitive and perceptual skills (Rymer, 1994)[13].

It seems, then, that what is meaningful to a human being is, literally, realized in the microprocessing structure of the brain as inscribed by practices where we interact with one another as people (some of whom are immature and need nurturing). Those practices are themselves structured by rules dictating what conditions license the application of a concept and how that concept is articulated in thought so that it holistically interacts with skills used 'around here' to adapt to and exploit the environment, and some of them may not transfer successfully into a new context of use (think, for instance, of the infantile habits of dependency and the adolescent context of social interaction). Because discursive skills are engaged with and structured by the meanings we are immersed in, they are part of intentional explanation and demarcate the domain of mental activity so that the mental (as a complex of situated skills and socially structured configurations of information) is ineliminable from an understanding of cognition and brain function, a conclusion with profound implications, already hinted at, for neuroscience, psychology, and psychiatry, particularly when we confront the claim that 'there is no such thing as a psychiatry that is too biological' (Guze, 1989).

In neuroscience, we are concerned to explain why the brain functions as it does, recognizing that it is designed to be modified by experience as part of the equipment of an active organism seeking out significance in the environment and finding it in ways partly learned from others. The child has a natural propensity to respond

----

[12] Bolton and Hill (1996) make exactly the same point (see especially Chapter 6.3 of that work).

[13] We shall explore these thoughts further in discussing autism and its implications for epistemology.

'congruently' with other human beings and is biologically equipped with similar sensitivities—to warmth, faces, movements, bright colours, and so on—but evinces, in Lacan's (1977) terms, 'a primordial discord', 'anatomical incompleteness of the pyramidal system', and 'a real *specific prematurity of birth*' (p. 4). It is not supposed to be self-contained but to be formed and informed through discourse so that it is made in the 'image of the human' prevalent 'around here' (a historicocultural context). In fact, the brain receives information that is weighted, or classified, in terms of what the organism has learned to detect so that the experience and cognition of the individual is articulated (based on natural propensities) dynamically within a discursive setting (Gillett, 1989). Therefore, when we look at the thought life of a person or a human group, we note that their reasoning, structured by their concepts and the rules governing them, permeates their intentional activity including their relationships to the world and each other (Winch, 1958). Thus, we are led beyond the irreducibility of the individual mind (as in varieties of non-reductive monism such as supervenience of the mental on the physical) to the role of a situated embodied subject, understood holistically, in understanding human experience.

This conclusion is strengthened by experimental work in neurochemistry showing that stress, induced in diverse ways, causes effects such as gamma-aminobutyric acid (GABA)-binding changes on neuronal membranes and changes in LTP and Long Term Depolarisation (LTD) in hippocampal *N*-methyl-*D*-aspartate (NMDA) receptors (Akinci & Johnston, 1993).

> Rats exposed to uncontrollable stress . . . show an impairment in long-term potentiation (LTP) in the hippocampus . . . Rats able to control shock schedule do not show LTP impairment unlike 'yoked' animals receiving the identical shock schedule without control.
>
> (Kim et al., 1996, p. 4750)

Thus, a psychological variable (albeit simple)—the degree of control over aversive events—is causally responsible for a neurochemical change in the brain (here, the hippocampus of a rat). In human beings, the psychological stressors are not simple (such as physical pain induced by electric shock, hunger, or schedule-sustained physical activity) but, as one might expect from our 'specific prematurity and dynamic engagement in discursive relations' (Lacan), are often social, cultural, and psychological. Why should a high-performing executive show similar physiological changes to a swim-stressed rat? To explain that, we need to invoke psychological influences such as the person's apprehension of the social context, his (or her) thoughts that he (or she) is responsible for others, and his (or her) future-oriented thoughts about himself (herself). Or, to use an analogy between rat and human behaviour, we coin the term *learned helplessness* and use it to understand human responses to certain discourses, power relationships, and positions within them; in both cases, the social and inter-personal aspects of the context have profound effects on changes in brain function.

1.9 Explanation, reduction, and genealogy

This anti-reductive (or holistic psychosomatic) theme is strengthened when we scrutinize discursive explanations. Explanations reflect our interests and capabilities, and causal explanations correlate with the kinds of things we can achieve through physical interactions with things (Strawson, 1985). Discursive explanations might therefore be expected to relate to non-mechanical interventions, for instance, in the political or relational milieu of the human life-world, and so they do.

Imagine, for instance, the 'competing' explanations of the behaviour of gulls in the breeding season. The molecular biologist claims, 'All genetic traits are based on processes by which genetic material determines changes in proteins and through them the structure and function of organisms; that is the fundamental explanation of this behaviour!' 'Wrong!' says the neurophysiologist: 'Of course there are cellular mechanisms underlying behaviour but the behaviour itself is best understood and explained by the way the brain of the gull processes information through its neural circuits, their structure, and their dynamic changes.' 'You are both wrong', says the ethologist, 'because you do not ask why the animals behave that way. They do so because there is a parent–child interaction in the context of a large breeding colony that necessitates the neural and genetic machinery you find.' The ecologist calmly puffs his pipe. 'Small minds', he laments; 'none of you look beyond the individual to the ecological niche being exploited. The parent–child bonding, the behaviour cementing it, the neural circuits producing that, and the genetic mechanisms encoding those are all there because these are essentially migratory colonists exploiting a food chain with geographic and climatic characteristics causing large groups of animals to reproduce at the same time and place. That is the real explanation of this behaviour.'

The example exposes the tendency to fixate on a fundamental right answer to any given problem (varying according to the scientist concerned). Different explanations serve different purposes, each trades in its own set of categories linked to specific interventions (genetic manipulation, brain stimulation, modification of behaviour, or ecological measures), and seeing a phenomenon in terms of one set of categories precludes seeing it otherwise. But should the terms of one kind of explanation be eliminated in favour of a more complete and generally useful one to determine the 'best' way of understanding a given phenomenon? (Churchland, 1986) Two constraints apply:

(1) We should not lose sight of important truths about the world by replacing one explanation with another.

(2) We should not deprive ourselves of useful explanations by making the switch.

For instance, in the gull example, a focus on molecular genetics should not blind us to ecology. By analogy, if the present account of thought and concepts is correct, explanations in terms of meaning and the human soul should not be eliminated in favour of explanations in terms of brain function. The argument is as follows.

(i) Explanations of meaning make essential reference to the rule-following practices or discourses in which an individual's soul or psyche has developed.

(ii) What is meaningful has a formative influence on information-processing structures in the brain because it structures the experiential history of the person in important ways.

(iii) Even if we were to accept a strictly neural and neurochemical basis for all psychiatric disease, we would still need to take some cognisance of meaningful patterns of events in the individual's life in order to rebuild the connections in the psyche.

(iv) We lose truth and explanatory power in attempting the eliminative reduction from mind to brain in that concepts and the discourses producing them involve norms for persons to follow and not merely functions in subpersonal processes (Peacocke, 1986, p. 50–51).

The claim that descriptions of brain function are more basic than psychological explanations loses sight of what is meaningful to the individual, plausibly part of the genesis of a psychological problem and of the explanation of its subjective contours. Given that meaning arises in discourse and discourse is affected by culture and history, psychological explanation should embrace sociopolitical issues and a broad concept of genealogy (Foucault, 1984; Nietzsche, 1887/1956).

A discursive account examines the way that meanings develop and become formative in shaping individual subjectivities. Discourse, as we have noted, imparts (along with imperatives or evaluations associated with various ways of thinking of things) those concepts allowing an individual to understand and assign value to his or her experiences (as Lacan notes). The word *signification* makes that explicit; signifiers such as 'weak', 'strident', or 'wounded' convey ways of thinking replete with evaluative colour as do words such as 'disorder' in psychiatry and psychology. A human being, positioned discursively, for instance, in the discourse of academic success or the social life of middle-class suburbia (with its complex, often unspoken, norms), is influenced by the evaluations pervading that discourse in regarding certain things as worthy or worthless. Evaluations such as 'doing well', 'failing', and so on have normative significance and position the individual (for self and others) according to the way that he or she receives those judgements; professionals should note that for those in power the hidden presuppositions and evaluations may be invisible whereas to the vulnerable they are likely to be highly salient.

In any person's life, multiple discourses overlap and interfere with each other (similar to waves creating interference patterns or currents creating vortices), and when this occurs, the subject in whom they coalesce may become conflicted. The conflict concerns what is legitimate, normal, or good and true. Somehow, the individual subject must integrate and adapt to the resulting interpersonal and intrapersonal forces. Because each person is uniquely placed in terms of the configuration of discourses shaping him or her, each of us is, necessarily, unique. What is more, each individual acquires a range of discursive skills to deal with the various challenges that arise in his or her interpersonal, cultural, and historical setting (and individual life trajectory). Thus, Kristeva (1995) remarks that the therapist who does not recognize a new *malady of the soul* in every person he or she sees is missing something of vital importance.

A genealogical orientation (as in Nietzsche and Foucault) overturns the thesis that any particular discourse (with its embedded significations) is privileged. There is no progressively refined story, based on a single view of the nature of reality (as is assumed by traditional metaphysics in general and scientific realism in particular), to tell about the human condition. Instead, the truth is 'a mobile army of metaphors' that allow us to see the world in diverse ways. Some of these, for various reasons arising within human discourse, come to be widely seen as legitimate or privileged. The view of the world that results reflects the rules governing the production of statements (Foucault, 1984, p. 74) and, particularly when we try to understand human beings, a much more fluid formative environment than conventional physical (or natural) science is needed. This is evident when we deconstruct human practices of knowledge creation and validation rather than try to discover some preordained harmony or 'fit' between our (privileged) representations and the real world.

We need not subscribe to postmodern ways of thinking to observe that our conceptions of the mind and human beings influence the way we are. This 'looping effect of human kinds' (Hacking, 1995) highlights the formative role of myths and images in one's conception of what (type of thing) one (as an individual) is. Human beings shape their life stories in the light of the attitudes and evaluations that surround them and to which they commit themselves. For this reason, medicine in general and psychiatry in particular not only describe human nature and its variations but also influence or shape it (and thereby participate in human evolution).

The ineliminability of mind and the nature of persons from the world is a conclusion strengthened by the realization that neuroscience itself is a project undertaken by human thinkers and dependent on their 'ordered procedures for the production, regulation, distribution, circulation, and operation of statements' (Foucault, 1984, p. 74) to determine what is true and, in particular, the truth of reductive and biologically based accounts of human reality and subjectivity.

Analytic tools such as discourse, subjectivity, position, power, signification, evaluation, legitimation, and so on make visible the interaction between human thoughts and the nature of the human beings thinking them. This crucial feature of the moral sciences is important in any analysis of psychiatry as, itself, a hybrid product of the mixing of moral and natural science.

1.10 **Psychiatry revisited**

If it is useful to consider the meaning of certain events for the person concerned to explain the psychological malady being suffered, then it follows that a purely biological approach to psychiatry deprives us of valuable clinical tools. Examples where that seems to be the case are not hard to find; consider, for instance, a young man, Bob, who is refusing to communicate with anyone.

> When assessed in hospital, Bob remains silent, passive, immobile, and refuses both conversation and food. During the next few days, he makes two attempts to overdose on drugs taken from the ward office. After three days, he is identified as the brother of a young woman who has been murdered by her father with an axe. Bob and his father have a marked physical resemblance, the same name, and work at the same factory. We find out from Bob's friends that he has been reacting in an increasingly sensitive and downcast way recently, particularly when likened to his father. One such incident resulted in him going missing for several hours.

It is difficult to maintain that Bob is in his present state for reasons completely apart from the perceived relationships between himself, his father, and his sister, even if he and his father both have a genetic predisposition to bipolar disorder.

> Carol is a young Roman Catholic woman who has a psychotic episode. She has heard voices prompting her to run through the streets naked and shout obscenities. She is admitted for acute assessment and claims not only that the autumn leaves and the wheels of passing vehicles speak to her but also that her thoughts are being put in her head. We find out that she is in a relationship with an atheist university lecturer and that some of her voices are accusing, abusive, and linked in her mind to images of her mother and father. Others say sceptical, disparaging, and even obscene things about her parents and her own beliefs.

Perhaps, we should accept a primarily biological model of such psychotic breakdown and treat Carol with appropriate medication, but does she need any other kind of help? That turns partly on whether the meaning structures inscribing her are causing stress that has a role in explaining her mental disorder or whether they are merely articulating a disorder that should be dealt with by biological means. We ought at least to consider the question, if for no other reason than the fact that there is an intimate relationship between the functions of the brain and the control of internal biochemistry so that their mutual influence is subtle and profound. The importance of the meanings articulating her suffering also emerges when we realize that she will have to reconstruct her life once a therapeutic intervention has given her a hope of doing so. Any intervention in a broken story should therefore be accompanied by help in the healing process of narrative reconstruction.

In fact, Bolton and Hill (1996) develop a detailed theoretical basis for the inclusion of the meaningful (or intentional) in the explanation of psychiatric disease through a consideration of social interactions and learning history (in terms of rule following) as key features of human development (a point to which I shall return in discussing the Unconscious).

> Dave is morbidly jealous. The worst episode occurred when he was 800 km from home and phoned his wife. He formed the impression that she had been a little too quick to get off the phone and concluded that she had another man with her. On reflection, he realized he was being irrational but became increasingly tortured by lurid images of her in fla-grante delicto and resolved to drive home. He left his motel at 2 am and arrived home at 12 noon the next day to find an empty house. He felt very foolish.

We cannot explain Dave's behaviour without considering the causes of such jealousy and the patterns of meaning that have led him to form the thoughts and images that fuel it. He clearly suffers from a profound and disruptive disorder of his intentional and relational life (A Freudian might guess as to the genesis of his problem.) For such problems, we need to draw on both biological (perhaps impulsivity) and meaningful understanding to disclose the effective influences on him.

Therefore, even if human thinking is realized in brain function, we cannot proceed from that conclusion to the claim that mental life is explained by a subtype of the causal explanation found in biology. The terms in one type of explanation (interpersonal relations, meanings, myths, metaphors, discourse, culture, and history) are not visible in the other (neuronal connections, synaptic transmission, action potentials, biological mechanisms, and so on). Significant truths about human beings evident in one type of explanation and description are blind spots for the other and there are many reasons to believe that the 'blind spots' may be important in understanding mental disorder.

Griffiths (1997, p. 171) argues that scientific explanations of phenomena should capture the forces maintaining a type of thing in the form that underpins our best classification and useful generalizations. For biological species, those explanations concern descent, cladistic location, and ecological niche, but for complex human phenomena, the productive and maintaining forces are both biological and sociocultural. The current approach to mind and brain draws on both types of knowledge, but the more general point is that any phenomenon should be located in the nexus of significations that yield an adequate understanding (or circumspective knowledge) of it[14].

1.11 **Mind and brain in practical psychiatry**

I have argued that mind is a mode of functioning linked to rules, discourse, and interpersonal relationships through which certain things come to be valued and have a profound influence on the thoughts and feelings of a human individual. The complex information processing of the brain enables these forces to inscribe the individual and the mind that is an abstraction from the extended and narratively integrated (to some extent) life of such a 'rational and social animal' (Aristotle).

The present view implicates meanings both in the empathic understanding of mental disorders and in their genesis because it suggests that the mental life of an individual can be distorted in its workings both by the content of the thoughts involved and the biological processes realizing them (this would be the case, for instance, with Manic-Depressive Psychosis or Bipolar Disorder.) Where we can only understand the genesis and maintenance of a pattern of behaviour by appealing to the meanings connecting present events with life history, we must examine those connections to understand the disorder we find. Explanation and treatment based on that orientation incorporate Jaspers' (1913) understanding that the 'psychology of meaning has possibilities of extensive growth by bringing material of which one has been unaware into clear consciousness' (p. 89) and imply that certain disorders arise from meanings that influence the patient's thought in ways that are not acknowledged by the patient. Consider the case of Eva.

> Eva is a psychopathic liar. She has, it turns out, a mother who became jealous of her from as early as she could remember and a father who overtly derided her in her mother's presence but secretly sexually abused her. She has a tendency to ingratiate herself with people by telling elaborate and pathetic stories about her life, all of which dwell on the cruelty of various male acquaintances. Having won the trust of her confidantes, she then abuses it, for instance, by stealing from them or trying to create discord between any couple who have the misfortune to become entangled with her.

---

[14] The term *circumspection* is, as I have noted, from Heidegger (1953/1996) and the general point is found in structuralist or post-structuralist analyses.

Interpersonal dynamics figure largely in Eva's problem and her need to test, indeed attack, those who care about her so that she destroys relationships that (subjectively) threaten to involve her too closely. Her love–hate relationships with her father and mother and her guilt concerning them are clearly important in trying to help her deal with her problem.

A dynamic methodology can, however, only constitute part of our understanding of the origins of mental disorder because the meanings that guide and direct behaviour are realized in a biological system that is vulnerable to causal and 'essentially extraconscious' (because physiological not psychological) influences. Such disordering causes, even if they have been potentiated by meaningful connections, have a 'surd' (or meaningless) effect not based in our understanding of persons as beings shaped by meaning. These intrinsically meaningless influences nevertheless affect meaningful processes by disordering, distorting, driving, or fragmenting them as in schizophrenia or Manic-Depressive Psychosis. In the latter disorder, the sufferer may be fascinating, creative, and personally mature in between the manifestations of a primarily biological disorder. Thus, in addition to the effect of abnormal meaningful aspects in the life history, causal influences present and unrelated to the meaningful structure of the person's life can produce a state that expresses itself through channels of meaning realized by the microstructure of the brain.

What is more, when we turn the spotlight on phenomena such as institutional neurosis, multiple personality disorder, or suicide, the need to take in the contextual effects of discourse and culture is writ large. In practice, it may well turn out that many syndromes are mixed so that an individual's mental function reflects the interplay of mood-generating thoughts, perhaps shaped by cultural contexts, and mind-affecting physiological changes. The mood-generating thoughts may be empathically understandable, as Jaspers suggests, but quite particular to the psychology of the individual being addressed or they might form a recurring theme understandable in historical or political terms by examining the structure of certain discourses.

The mind, however affected, itself causes effects, for instance on mood, empirically discernible by natural scientific methods and the cultural realities may be so accepted that they are seen as part of the nature of human beings in that setting (Barthes, 1972). The singular patterns of thought and meaning that result are likely to require careful interpersonal and longitudinal analysis so that we encounter, as Kristeva (1995) claims, 'a new malady of the soul' in each patient. Many disorders arise when a range of thoughts (or learning set) dominates and distorts the personality of the individual in ways that are explicable on the basis of the individual's learning history (Bolton & Hill [1996] take this view). But psychosis seems to arise in a surd (or meaningless), disease-like, way. The 'surd' influences on a human being reveal themselves to be so when we learn to detect a pattern of events befalling creatures similar to us.

> Fred has a manic-depressive psychosis. He first comes to medical attention in the full throes of a manic episode, having disposed of $74,000 during a spending spree, sexually assaulted his neighbour's wife, driven a car at high speed to evade the police, and then run to the top of a parking building reciting 'The Charge of the Light Brigade'. Fred's father is

on lithium for a bipolar disorder and his older brother committed suicide during a severe depressive episode. Fred usually functions well as a real-estate salesman on a moderate dose of lithium.

Fred, one could safely reckon, has a physiological disposition to develop psychotic episodes best managed by appropriate doses of a pharmaceutical. However, the detection and correction of biological abnormalities is only part of the restoration of integrity and meaning that engages us with the patient as a person and helps restore a person's humanity. The land of the clinic, however, is not marked out in straight lines and, in practice, we need weighted rather than exclusive explanations for most psychiatric phenomena.

The meaningful connections in a patient's psyche are discerned through empathic understanding even if we are looking at the person as an example of an organism with a cognitive system played upon by certain impersonal effects. Empathy is likely to be both revealing and restorative as it draws a person back into a world of interpersonal activity and potentiates ways of being-among-others. Kay Jamison (1996) remarks, 'But, ineffably, psychotherapy heals. It makes some sense of the confusion, reins in the terrifying thoughts and feelings, and returns some control, hope, and possibility of learning from it all.' (p. 88–89)

Once meaning, arising in the cultural, social, interpersonal, symbolic, or discursive milieu, is admitted as a component of psychological or psychiatric description and explanation, we can glimpse the phenomenology of psychological disorder and discern aspects of human life as things of the 'spirit' (Sims, 1994). These are proper to the *psuche* and not merely 'spooky'. The meanings of life events as interpreted by the patient and the experiential world of the patient as a spiritual dwelling place are, in part, revealed by a discursive inquiry. That revelation is responsive to the patient's situation and allows us to discover genuine insights about ourselves in the psychiatric clinic.

We can close by considering a case discussed by Drury from his own practice (p. 117).

> A man aged fifty-four, a priest . . . a few months prior . . . had begun to feel very depressed about his work . . . He could no longer put any feeling into what he was preaching; that he was asking people to believe and do things which he himself had lost faith in. It was a great burden for him to say mass or read his daily office. He felt that he ought never to have been ordained, that he had no vocation . . . He began to lose weight and to have very disturbed sleep . . . worrying about his spiritual state . . . He could not eat . . . A psychiatrist was called in who diagnosed an involutional depression . . . When I first saw him he was resentful and suspicious. His condition was a spiritual one, he stated, and no doctor could help him.

Drury 'gave him a course of what is known as electroconvulsive therapy'; by the time he had had seven such treatments, 'his spiritual problem had disappeared' (p. 118). The case is interesting and shows, if anything further was needed than ordinary psychiatric practice, that we are psychophysical creatures (to use Husserl's words). We are each a mixture of spirit, word, and flesh in which the vehicle of the *soma* is also the stuff of the *psyche* and is transformed into that which connects us (in the human life-world) to meaning and significance by the influence of discourse with its layers of meaning and its intensely relational character. The art of the psychiatrist is to discern how the psyche is being affected and what mode of address to its discontent is appropriate in relation to the 'new malady of the soul' presenting to him or her in the clinic.

1.12 Conclusion and arguments about the nature of mind and psychiatry

Our biological propensities, discursive context, and our meaningful experiences together contribute to the development of the soul or psyche. The brain is the substrate of thinking and our concepts, articulating our (second) nature as human beings, clothe experience with meanings or significance. Those significations become available to us through interpersonal contexts heavily influenced by culture and history and entangle us in the world as beings-among-others.

> The next theoretical debates in this field should be more on *how* the social and embodied are connected, how the process of mediation between culture and biology works. (Lewis-Fernandez & Kleinman, 1995, p. 440)

The current account, combining connectionism, discursive psychology, and post-structuralism connects culture and biology through the information-shaping brain processing networks and shows how the philosophical arguments justifying a more reductive biological approach all fail.

1.12.1 The argument from underlying reality

1.1 The underlying reality of the world is a set of physical objects and their relations.

1.2 Any plausible scientific account of human life must be in terms of the underlying realities.

1.3 The most scientific and basic accounts of human phenomena are in physical terms.

Such arguments can convince psychologists and psychiatrists to regard neurophysiological or neurochemical accounts of psychiatric phenomena as 'real' or basic. But the fallacy, exposed by Wittgenstein, is the belief that there is a way that things are similar at some fundamental level. At a certain point, our metaphors and images, based on 'middle-sized dry goods' such as billiard balls, levers, lines on paper, and waves at the seaside, all fail and we have gone as far as our Newtonian understanding of the components of reality and the mechanisms connecting them can take us. Electrons are not particles and not waves, but both metaphors (or analogical characterizations) help us in certain ways. Similarly, synapses, neurotransmitters, neural networks, brain pathways, cognitive representations, concepts, thoughts, personality traits, and symbols each (in their own way and in their proper context) are very useful, but no one set of descriptions tells us what reality is *really* like. There is no such absolutely basic understanding; each set of descriptions has its usefulness and serves some purposes well but systematically devalues and obscures others. Beyond that we cannot go, and metaphysical conclusions are (generally) unhelpful. Thus, the argument from underlying reality fails because the whole idea is a mistake.

1.12.2 The argument from basic explanations

This is an argument focusing on the idea that fundamental scientific explanations must deal with the physical or biological level.

2.1 The mind is a set of functions crucially dependent on brain mechanisms for their integrity.

2.2 The underlying events are connected by causal links.

2.3 The fundamental explanations of such links are in physical or biological terms.

2.4 Therefore, the connections between physical events explain mental events but not vice versa.

I have attacked 2.3 by noting that some of the links between brain information-processing events are affected by social and historical contexts replete with discourse and signification. If meaning enters into the explanation of brain configurations, then the search for an (internal and) sufficient set of brain-based explanations of behaviour is a will-o'-the-wisp and 2.4 is false. There *are* genuinely explanatory connections between meaningful (social, cultural, or discursive) events and physical events, and exploring them helps us understand the brain events realizing mental function.

1.12.3 The argument from effective intervention

This is an argument based on the nature of effective interventions in mental disorder.

3.1 We can change states of mind and thought patterns by physical means.

3.2 We cannot change states of mind and so on by mental means.

3.3 Therefore, the physical level causes changes at the mental level but not vice versa.

3.4 Therefore, the mental is a causal by-product of the physical.

3.2 is false: a state of grief that results from being told that one's partner has just died can cause profound physiological effects. I can change your behaviour by telling you that Cambridge is to the north of London because, if you want to go to Cambridge, the resulting belief explains your bodily location during the next few hours. I might also persuade you to take medication, change your diet, and exercise if I convince you that you are likely to have a myocardial infarction and so change your physiology by changing your attitudes. I can defuse your anger by explaining that your wife told her best friend rather than yours to call in while you were at work tomorrow so that they could be alone. In each instance, a mental intervention causes physical effects. Cognitive restructuring or analysis in psychotherapy are examples from clinical psychiatry in which mental interventions can have real effects (despite the fact that telling a psychopath that he needs to treat others differently does not work). A simple logical fallacy connects 'Some mental interventions do not work on some patients' to 'All mental interventions are ineffective', however attractive that conclusion might be to health-system managers.

Thus, even though biological function and, in particular, brain integrity are important in the understanding of the psyche, human mental life is not an epiphenomenon of biology (in particular, neurobiology); it has an essential link to the sociocultural activities and relationships of persons as one might expect from the colloquy of skills that we use in adapting to a human life-world. Aberrant mental function may, therefore, draw on a combination of three types of explanation:

(1) Those invoking the individual subject who classifies and organizes his or her experience,

(2) Those drawing on the position of an individual in culture and discourse, and

(3) Those invoking the biological system that realizes human experience.

Psychiatric disorders, differing radically in their phenomenology and genesis, may range from, at one end of the spectrum, delirium caused by meningococcal pneumonia to, at the other, a personality disorder in a teenage rapist with an alcoholic mother and a violent father. In between, conditions such as Manic-Depressive Psychosis, acute schizophrenia, cycloid psychosis, endogenous depression, psychopathy, anorexia, obsessive-compulsive disorder, pseudologia fantastica, morbid jealousy, reactive depression, borderline personality disorder, and so on may each have a particular type of genesis. And treating any given disorder may involve releasing the person from distorting causal influences (such as porphyria) or from aberrant ideas and habits of the heart arising in the individual's development as a person, because the function of the brain as the substrate of thought is changed by many different types of intervention in the complex nexus informing it.

The next chapters concern the moral and interpersonal effects of certain discourses and practices in psychiatry affecting the human person at both conscious and unconscious levels. In them, discursive psychology and an understanding of human subjectivity as located in relations of power jointly ground an analysis in terms of self-understanding and the narrative project of care-of-the-self.

Chapter 2

Categorization and stigmatization

> Every mental patient is an individual enigma, and we should always think of him as such. There is something more disturbing and puzzling in a dissolution of the personality than in any bodily disease.
> *(Drury, p. 89)*

The very idea of a disease of the psyche is problematic, and the extension of the idea to posit categories of disorder instanced in sufficiently stereotyped ways to fit into groups susceptible to off-the-shelf treatments based on the study of natural or typical human function is also disputed. These facets of psychiatric categorization are illuminated by a case subject to review after complaints were received about the patient's diagnosis and treatment.

Kate Herring (not her real name) was 17 and had lived in rural New Zealand. Raised as a Roman Catholic, she had originally attended a Roman Catholic School. She was fostered and worked on the foster parents' farm until, in 1977, her mother arranged her admission to a psychiatric hospital, Cherry Farm Hospital, as a result of child and adolescent troubles. In 1973, a young friend had committed suicide. In 1974, Kate herself was expelled from high school for disturbed behaviour after a self-inflicted injury. In 1975, she was treated for an overdose and, later the same year, for self-inflicted injuries to her head and arms. The diagnosis of the admitting doctor at the time is unclear, but the word 'depression' is found in the notes and at no point is a more definitive diagnosis given. Another doctor considered that she showed evidence of 'inadequate personality with poor emotional control' (none of the expert commentators have subsequently disagreed with that diagnosis). A friend who visited her recalls, 'We spent the next hour walking, talking, and catching up on what has been happening in our lives.'

After admission, Kate received 'full narcosis treatment'. Only poor records exist of the drugs used, but it seems that very high doses of drugs including clonazepam, lorazepam, sodium amytal, thioridazine, and doxepin were given sufficient to induce a drowsy state and to require a 'full narcosis chart'. This regimen produced a 'confused and unhappy state' and was 'the likely cause for seizures, confusion, urinary retention, and complete constipation' requiring 'the degrading need for manual evacuation of stools and repeated urinary catheterization'. The same friend that met her before admission recalls, 'After admission, I went to see [Kate] in the narcosis unit of Villa A. She looked terrible, pale with bloodshot eyes, and she did not recognize me, or another couple that were also visiting her.' A later commentator calls this management 'incompetent, excessive medical treatment', which led to serious physical, psychological, social, and vocational damage. Yet another commentator stated , 'the way in which the antidepressants, antipsychotics, anti-epileptics, and tranquillizers were prescribed, in my opinion, fall outside the range of acceptable prescribing.'

During early 1978, electroconvulsive therapy (ECT) was added to Kate's regimen to counter increasingly suicidal behaviour; later in that year, having been repeatedly treated with large doses of medication and while attempting to escape during a readmission to hospital, she was hit by a car on the main highway and sustained a fractured leg that left her with a permanent arthrodesis of her knee.

Should Kate have been treated in the way she was? In view of her immature behaviours and self-harm between 1974 and 1977, her 1977 admission is understandable; however, her problem would not be treated by the methods used in her case, and in many places would not warrant inpatient care let alone long-term stay.

So how well grounded was her original diagnosis and what does it mean? Does a psychiatric diagnosis name a disorder that afflicts an individual or reflect a mismatch between the individual and the setting in which he or she lives? Kate's story makes vivid questions at the centre of some long-running debates in psychiatry. I will argue that psychiatric disorders form a 'messy' category (Cooper, 2007) in which a human being as a 'being-in-the-world-with-others' is caught in a situation that reacts with his or her psyche in a distressing and malapative way. Deconstructive critique and qualitative or autobiographical data can therefore help to unravel the questions of illness and disease surrounding psychiatric categories and the role of individual (or biological) factors in their genesis.

Psychiatric illnesses are delineated by taking note of behavioural syndromes, presumably underlying organic changes that, in part, explain them, and responses to therapeutic agents. Data of the second type are often missing in the case of mental disorders so that the weight of diagnosis falls on the first and third. The lack of an underlying pathology has given rise to claims that mental illness is nothing but a social construct designed to deal with individuals who do not fit into the dominant discourse and as a consequence a frantic search for some particular brain abnormality or system dysfunction producing each type of disorder. We therefore need to examine the key concepts in play and find a phenomenologically adequate view of the diverse phenomena encountered in current psychiatric practice.

2.1 The idea of psychiatric illness

A commitment to the reality of mental disorders and the need for clear diagnostic categories is quite explicit in the *Diagnostic and Statistical Manual of Mental Disorders IV* (DSM IV; the leading guide to psychiatric classification; APA 1994a):

> Each of the mental disorders is characterized as a clinically significant behavioral or psychological syndrome or pattern that occurs in an individual and that is associated with present distress (e.g. a painful symptom) or disability (i.e. impairment of one or more important areas of functioning) or with a significantly increased risk of suffering death, pain, disability, or an important loss of freedom. In addition, this syndrome or pattern must not be merely an expectable and culturally sanctioned response to a particular event, for example, the death of a loved one. Whatever its original cause, it must be considered a manifestation of a behavioral, psychological, or biological dysfunction in the individual. (pp. xxi–xxii)

Notice that a psychiatric disorder is seen as an individual problem of which certain behaviour is a manifestation. Some would immediately object, claiming that all the relevant behavior is to some extent interpersonal so that there is scope for the abnormality to be located in any of at least three places: the person, the situation, or the relationship between them; others would add the sociocultural context of the interaction, arguing that 'a practice must not be severed from the social relations of which it is a part' (Kovel, 1988, p. 129). Some contexts are intrinsically disordered, such as war, prisons, or asylums, and arguably, in such situations there are no good actions and choices, only least worst alternatives. Post-Traumatic Stress Disorder, for instance, is a psychiatric condition causing distress and disability but is arguably produced by a normal response to a highly abnormal situation. And the same might apply to 'institutional neurosis' or 'the sick role'.

Over and above the implicit individualism of most diagnostic schemata, the attempt to classify disorders by reference to patterns of manifestation also strikes the problem of observation and interpretation (Kovel, 1988; Lewis-Fernandez & Kleinman, 1995). This might be a relatively slight problem when the categories are easily recognizable kinds such as rabbits and foxes, but genuine psychiatric disorders are a little more problematic in that setting and presupposition may play significant roles as it did in the famous study involving healthy volunteers who were admitted as patients (Rosenham, 1973). But, we should also notice categories that are closely related but radically different in their implications, such as simple schizophrenia and cycloid psychosis, in that here we see the nature and importance of psychiatric diagnosis writ large.

Cycloid psychosis is a controversial mental disorder usually described in the following terms:

(1) A psychotic state

(2) Complete resolution

(3) Mood swings during psychotic state

(4) At least two of the following five features

    (a) Paranoia-like symptoms

    (b) Motility disturbance

    (c) Confusion

    (d) Pananxiety

    (e) Ecstasy (Cutting, 1990)

A typical patient is described as follows:

> A 43-year-old woman had several incoherent excited phases and perplexed inhibited phases. When excited, she was admitted screaming with incoherent, pressured speech with the reiteration of certain words, and with gesticulation, dancing, monotonous hitting, and erotic tendencies. When inhibited, she said everything was so strange, colourless, and empty. . . . She made a complete recovery.

> (Brockington et al., 1982, pp. 652–653)

The condition is often, or even usually, diagnosed as acute schizophrenia or, on occasion, bipolar disorder. The latter reflects the generally favourable prognosis of this condition compared with others in the schizophrenia group. Believers in the cycloid psychotic disorders tend to stress that the clinical picture is, on the one hand, unlike an affective disorder and its course, on the other hand, is unlike schizophrenia, suggesting that it should be distinguished from both. When we turn to the DSM IV (APA 1994a), we find 'Schizophrenic Disorder: Episodic Type with No Interepisode Residual Decisions, Schizoaffective Disorder, Brief Psychotic Disorder, and Schizophreniform Disorder', any of which would fit the presenting picture. But the debate assumes what could be called, after Foucault, an *Essentialist* position, according to which each diagnostic category marks an entity with a distinct nature or essence and it sidelines the possibility that we are, in diagnosis, imposing evaluatively loaded categories and discursive constructions on a continuum of mental discontent featuring schizoid and disorganized tendencies in the human psyche.

The DSM IV (APA 1994a) notes the need for training and clinical judgment in the use of its diagnostic criteria and rejects the idea that 'each category of mental disorder is a completely discrete entity with absolute boundaries dividing it from other mental disorders or no mental disorder' (p. xxii). It claims that the categories are not meant to be applied 'in a cookbook fashion' so that there is flexibility in interpretation by different skilled judges and it does not pronounce the causes of any disorder nor the degree of control exercised by the individual over their symptoms. But this tolerance raises other questions.

What, in the face of this 'messiness', is the purpose of a diagnostic system such as that in the DSM IV or the *International Classification of Diseases 10* (ICD 10)? If it does not always allow clear-cut categories, some disorders will have fuzzy boundaries. If it does not make aetiological or therapeutic suggestions and does not enter the debate about malingering, factitious disorders, and 'genuine' illnesses, then should it be taken realistically (in the sense of delineating diseases)? Even though these may be serious flaws from the position of a philosophical realist, they should not worry more pragmatic or everyday realists, a difference that emerges from serious (metaphysical) philosophy of science (the kind of thing pragmatists, Wittgensteinians, phenomenologists, and other low-life thinkers generally bypass).

Philosophical realists concern themselves with *natural kinds*, more or less the categories we use when we aim to 'cut nature at its joints' in pursuit of a metaphysical quest to discover the real nature or essences of things (their properties independent of our ways of thinking about them)[1]. I have already noted a more modest task whereby we search for the mechanisms securing *causal homeostasis* in a given domain to guide us in taxonomy (Griffiths, 1997). The problem is that the production of complex human phenomena such as mental disorders is misleadingly assimilated to biological or physiological processes (as I have noted). Genuinely informative and projectable generalizations need to take account of the sociocultural and discursive forces in play, including moral and intersubjective influences, best understood, for some purposes, 'from the inside' rather than from the detached vantage point of the clinical observer (Lewis-Fernandez & Kleinman, 1995). It is therefore worth revisiting the critique of psychiatry from the point of view of discursive psychology and deconstruction.

---

[1] I will discuss this in Appendix B.

Similar to all metaphysical quests, the quest for natural kinds in psychiatry is fuelled by a type of realism that rests on two postulates:

> Illness is an essence, a specific entity that can be mapped by the symptoms that manifest it, but that is anterior to them and, to a certain extent, independent of them.
>
> Side by side with this 'essentialist' prejudice . . . there was a naturalist postulate that saw illness in terms of botanical species; . . . thus, dementia praecox was like a species characterized by the ultimate forms of its natural development and which may present hebephrenic, catatonic, or paranoid variants.

(Foucault, 1954/1987, p. 6)

These (realist) commitments have two corollaries. The first is a *bivalence* claim, according to which any candidate for a given category either does or does not belong to it. On that basis each patient presents with a genuine case of 'X' or not, despite any difficulties in making the judgement because the categories in question are independent of our judgements about them (fallibilism, for instance, holds that there may be examples of X about which, given our epistemic limitations, we cannot be sure, but that nevertheless there is a truth of the matter). The realist or essentialist cannot tolerate fuzzy boundaries (unless the fuzziness is confined to our ability to judge on the basis of the evidence we have) because if our categories correspond to the way that nature itself is in itself, we should be discerning real regularities connected by natural laws open to scientific investigation.

Secondly, the naturalist programme aims to find typical examples of each disorder and to identify the causal regularities underpinning it. Genuine regularities, marked by terms linked to real features appearing in natural laws (such as those of biology), explain how things work (causally), as in the rest of medicine. For instance, embolic strokes are caused by blood clots from major blood vessels such as the carotid artery detaching from the vessel wall and blocking a more distal artery (such as the middle cerebral or one of its major branches). The object of explanation—a stroke—is seen to result from a natural process and the causal chain seems to be understood (in part). Such a beginning grounds further study of and intervention in the phenomenon of interest (we know what processes have to be changed).

Unfortunately, the requisite certainties in clinical observation are not easily had in psychiatry despite instruments such as the DSM IV (or the magnetic resonance imaging [MRI] scanner). There is no general agreement about the processes we are studying and whether there are (biological) causal chains with a discernible relationship to psychiatric disorders. Thus, a story of obsessional neurosis or even catatonic schizophrenia from a dynamic or object relations theorist works with clinical descriptions that have dynamic overtones. That theory-laden descriptions abound more in psychiatry than in most sciences is almost inevitable because descriptions of behaviour occur against framing presuppositions. For instance, even basic intentional language—as in 'He reached for the door handle', 'He started at her name', 'She looked up suddenly', 'She saw her mother walk in'—embeds a person in a situation full of perceptions, desires, attitudes, and so on. Indeed, many philosophers argue that it is impossibe and irrational to try and provide behavioural descriptions without colouring them by relating them to the kinds of things people usually think and do (Hornsby, 1985; Merleau Ponty, 1964) so that the events and the story giving them their significance are hermeneutically interwoven. Change the story so that different (contextualizing) events emerge and the patterns of behaviour become significant in a different kind of way. Consider the following case.

> The wife: 'I arrived home and found my husband with that woman and I was just overcome with anger; I was so shocked and surprised. I reached into my bag and my hand came across my gun and I pulled it out and he ran towards me and I squeezed the trigger.' The detective: 'You know I believe almost all of that story. I believe you went inside the house, I believe you saw your husband embracing Ms. Scarlet, I believe you pulled your gun out of your handbag, and I believe you pulled the trigger and shot him dead. But Mrs. Oates from down the street saw you parked in your car and watching as your husband got out of the car and took Ms. Scarlet inside.'

The observation changes our understanding of the wife's behaviour, not in respect to what she did, only in regard to the self-ascription—'I was so shocked and surprised'— crucial to our interpretation of what happened. Mrs. Oates observation reorients the psychological explanation, connecting it differently to feelings and thoughts about the situation. The wife was not overcome by shock and surprize. Her actions must be explained differently and we do not need scientific psychology to tell us so; we need Verstehen and the messy (unlawlike) world of phenomenology and discursive reality. There may be neural correlates of her calculated cognition (perhaps dorso-lateral prefrontal rather than hypothalamo-medial temporal), but the real story is in the instantly comprehensible human story. Neurobiological precursors are not our best explanations of psychological events (and the phenomena producing certain types of mental illness) and are only credible insofar as they correlate with the real explanations. And, there are strands of philosophy, eminently suited to therapeutic practice, that support this tentative conclusion.

Pragmatism begins by assuming that humans approach the world with the attitude 'Here is a problem; how shall we solve it?' and it examines the cognitive tools that help us achieve our goals. Concepts are better if they are more *complete* (in terms of capturing the richness and connectedness of experience) and have the right mix of *transferability* (or generality) and *task specificity*. A really good system of concepts and beliefs is as wide ranging and exceptionless as possible and thus 'as near as dammit' to a set of true beliefs (as the realist sees it) and also closely articulates our activity with the fragment of the world it is aimed at. But the idea of cognitive tools raises a problem: 'To a hammer everything looks like a nail.'

We are all realists at heart and want to know how things really are with the world ('Does the world really comprise good and bad nails?') A pragmatist argues that we have ways of looking at things that are very good for some purposes and useless for others and that is as good as it gets and is on fairly solid ground. For instance, is a photon a wave or a particle? It depends what you want to do: if you want to understand the quanta of energy needed to make a sensitive radiation counter work, you better believe electrons are little packages of energy; but if you want to understand diffraction patterns in slit experiments, then you had better believe that they are waves. In the end, the limitations of middle-sized dry goods language (replete with bivalence) should not mess us about too much in real science. We should just get on with the job of observing, theorizing, and explaining and set to one side the metaphysical uncertainties at the heart of what we are doing.

In a similar way, the growth of psychiatric knowledge is likely to be served by therapists communicating and pooling their observations. To do this, they need to use and agree about certain concepts: in the spirit of the DSM IV (APA 1994a), they can *bracket* questions about how deep those concepts go. Theory building about the nature and kinds of mental illness can wait until we have a rich and clearly articulated data set and can see patterns in it that really help us.

This, in one sense, is 'the phenomenological method' in that it first attends closely to the data of experience and then uses conjectures, metaphors, and models, without metaphysical prejudice, to try and get an insightful understanding of what is going on. We need to find descriptions adequate to characterize a broad range of clinical presentations and defer (perhaps indefinitely) a judgement about the ultimate truth of categorical statements regarding the 'illness' suffered by this or that person. The DSM 'slot' characterizes the disorder so as to group it with others showing relevant similarities, and holding lightly to the schema allows us to notice regularities that may not be in accord with our theories. Seeing patterns, some of which may indicate unifying explanations (such as the thought that psychopaths are disconnected from others in some respects like autistic people), may show us ways of helping people who are 'alienated' in ways that cause distress and misunderstanding.

The DSM IV (APA 1994a) need not, therefore, be part of an essentialist and individualist programme in psychiatry but should be seen as providing an aid to clinical communication about the varieties of mental disorder. It does trade on the idea that common configurations in the discontents of the mind show us *mental disorders best thought of as diseases*, but one need not buy into the metaphysics to use the tool (Cooper, 2007). The DSM IV might best be regarded as serving an interpersonal conception of truth so that different observers can pool and compare their observations to produce provisional revisable conceptions of the types of mental disorder. Such a pooled and intersubjective view can accept a more humble phenomenological and pragmatic basis for its use. The need for categories, on this modest conception, amounts to no more than an agreed set of judgements grounding, in Wittgenstein's terms, a language to map out a domain of activity in which we deploy certain quasi-medical and quasi-juridical skills to gain insight into the experience of and deal with those whom our society calls mad, a theme developed by Foucault in his seminal works on mental illness.

2.2 Foucault on mental illness

Foucault is a post-structuralist who examines not only the linguistic but also the discursive roles of domains such as medicine, psychiatry, and mental illness, subjecting them to the anti-metaphysical and deconstructive tendencies of postmodern thought[2].

---

[2] See the appendix (G) on structuralism and post-structuralism.

At times, he reads like Freud, focusing on the dynamic reality of the psyche:

> The illness then proceeds like a vicious circle: the patient protects himself by his present defence mechanisms against a past whose secret presence arouses anxiety; but, on the other hand, against the possibility of a present anxiety, the subject protects himself by appealing to protections that were set up in earlier, similar situations.
>
> (Foucault, 1954/1987, p. 41)

At times, he hunts with the hounds of sociohistorical critique and deconstruction:

> For a long time now, one fact has become the commonplace of sociology and mental pathology: mental illness has its reality and its value qua illness only within a culture that recognises it as such.
>
> (Foucault, 1954/1987, p. 60)

The first tendency fosters theories about the intrapsychic origins of mental illness:

> Imagination is not madness. Even if in the arbitrariness of hallucination, alienation finds the first access to its vain liberty, madness begins only beyond this point, when the mind binds itself to this arbitrariness and becomes the prisoner of this apparent liberty.
>
> (Foucault, 1973, p. 92)

He invokes a 'vain liberty' unconstrained by the discourse of embodiment and the discursive context of thought to distinguish between ordinary distraction and internal distress and insanity. Madness is a surd quality or disorganization of the relationship between external discourse and the image imprisoning the individual within a profound disruption of embodied experience so that he or she is alienated from the world of others (and from himself or herself). 'The body and the traces it conceals, the soul and the images it perceives, are here no more than stages in the syntax of delirious language (Foucault, 1973, p. 97).

This is Foucault in a phenomenological mood, but the second theme in his work locates the origins and delineation of mental illness in a cultural milieu that marginalizes and labels certain human beings as mad or mentally ill because they transgress or resist the legitimated discourses of their sociohistorical context.

> More effectively than any other kind of rationalism, better in any case than our positivism, classical rationalism could watch out for and guard against the subterranean danger of unreason, that threatening space of absolute freedom. (Foucault, 1973, p. 84) . . . The savage danger of madness is related to the danger of the passions and to their fatal concatenation. (p. 85)

Foucault traces the distinction between reason and passion in the classical period and the internal link between reason and the orderly conduct of social life (the Soul mirrors the Republic). Against that context, the beast within rages (as in Freud's *Civilisation and Its Discontents*) and the discourse of the human being tortured by excess passion beyond the control of reason begins to shape conceptualizations of the psyche. The person who falls into 'violent liberty' or '*liberum brutum*' (Kant) must be curbed, constrained, and disciplined by the order intrinsic to reason, an interpersonal and social task. 'It is . . . the exactitude of a social order, imposed from without and, if necessary, by force, that can gradually restore the minds of maniacs to the light of truth.' (Foucault, 1973, p. 186)

This second theme gives rise to Foucault's widely known (sociohistorical) claims about medicine in general and psychiatry in particular:

> If the medical personage could isolate madness, it was not because he knew it, but because he mastered it; and what for positivism would be an image of objectivity was only the other side of this domination.
>
> (Foucault, 1973, p. 272)

Here, Foucault both summarizes and castigates contemporary scientific realism in psychiatry, observing that our medical attitude (widely promulgated) is that madness is a kind of *otherness* from right thinking and therefore incomprehensible and needing containment. As *other*, the insane are cases or instances of human aberration to be studied from the (objective, rational) vantage point of 'normality', distanced from madness or unreason and part of the mechanisms of domination. Positivism or rational scientific realism is part of this view, available to the clear thinking when they gaze upon the afflicted, and it canonizes the exclusion and categorical distinction between us and them. Foucault deconstructs the truths or 'images of objectivity' that legitimate the domination imposed on those who undergo psychic suffering.

The second strand of Foucaultian thought can give rise to social constructionism and the labelling theory whereby mental illness is thought to be no more than the result of social norms acting on individuals who are 'different' (and therefore excluded) in various ways (Foucault, 1984, p. 147). This orientation vastly extends 'the element of value that is present in any definition of health' (Wing, 1978, p. 29) and can threaten (by excess) to taint by association any insights into mental disorder arising from a discursive inquiry.

We ought to avoid the extreme claims associated with either aspect of Foucault's work and attend to both perspectives, seeking to appreciate the interpersonal dynamics of mental disorder and the sociohistorical context that allows a particular disorder (such as 'mad travelling') to thrive at a given time in a given place (Hacking, 1998).

2.3 The anti-psychiatrists—Thomas Szasz

Szasz (1962/1972) argues that mental illness is not a variant of physical illness as reflected in essentialist and classificatory models found throughout medicine, but is a discourse in which the meanings attached to illness are appropriated and enable certain kinds of transactions to go on between people. In these transactions, one player or set of players has a quasi-juridical function and other people can apply to (or be referred to) that player to be judged ill. Once judged to be ill by someone with 'the social power to make their judgements heard and to implement them' (p. 27), a certain pattern of discourse or complex set of roles is played out by the participants in subsequent transactions. For a post-structuralist, this looks exactly like the deployment of meanings to change our attitudes and activities in a situation.

Szasz (1962/1972) is at his best in the phenomena associated with hysteria, but he holds a radical view of mental illness in general, arguing that psychiatry, unlike medicine, deals with 'moral and personal conflicts' (p. 44) and 'problems in human relationships' (p. 47). He observes the difficulties in psychiatric classification and attributes them to two quite distinct sources:

(i) The epistemological problem, compatible with realism in all its guises but with twists that are evident in Multiple Personality Disorder (MPD);

(ii) The human propensity for 'intelligent goal-directed participation in the events that shape his [or her] life' (p. 51), which is seen in both role playing and coun-terfeiting, but is perhaps better linked to 'the looping effect of human kinds' (Hacking, 1995).

Hacking (1995) notices,

> People classified in a certain way tend to conform to or to grow into the ways they are described, but they also evolve in their own ways so that the classifications and descriptions have to be constantly revised. (p. 21)

Hacking notes that every self-conception has a formative and not merely representa-tional relation to the human being using it so that, 'in the social sciences, we are faced with a full and complicated interaction between observer and observed' (Szasz, 1962/1972, p. 22). Szasz locates psychiatry among the social sciences rather than the natural or medical sciences because it 'consists in the study of personal conduct' (p. 24) and draws not only on biology and physiology but also on 'anthropology, ethics, and sociology' (p. 29). He argues that in psychiatry or psychology the investiga-tors and the persons being investigated each assess and react to the other according to conceptions of what is happening between them[3].

Szasz's analysis of interpersonal relations and conduct, in terms of rule following, draws heavily on Wittgenstein, as do Bolton and Hill (1996), who examined our hab-its of rule following to find cognitive learning sets that are the basis of inappropriate and maladaptive behaviour. For Szasz, rules are normative in the non-biological or moral sense, arising within 'the games people play' and the narrative work of self-formation (Wittgenstein, 1953, ¶202ff)[4].

Szasz also draws on Mead (the anthropologist) for whom language and the definition of self within a social process are the features of human natural history distin-guishing us from other animals. The social process is viewed as a loosely interwoven set of games allowing a person to take different roles that help each of us answer the ques-tions, 'Who am I?', 'How should I act?', and 'What is it OK to do around here?' These questions and their answers articulate the complex interaction between subjectivity, agency, and the background discourse structuring one's form of life. Szasz (1962/1972) concludes that 'Mental illnesses thus differ fundamentally from bodily diseases, and resemble, rather, certain moves or tactics in playing games.' (p. 208) Szasz echoes a point made by both Kant and Wittgenstein, that human beings obey rules because they are rules (normative requirements, prescriptions, or imperatives) and not merely

---

[3] Vygotsky and Donaldson (1979) have shown how important this is in developmental psychology.

[4] ¶ denotes paragraph or section numbers in Wittgenstein's work

because of causal processes obeying natural laws (although we have noted that humans develop a second nature as a result of being configured by culture and discourse).

The fact that we can reflect on the rules we are shaped by and the roles they define for us brings to the fore intentional or conscious rule-following behaviour. A human being is, at any given time, both trying to conform to the rules of a given discourse (in part through trying to answer a question as to who she or he is and what is expected of her or him) and also subject to inclinations of a less discursive kind. One could picture this as a complex psychic juggling task performed by the narrative self not as an idle pastime but in order to exist in a way compatible with a coherent sense of self and identity. The existential *angst* and bewilderment when one lacks the (psychic juggling) skills required strikes at the heart of one's being-in-the-world-with-others, and that is the only kind of being a human being can live. The hysteric is, on Szasz's account, a clever player with a distorted view of the point of the game who manipulates others for ultimately dysfunctional ends, but any acquaintance with the realities of the clinic reveals that the psychotic patient is otherwise. Szasz might be able to justify the claim that one should treat hysteria in moral rather than pathological terms, but the moral intricacies of hysteria both deserve and reward close scrutiny in discursive terms and illustrate how subtle and shifting the boundary of madness is for any of us[5].

What we can take from Szasz, of general relevance, is the thought that the expectations and norms of a social setting and the unwritten rules by which we all live can yield genuine insights into the experience of madness. However, a more generally adequate account of psychiatric illness must accommodate the fear, bewilderment, and distress characteristic of psychosis, insights that did not escape Foucault and take us beyond the moralistic horizons of Szasz's anti-psychiatry and towards his contemporary Ronnie Laing.

2.4 The anti-psychiatrists—R. D. Laing

R. D. Laing, in his attack on psychiatry in the 1960s and 1970s, undertook the task of understanding schizophrenia and attempted to include the psychotic in a discursive understanding of diverse and tortured subjectivities by championing two main theses. The *first* is that psychotic phenomena are a response to an *existential challenge* threatening the patient's identity and integrity (as a being-in-the-world or *ipseity*). The *second thesis* is that many of the 'symptoms' of schizophrenia represented an attempt to cope with an *intrinsically mystifying and internally contradictory set of demands* arising in an aberrant social context. Both theses indicate important insights not only into the discursive reality of some patients diagnosed as schizophrenic but also into psychiatric phenomenology in general.

The first thesis appeared in *The Divided Self* where Laing (1962/1965) pursues Sartre's (1958) 'existential psychiatry' (gestured at in *Being and Nothingness*): 'In the context of our present pervasive madness that we call normality, sanity, freedom, all our frames of reference are ambiguous and equivocal.' (p. 11) Laing captures the spirit of the sixties anti-establishment values and rebellion against polite society and

---

[5] I shall return to this in Chapter 12.

suburbia, the context of life for many in the West, and asks us to shift our perspective in order to understand the phenomena of schizophrenic subjectivity.

Laing-style anti-psychiatrists summarize the claims of psychiatry as follows:

(1) The mad things said and done by a schizophrenic will remain essentially a closed book if one does not understand their existential context. (Laing, 1962/1965, p. 17)

(2) [T]he concretum is seen as man's existence, his being-in-the-world. (p. 19)

(3) It is the task of existential phenomenology to articulate what the other's 'world' is and his way of being in it. (p. 25)

(4) A man may have a sense of his presence in the world as a real, alive, whole, and in a temporal sense, a continuous person . . . an existential position . . . I shall call *primary ontological security*. (p. 39)

(5) This study is concerned with . . . anxieties and dangers that I shall suggest arise *only* in terms of *primary ontological insecurity*. (p. 39)

(6) The ontologically insecure person may feel threatened by engulfment, implosion, or petrification and the consequent loss of self by any one of these means. (p. 43ff)

(7) Existential psychotherapy listens to the patient engaging with him or her as a real person whose conduct of his or her own life is to be affirmed and strengthened.

This last statement seems largely to have been accepted by contemporary psychiatry, but its framework of existential psychoanalysis is less widespread. Sartre and Jaspers derived the ideas from Heidegger but Laing, in applying them to real patients in the British psychiatric system, brought them to the fore. Contra Jaspers' claim that psychotic thought was bizarre and incomprehensible, Laing argued 'that we require to orientate ourselves to this person in such a way as to leave open to us the *possibility* of understanding him' (p. 32) so that basing a moral stance to the patient on a contrast between the meaningful and causal origins of the disorder was problematized and seen as inherently alienating.

Laing takes seriously the interactive reality—comprising the psychiatrist, the patient, and the context—and examines the mismatch or maladaptation of the patient as someone who is living a desperately complex, bewildering, and threatening experience and who does not share an important and existentially basic feature of the human life world—congruence with his or her fellows. Laing is critical of the orthodox psychiatric attitude to psychosis and remarks, 'the existential phenomenological construction is an inference about the way the other is feeling and acting' (p. 31), a projective or imaginative approach recreating the lived experience of the world in which the psychotic patient finds him or herself.

Laing's second thesis is that one can understand schizophrenic patients in the context of their families. He argues that psychosis is a response to intrinsically mystifying and internally contradictory contexts accessible from a phenomenological and existential orientation. In *Sanity, Madness and the Family* (Laing & Esterson, 1970), the case is argued and illustrated:

> It is most important to recognise that the diagnosed patient is not suffering from a disease whose aetiology is unknown unless he can prove otherwise. He is someone who has queer experiences and/or is acting in a queer way, from the point of view usually of his relatives

and ourselves. Whether these queer experiences and actions are constantly associated with changes in his body is still uncertain, although it is highly likely that relatively enduring biochemical changes may be the consequence of relatively enduring interpersonal situations of particular kinds. (p. 18)

This last claim—that social arrangements can affect the chemistry of the brain—has been noted already in relation to animal experiments (see Chapter 1) and underpins the realization that social and interpersonal relations affect the microprocessing structure of the brain. However, even if one were to concede that disordered interpersonal arrangements could, through stress, internal conflict, fear, and anxiety, affect the biochemical reactions in the brain, it is a further step to claim that it would affect the biochemistry enough to produce some of the more florid disorders seen in the thought, affect, and motor function of the psychotic patient. The motor problems, well recognized before the advent of neuroleptic medication, include retardation, echopraxia, incoordination, tics, restlessness, spasms, choreiform movements, and so on. They seem to indicate a basic dysfunction in cerebral systems unassociated with intentional content. However, even if the primary aetiology of schizophrenia is not always familial or social, understanding intrafamilial dynamics may well illuminate schizophrenic behaviour as in some of Laing and Esterson's (1970) claims:

(i) Interactions within the family nexus reveal that some features of schizophrenic thought and behaviour, such as thought insertion, influence, and withdrawal, have an adaptive psychological or discursive function.

(ii) The meanings of certain symptoms in terms of the patient's lived experience are revealed by family dynamics.

(iii) Certain phenomena, such as blurring of ego boundaries, impoverishment of affect, and paranoid delusions, may be produced as reactions to aspects of family interaction.

These claims are successively stronger, the last implying that at least some schizophrenic phenomena are shaped by or even result from family dynamics. The strongest thesis is that schizophrenia is entirely a social product, but a more nuanced philosophical attitude is also consistent with their data.

A. S. Byatt (1984) makes vivid the (existential phenomenological) possibility that a coherent but alienated story lies behind even the most bizarre encounters:

He had no faith in Mr Rose's ability to help him. This may have been because he defined 'help' to himself as a putting right of something that had gone wrong, a restoration of some earlier good, 'normal' state, and he was not sure that such a state had existed or could exist. Normal was what people said some of their actions and relations were, from time to time, and in Marcus's experience what they said they were bore only a vague relation to their actual forms and configurations. . . . It did not occur to Marcus to say any of this to Mr Rose. (pp. 30–31)

Such stories are abound in Laing and Esterson's (1970) intriguing exploration of 11 quite dysfunctional families in which the patients are subject to mystification threatening their existence by constantly discounting and undermining their attempts to understand what is happening to them: 'To what extent is the experience and behaviour of that person who has already begun a career as a diagnosed 'schizophrenic' patient intelligible in the light of the praxis and process of his or her family nexus?' (p. 27)

A discursive approach sidelines the biological and natural and aligns itself with patients as authors: 'It is precisely each person's perspective on the situation that he shares with others that we wish to discover' (p. 19). The resulting perspectives are not only intelligible but also persuasive and contribute to our appreciation of the phenomenology of psychosis.

> An idea of reference that she had was that something she could not fathom was going on between her parents, seemingly about her. Indeed there was. When they were all inter-viewed together, her mother and father kept exchanging with each other a constant series of nods, winks, gestures, knowing smiles, so obvious to the observer that he commented on them after twenty minutes of the first such interview. (p. 40)

The 28-year-old woman concerned was trying to assert herself as an adult but her parents attributed such attempts at independence to her 'illness'. The therapist remarks: 'The close investigation of this family reveals that her parents' statements to her about her, about themselves, about what they felt she felt they felt, and even about what could be directly seen and heard, could not be trusted.' (p. 43)

This is *mystification*, because her thoughts and feelings are discounted, denied, or ridiculed so that she cannot name and articulate significant aspects of her interactions with others. Such a milieu leaves a person uncertain about their own thoughts and feelings, alienated from self and others, and likely to resort to strange images and expressions to explain that predicament. The images are born of desperation and reflect the subject's existential insecurity and sense of threatened identity (an *ipseity* disrupted) rather than revealing biologically generated delusions and misperceptions of what is going on around them.

In each case, the patient's words are located in a discursive situation where discon-nections and disruptions separate the patient's avowals of certain thoughts and feel-ings and the parents attributions undermining them. This process of discounting and invalidating or projectively distorting a person's thoughts and feelings shows up time and time again in Laing and Esterson's (1970) case histories: 'The mother and father did not simply tell her to be afraid of crowds, to fear men, etc.; they told her she was and is afraid of crowds and men.' (p. 87)

They also describe situations in which the adage 'just because I'm paranoid it doesn't mean that people aren't picking on me' is graphically instanced:

> On one occasion, when Sarah left the room, her mother, father, and brother began a furtive whispered exchange about her. As Sarah re-entered, she said uncertainly that she had the impression they were talking about her. They denied this and looked at us significantly, as though to say: 'See how suspicious she is.' (p. 114)

The authors contend that false, mystifying, and confusing communications of this kind induce a kind of paralysis in which such things as paranoid delusions, thoughts of influence or thought insertion, and 'impoverishment of affect and incongruity of thought and affect are here intelligible as social praxis' (p. 106). They are intelligible because there is no right way to act or think for the psychotic person trapped in the middle of contradictions and condemnations or what, after Lacan, we could call systematic *meconnaissance*. 'If, whatever I see or think, things are not the way I think they are, and however I act, I do the wrong thing; what more can a poor boy do?'

The same revelations emerge from subjective reports by ex-inmates of institutions:

> I felt increasingly like a guest who is given every hospitality in a country mansion but yet who finds in unexpected moments a trace of a mysterious presence: sliding panels; secret tappings; and at last, surprises the host and hostess in clandestine conversations and plottings with mention of prison, torture, death.

(Frame, 1961/1980, p. 75)

These are classic paranoid thoughts, but a single incident shows them in their true light; they are astute perceptions of a situation where, indeed, much was hidden and where existential *angst* was in fact a realistic response to a highly abnormal environment and set of praxes. The incident erupted when a patient defied the Matron of the hospital.

> Matron Borough's glance sent her into a fury. She began to call Matron names to swear at her. 'You big fat bloody bullock, don't you stare at me.' Matron's face and neck reddened; she too was sensitive about her appearance. 'Out of here', she said. . . . Mrs. Dean refused to leave the bathroom. . . . 'Right', snapped Matron, beckoning to a nurse; and moving towards the door in the bathroom which was always kept locked and which I had never seen used, Matron Borough opened it and, with three other nurses who had arrived, dragged the struggling Mrs. Dean through the door. She never returned to the ward.

(Frame, 1961/1980, pp. 76–77)

Some days later, the 'mysterious disappearance' of her fellow patient is illuminated for her.

> Returning past the conglomeration of old buildings which seemed unreal in their lack of relationship to our bright admission ward, we met two attendants carrying out the back way from Four-Five-and-One, a corpse, bloated looking under its canvas. 'That's Mrs. Dean,' the nurse said indiscreetly. 'She died.'

The 'paranoid' impressions clearly demonstrate a perspicuity beyond that expected of a psychotic patient reporting her 'mad' experiences. There are secret goings on, some with lethal significance for the patients; they occur in places known only to selected participants in the discourse, and are systematically hidden from others. The discourse of the institution renders certain realities invisible and silences certain voices so that some observations are never legitimated and are therefore 'not real'. Whatever we think of the implausibly strong social production thesis, the praxes and discourses explored by Laing and Esterson (1970) might be expected to exacerbate and account for many of the symptoms and signs of psychosis. And looking past the 'flagship' psychoses—schizophrenia and bipolar disorder—to the whole gamut of maladies of the soul, it is plausible that disordered family and institutional dynamics do affect clinical phenomenology.

This relatively modest thesis about context (and family praxis and process in particular) together with the existential insecurity made vivid by Laing make the suffering, helplessness, and confusion of a psychiatric patient all seem much more comprehensible than the descriptions of psychosis in standard texts otherwise suggest. Vulnerability and existential danger are marauders on the journey of life threatening to destroy or viciously wound the psyche as is seen in the study of Oscar (Wilson, 1974).

2.5 **Oscar**

Oscar, an inhabitant of Providencia, in the Caribbean, was an itinerant carrying a sack of 'valuables', (actually the detritus to be gathered at the edges of human life like all such). 'My study is of a single and singular individual. It is the story of his struggle for life as a person—a struggle pursued at every turn with those among whom he lives: his society.' (Wilson, 1974, pp. ix–x)

This 'study of the relationship between an individual and his society' begins when Wilson first arrives in Providencia and is welcomed by 'Professor Oscar Bryan de Newball,' who rows out to the ship, comes aboard, and asks 'who I was and what brought me to these parts' (p. 8):

> My ferryman explained to me not to mind, for it was only Oscar who was mad. Then he quickly added, as if he had given a false impression, that I must also remember that Oscar was very intelligent.
>
> Oscar was quite short, and his habitual stoop and rounded shoulders made him appear even shorter. There was a certain chunkiness about his build and firmness to his skin and muscles, which gave notice of great strength and toughness. He stooped but he did not sag. His head was large and crowned with tightly curled silver hair. His face was strikingly handsome: deep brown eyes twinkled in their sun-creased sockets . . . Finally, there was his voice: strong, clear, and resonant, it established his authority. (p. 9)

Oscar had compendious knowledge of the island and its inhabitants, but Wilson began to notice a strange aspect to his dealings with Oscar: 'It seems as if we were two characters acting scenes written by Samuel Beckett or Harold Pinter' (p. 10). Oscar is, in some elusive way, alienated within the shared human world. Despite his alienation, Oscar seems well aware of his own position in society and of what was said about him, revealing reflection and insight similar to that seen in the works of Janet Frame.

> I cannot understand why the people say I am mad. I feel free to do what I want to do. If I want to refrain, I can refrain. I feel I am in possession of my mind. I become despondent thinking on things of the past. The best thing is to be busy night and day. I forget some of the stings.
>
> (Wilson, 1974, p. 16)

The 'stings', in Oscar's case, were considerable. Caribbean culture, according to Wilson (1973), is a culture in which twin values are in a schizoid tension: *respectability*, a value derived from middle-class European culture, vies with *reputation*, which 'emphasizes egalitarianism and opposes class heirarchy' (Wilson, 1974, p. 116), rooted in the island community. Respectability is found where the people who hold positions of discursive power and status say it should be and is derived from certain values reflecting an idealized society displaced from its European middle-class origins. Reputation, on the other hand, is based on fathering, both biological and social, a much more tribal construct, but is also built on the willingness to defend one's honour, the mastery of certain verbal and rhetorical skills, musical ability, knowledge of local lore, and experience of foreign lands (1974, pp. 116–117).

Oscar was born illegitimate and therefore, in a society structured by respectability and reputation, certain expectations and categorizations informed his subjectivity or lived experience. For instance, the highly significant path to respectability could only be traversed by becoming a good father and achieving a 'notably respectable position'.

> Oscar not only failed in this, he failed miserably. He married out of a misplaced sense of duty to respectability. He got his girlfriend pregnant and married her because it was the 'right' thing to do. Then she was unfaithful, beginning with when he left the island to begin his training for ministry. Though she bore him five children, he has lost touch with all of them. (p. 121)

Oscar understands the course of this tragedy fully well:

> My father-in-law, nourishing old grudges of eight years ago—for that I took his daughter and he would have had it but she was impregnated—went from office to office advertising the limitations of his son-in-law on the scale of madness. . . . Many others also join in this conspiracy, a conspiracy second to none against a man that was ready to risk everything for the defense of his family and a liberal education.
>
> They block and trip me, block my progress to have me tripped.
>
> *In my concept, I made good until the brethren decided my aspiration is too high for my complexion, and a boy who is scarcely known among his father's sons.*
>
> But now they were trying out a scheme of extinguishing me behind bars and asylum walls.
>
> When I returned to my island home, I wrote back to those headhunters: 'I am back to normal. You ought to be ashamed and throw away your Bibles.'
>
> While confined in the asylum, my wife went into open prostitution, taking one Andreas O'Neill into my home and defiling my marriage bed. (pp. 101–104)

The comments refer to Oscar's move to Panama to further his theological education. But he was admitted to a mental hospital so that his intention to pursue theological studies was thwarted and he returned home to Providencia to find his wife living with another man.

> Just what happened during his stay in Panama will never be known. But it was there that he broke down, and I suspect it was there that the impossibility of his ever being able to pass from reputation to respectability became apparent to him. And to this failure to be accepted into the ministry was added his failure as a son, as a husband, and as a father.
>
> (Wilson, 1974, p. 122)

This tragic story is a dynamic vehicle for a subtle analysis of sanity and madness. Wilson notes that Oscar's colourful reputation 'extended beyond the borders of Providencia' (p. 123) and also that the community had a markedly ambivalent attitude towards him: he was mad, but also intelligent and knowledgeable, worthy of respect, but also of fear. The attitude reflected Oscar's reputation for ironic and quasi-heroic exploits.

Oscar fashioned for himself a unique life, his exploits the stuff of anecdotes and local legend as when Oscar absconded with all the records of the government office and hid them in a garbage tin. Further mayhem occurred when Oscar played tricks on several fellow citizens.

> Ovideo and Maria had awakened to find all their clothes and utensils gone! Yet the doors were still shut and the windows shuttered. At the same time, Mr Forbes and his household had awakened to find somebody else's cups and plates on their shelves . . . and . . . somebody else's clothes hanging on their line. But their own clothes were no longer there! . . . Reyaes, who lived alone, stormed out of doors carrying a pile of ladies' clothes and yelling, 'What de goddamn is dis?' and Cissy, a spinster, began screaming her head off and wouldn't come out because, as it turned out, Mr. Forbes's trousers and shirts were lying at the end of her bed. (pp. 41–42)

The incidents are humorous, full of irony, and represent a deep satire on the respectability of society in Providencia and the fragility of the pattern of perceptions and social conventions supporting the prevailing discourse. This is Oscar, the gadfly, offering active and eccentric commentary on his fellows, both like and yet unlike his Athenian forerunner.

Oscar adapts to his blighted life, and the schizoid society with its two central values in an uneasy tension and responds, in part, through self-imposed abstention from the normal *interpersonal reciprocity* and entanglements with others. Oscar observed, reported, acted, formed temporary associations, preached sermons, took part in some significant community activities such as the sugarcane harvest, and had a recognized place without being fully engaged. Wilson accompanied Oscar on some of his lonely expeditions, spending days in solitude: 'When he took me on these trips, he was allowing me to enter into his real world, where words were not necessary.' (p. 97)

The silences and moments of quiet companionship that made these occasions memorable and distanced them from Caribbean discourse reinforced the point that signification and narration and language itself are selective tools used for many diverse and loosely connected purposes. On Oscar's journeys, he and Wilson were in a world apart from mundane human interactions and the everyday discourses structuring and focusing them.

Wilson suggests that, in the Caribbean, the colonizer's *language* is used subversively in black subculture: 'Stories, insults, boasts, toasts, poems, allusions, parables, jokes, irony, satire, mimicry, puns, and style evolved to heights and extents unknown to the speakers of English' (p. 126). The 'honkey' (note the relation to donkey—loud, determined, and slow), in Caribbean- based societies, therefore often finds himself excluded from an elaborate game in which conventional hierarchies are overturned and concepts of knowledge and ignorance no longer have their established meaning: 'The strength and wit of Oscar's language earned him respect in the eyes of his fellow-men' (p. 127)—or 'reputation'.

Wilson also explores *the use of power*, in society. In Providencia, the power to reveal or conceal details of the lives, actions, and hypocrisies of others runs in channels carefully regulated by dominant social groups, a system that has no hold on Oscar. He is a wild card, his knowledge and intelligence provoking respect and even fear and reversing his marginalization to give him a standing and power otherwise unattainable.

Out of this cocktail of ingredients, Oscar fashions an identity: 'The search for identity rests squarely on the freedom of choice we can exercise in entering into and conducting relationships with others. By seeking total divorce from others, we can achieve nothing except complete alienation and total negation.' (p. 139)

Oscar's identity emerges out of the schizoid tragedy of his history and strikes a balance between individuality and belonging, an autobiographical task difficult for any of us but especially difficult when the normal milieu of interpersonal relationships is in some way distorted or fractured by a psychiatric diagnosis.

2.6 The burden of a psychiatric diagnosis

A number of my patients had subarachnoid haemorrhages (SAH) and some had multiple berry aneurysms unable to be clipped at a single operation. In the period after their acute bleed and their aneurysm operation, they had to carry on their lives aware of the small but definite chance that another of their aneurysms might rupture at any time. Some found the uncertainty difficult to live with and pressed for the second operation as soon as possible after their first, living, meanwhile, a 'suspended' life that precluded meaningful plans and the re-establishment of life structures. Note the similarity with the person suffering schizophrenia, or bipolar disorder, and living with uncertainty about when or if they will next become ill. Other burdens of a psychiatric diagnosis (quite apart from the illness) include stigmatization, marginalization, loss of autonomy, and the consequent vulnerability of the patient to the actions and attitudes of others.

2.6.1 Stigmatization and marginalization

One patient observed, 'Once you have been a psychiatric patient, people often refer to you as an ex-psychiatric patient but they don't refer to other people as, say, ex-orthopaedic patients.' The stigma of a psychiatric diagnosis is often a major life burden because the idea that you have something slightly wrong in your head is hard to carry around with you. It can make people think that you are 'alien' or 'other', excluded in diverse ways.

> Prior to the twentieth century, persons suffering from mental illness were thought to be 'alienated', not only from the rest of society but also from their own true natures. Those experts who studied mental pathologies were known as alienists.
>
> (Carr, 1994)

Janet Frame (1989) reports a common attitude:

> We had no loonies in our family, although we knew of people who had been sent 'down the line', but we did not know what they looked like, only that there was a funny look in their eye and they'd attack you with a bread knife or an axe. (p. 150)

She describes her reactions on passing Seacliff, a mental hospital, on her first journey from home to Dunedin. Similar to all such places, it was sited well away from the milieu of normal life and she is curious, as the train pulls into Seacliff station, in case any of the 'loonies' are on view. The term 'loonies' (reflecting the fabled link between madness and the moon) demarcates the inmates of Seacliff as 'other' with thoughts that are opaque to us, lacking sense, crazy. A person whose mental life is inexplicable (or alien) in this way makes us feel at sea, threatened: we cannot interact with them in the myriad ways that normally affirm or reflect our own hold on sanity and solidity.

Even a community used to psychiatric patients evinces the same exclusions and alienations (Jodelet, 1991).

> Nowadays they are very well dressed. But . . . you can still identify them in spite of everything. If one walks down the road, 'look there's a new one!' (p. 70)
> No, they're not like the rest of us. They've all got something, all of them; they're all abnormal somehow or another . . . Some of them seem all right for a little while and then later you hear them say something which shows they've got something. (p. 155)

All behaviour has a context, a thought prominent in the work of Szasz and Laing; that context is needed to make sense of the apparently absurd behaviour of mental illness and it often illuminates apparently senseless phenomena in an arresting way.

> Sometimes, with our share of stodgy apple pie in front of us, we were seized with an unreal extravagance and exuberance and would suddenly hurl our meal in the air and onto the wall behind us where it stuck and stained. This desperate rejection of what was so dear to us was infectious, as is self-sacrifice in wartime; I joined in the throwing of the food.
>
> (Frame, 1961/1980, p. 111)

This behaviour is clearly insane, perhaps one of the most striking manifestations of chronic insanity found in any institution, but something very similar is observed in an Oxford or Cambridge college dining room, often to a mindless chant such as 'Shop! Shop! Shop!'

> We flicked; we banged our crockery on the table; we sang rude rhymes about 'I took my girl to the pictures and sat her in the stalls and every time the lights went out . . .'
>
> (Frame, 1961/1980, p. 111)

One context is structured by diagnoses, the other nostalgic reminiscences of the life of young male undergraduates, but the phenomenon looks the same. In the context of a psychiatric system dealing with those suffering mental illness, the judgement has ontological and moral significance; such people are stigmatized, relegated to an alien status, and excluded from normal interpersonal interactions and terms of engagement.

Reich (1981), writing on this phenomenon of distancing and exclusion, remarks as follows:

> Diagnosis is perfectly suited to label, exclude, and dehumanise in both its informal and formal usages. Informally, the terms 'crazy', 'mad', and even 'schizophrenic' often serve as exclusionary labels that are used in everyday language to identify others who are annoying, discomfiting, and different. Formally applied—that is, by psychiatrists— diagnoses can make a person into someone who seems wholly other and who requires exclusion. (p. 79)

Stigmatization forms part of what-it-is-like-to-be a person seen that way (Goffman, 1968, p. 45) and inscribes the subjective body of the stigmatized. The inscribed subjective body (traced by language—'loonie', 'How are you, dear?'—and etched by ideas of mental illness) produces 'a dissociated self . . . a volume in perpetual disintegration' (Foucault, 1984, 83) as one learns to read oneself in the mirror that the world holds up through one's engagement with others (Lacan, 1977). The stigmatized soul carries that burden, a weight that grinds into one the malady of the soul.

Imagine, for instance, Jon, an ex-psychiatric patient who is despondent about his bank balance. Others, talk about him, are solicitous, treat him carefully, and so on, deploy the inscription: 'Jon is withdrawing into himself a bit,' 'Isn't that something we have to look out for?' and so on. The subliminal messages pervading human discourse can 'abnormalize' behaviour that in (the normal, included) people such as ourselves would pass almost without notice; they reflect meanings that profoundly affect many other aspects of life and relationships. They are poised to deprive the individual of autonomy catch him or her in the net of disability or incompetence, and create possibilities for abuse potentiated by that exclusion (a topic examined in more detail in the context of the moral attitudes informing the treatment of aliens).

With these thoughts in mind, we can return to Kate Herring (caught in the net).

2.7 Kate Herring revisited

Kate Herring's treatment is a disturbing indictment on a system more interested in diagnosis and categories than the psychic suffering of those who turn to it (or are put in its way) for help. The health authority looking after her was found to have provided inappropriate and unscientific treatment, but more serious problems lurk beneath that finding.

She seems to be a striking example of the medicalization of life problems in general and adolescent troubles in particular. The reports of the psychiatrists reviewing the case suggest that she was a difficult adolescent, at odds with her parents and protesting about her life context (she may even have been abused). But when she comes into contact with psychiatric services (in thrall to diagnostic categories and therapeutic regimes), this 'messy' reality is seen as an individual pathology and an internal disturbance of the organism (Cooper, 2007). She is given poisons, confined, and suffers enforced (chemical and social) silence. Her objections to this treatment are taken as further indications of her pathological state so that she is trapped in the dehumanizing cycle of a misapplied model of psychic distress as some claim is typical of a system of categorizations: 'Its whole weight is towards the totalization of an objectifying and dehumanizing attitude' (Kovel, 1988, p. 135).

> The mental disorder is the object wrought by the objectifying gaze; it is not so much what the gaze sees as what it constructs. (p. 135)

The subjective distress of the psychiatric patient should, however, give us pause in condemning psychiatric diagnosis as a socially devised system of categorization and remind us of the genuine causes of suffering not totally attributable to social praxis even as we explore conditions under which the objectifying clinical gaze which disregards discursive reality would be particularly worrying.

The use of the DSM and ICD systems would be sinister if the powerful figures in the system were under financial incentives to subdue the focus of the trouble, ameliorate the social disturbance he or she causes, and were rewarded for using expensive chemicals to do so. The rewards may vary from income related to 'throughput of patients' to more subtle and indirect funding streams, but the 'Kafka-esque' quality of what is going on lurks in the background, unnamed, throughout (Eisenberg, 1995; Elliot, 2004).

What is common to all the dehumanizing varieties of 'treatment' is their neglect of the lived experience, the story of the patient, who is trying to forge for him or herself a liveable narrative. That may require chemical modification of some of the worst effects of a disorder, but attention to the 'discursive lesion' is likely to be part of any healing intervention. Whereas production lines are good for machines, they may be damaging when human beings need help to become good enough individuals and, if even the president of the American Psychiatric Association is worried, perhaps it is a realistic concern.

> 'There is widespread concern of the over-medicalization of mental disorders and the overuse of medications. Financial incentives and managed care have contributed to the notion of a 'quick fix' by taking a pill and reducing the emphasis on psychotherapy and psychosocial treatments.
>
> (Sharfstein, 2005)

Production lines suit simplistic economic models currently driving medicine (which aims for maximum efficiency in providing health-care 'widgets') and so one fears for the fate of a sensitive and discursively based psychiatry if medical economics is allowed to shape clinical reality. In Ohio, a young mother of two was discharged after an acute psychiatric admission for severe depression, the length of which was mandated by managed-care funding arrangements. Her husband had to return to work having used up his compassionate leave to try and compensate for inadequate community-based care prior to admission. She called him at work to return home fearing that something awful might happen. Twenty minutes later, he arrived home to find that his wife had killed their two children. Only one case and perhaps the tragedy was inevitable, but the question must be asked about what we are doing to those who need our care.

2.8 **Philosophical problems**

There are philosophical problems in the very idea of psychiatric disease:

(1) What is a mental illness and to what extent is it a social production?

(2) Can we accept a version of scientific realism about psychiatric illness?

(3) Is the diagnosis of a psychiatric condition a value-laden or morally neutral determination?

Many have examined these questions (Cooper, 2007). A discursive analysis relates the discontents of the mind as individual, subjective works and introduces 'a consideration of the historical forces to which a work is subject as well as the historical role which the work is to play' (Kovel, 1988, p. 128).

2.8.1 **Mental illness and social production**

I have argued that social factors affect the presentation and phenomenology of psychiatric disorders and that psychiatric diagnosis often neglects social and interpersonal aspects of maladies of the soul. That is not to say that psychiatric diseases are merely social productions but to argue that, even if constitutional or biological predispositions are part of the aetiology of many of the discontents of the mind, the patient's subjectivity and the narrative arising from it is important in our understanding of any human being. What may look surd or ridiculous from the alienated point of view of a disease-oriented observer may be comprehensible through imaginative intersubjective discourse. This modest reading of 'social production' allows us to explore psychiatric dsorders in the context of a lived experience of being-with-others. We can then appeal to insanity and disorganization of thought only where it exists rather than consigning all unconventional discourse to a wastebasket of 'disordered thought form and content'.

2.8.2 **Scientific realism and psychiatry**

Do psychic conditions have essences fitting into matrices of natural law explaining their form and connections? This question is problematic. We are creatures who compose narratives and our life events must, if possible, be integrated into those narratives. Thus, when we discuss the human psyche, we are unlikely to discern a clear division between things that are true of us *simpliciter* and things that we make true of ourselves through believing in them. Our ways-of-being are historical, cultural, social, and psychological creations so that we are inescapably committed to engaging with personal and discursive realities when we consider the human mind and its discontents.

  We could capture this discussion in the following argument:

(1) Science aims for objective knowledge of the entities that actually exist in nature.

(2) Entities in nature are the way they are independent of our thoughts of them.

(3) Our thoughts about ourselves affect the ways we live our lives.

(4) The ways we live our lives affect the ways we become disordered.

So, either we can accept 1 and 2 *but not* 3 and 4 and go with

(5a) Psychiatric disorders are as they are independent of our thoughts about them.

Or, we can accept 1, 2, 3, and 4 and have to give up a form of naturalistic realism:

(5b) Psychiatric disorders are not real entities in nature.

But we can avoid the binary opposition by inserting 3a:

(3a) Some things in nature are products of the human mind (such as the Golden Gate Bridge) but can still be proper objects of science.

Then we can derive the following conclusion:

(6a) Psychiatric disorders are in part human productions but can still be the topic of objective knowledge.

6a accords with 'promiscuous realism' (Dupre) whereby a phenomenon is a confluence of multidimensional representations of similarity and difference resulting from a
dynamic process whereby one denotes a phenomenon and then refines and revises
one's knowledge of it through ongoing contact and reflection (Cooper, 2007). That
quite possibly reflects the fact that 'psychiatry is at the place where brains, behaviours,
values, laws, beliefs, society, psychology, and history seem to come together to make
humans what they are and what they believe themselves to be' (Pickering, 2006, p.
175). This is seen *par excellence* in the mad travellers whose mode of discontent was
informed by medical taxonomy, cultural polarity (between good and bad), the
distinctiveness and observability of their particular mode of (mal)adaptation,
and their need to escape a destructive and confining lived experience (Hacking, 1998).
The confluence of discourse, history, and a (di)stressed human psyche creates a
disease or malady of the soul the contours of which reflect the world of meaning and
the position of the subject engaged with it. These travellers in the journey of life then
go absent with leave—sick leave—which they desperately need.

The 'messy realism' (Cooper, 2007) resulting from discursive naturalism is accom-
modated if we see psychiatric illness or mental disorder as a metaphor (Pickering,
2006) that assimilates a complex breakdown in the relation between a human being
and the human life-world to a disease process. The metaphor is helpful because it
focuses us on the functions of the individual that adapt him or her to a sociocultural
milieu as a complex cultural artifact produced in an image (of the human and its
variations) under the imperative of the word (Lacan, 1977, p. 106), a realization that
carries with it both emancipation and responsibilities.

2.8.3 Facts and values in psychiatric diagnosis

To what extent are we able to keep the factual judgement that 'X' is suffering, say,
borderline personality disorder, separate from value commitments? Some writers
regard all diagnoses on the DSM model as morally objectionable because they embody
totalizing and dehumanizing attitudes and look instead for an emancipatory attitude.
Emancipation must be a laudable aim (just read the label) but perhaps does not require
rejection of psychiatric classification even though the threat of stigmatization and the
objectifying gaze are ever present. Kovel's (1988) remark ('The mental disorder is the
object wrought by the objectifying gaze; it is not so much what the gaze sees as what it
constructs' [p. 135]) reminds us of the discourse of the other and its damaging
effects—each of us is, in reality, a fragile enigma.

Discursive and deconstructive insights show that a psychiatric categorization does
more than detecting likenesses: it both judges the behaviour of the individual in relation to the validated conduct in a given sociocultural context and also has implications
for our treatment of a person. Diagnosis therefore always embodies a value—something is thought to be wrong; it is also focused on the individual inscribed by the
anomalous text that has been created as a performative device (or persona)
to fulfil a legitimated function related to the individual's social and legal status.
Therefore values pervade its origins, its effects, and its place in our meaning-world. To
say that somebody is psychotic, psychopathic, or anorexic is a moral act enmeshed in

a set of meanings and metaphors that influence the kinds of questions we ask about such persons and the problems causing their subjective distress or maladapation. The illness metaphor carries in its wake certain benefits such as an engagement with our modes of caring for those who suffer but also carries disadvantages such as marginalization and exclusion from the busy kingdom of ends and its human conversation defining moral structure and the commerce of its members (Jodelet, 1991). The worst effects of that marginalization and exclusion are revealed by the psychiatric abuse that has marred the history of our treatment of aliens.

Chapter 3

The treatment of aliens

The future accumulates like a weight upon the past. The
weight upon the earliest years is easier to remove to let
that time spring up like grass that has been crushed. The
years following childhood become welded to their future,
massed like stone, and often the time beneath cannot
spring back into growth like new grass: it lies bled of its
green in a new shape with those frail bloodless sprouts of
another, unfamiliar time, entangled one with the other
beneath the stone.
(Frame, 1989, P. 149)

I believe that we must let our psychiatric patients see that we understand that they are in a
state of affliction which is not comparable to a bodily pain however severe. To communicate such an understanding is difficult.

(Drury, 1996, p. 90)

Our futures are built upon our pasts in that our mental life congeals from inchoate
and multipotential beginnings into forms that are resistant to change. For most of us,
these forms are comfortable; they are part of a conscious narrative and give us personae
apt for the demands of everyday situations that express an identity. Everything in the
narrative, however chaotic, is structured or held in place by other things and some of
its strands, in terms of their emotive weighting, and their discursive connections are
deeply significant and resistant to change. The narrative is, in part, discursively
produced through significant moral and interpersonal encounters that condition attitudes to and images of self and others. The narratives of discontent distinguish their
subjects from others in ways that often cause discomfort: they are alienated and the
techniques of alienation (including exclusion and the physical treatments of madness)
work between and within people and exacerbate the distress suffered by 'the alien'.

For most of us, the valleys, mountains, public places, cobbled streets, familiar
haunts, and hideaways of self and personality are adequate for adult experience, but
for some, a few, the story and the world in which we travel congeals into oppressive,
entrapping, and self-alienating forms. For yet others, the narrative is fractured and
disrupted by the intrusion of surd and apparently malign influences, some of which

arise from human actions, some from congeries of chemicals, genes, and the internal milieu, and some from the singular interaction between the subjective body and its context.

Our reactions to human beings in such predicaments and their reactions to us have none of the familiar reciprocity of our relationships to 'normal' people. These *reactive attitudes* structure our life together as persons but go awry with 'aliens', those who are 'other'. Their stories may seem incomprehensible and our attitudes more appropriate to malfunctioning systems or beasts, *objective* rather than *reactive* attitudes (Jodelet, 1991).

> I had seen in the ward office the list of those 'down for a leucotomy', with my name on the list, and other names being crossed off as the operation was performed. My 'turn' must have been very close when one evening the superintendent of the hospital, Dr Blake Palmer, made an unusual visit to the ward. He spoke to me to the amazement of everyone.
>
> As it was my first chance to discuss with anyone, apart from those who had persuaded me, the prospect of my operation, I said urgently, 'Dr Blake Palmer, what do you think?'
>
> He pointed to the newspaper in his hand.
>
> 'About the prize?'
>
> I was bewildered. What prize? 'No,' I said, 'about the leucotomy'.
>
> He looked stern: 'I've decided that you should stay as you are. I don't want you changed.'
>
> 'You've won the Hubert Church Award for the best prose. Your book, *The Lagoon* . . .
>
> I smiled. 'Have I?'
>
> 'Yes. And we're moving you out of this ward. And no leucotomy.'
>
> The winning of the prize and the attention of a new doctor from Scotland who accepted me as I appeared to him and not as he learned about me from my 'history' or reports of me . . . enabled me to be prepared for discharge from hospital. Instead of being treated by leucotomy, I was treated as a person of some worth, a human being, in spite of the misgivings and unwillingness of some members of the staff. (Frame, 1989, p. 222)

The passage highlights the contrast between objective and reactive attitudes: those that negate the patient so that she or he is treated like a thing rather than a person—'*He spoke to me* to the amazement of everyone,' '*I've decided* that you should stay as you are,' '*We're moving you* out of this ward'—and those that are otherwise—'A new doctor . . . who accepted me as I appeared to him,' 'I was treated as a person of some worth.' The attitude types jostle for room in psychiatric practice (and the discourses surrounding it) and reveal the origins of and conflicts in our treatment of aliens.

3.1 Reactive attitudes and the self as a thinking agent

Peter Strawson (1974) delineates the contrast between reactive and objective attitudes with both economy and elegance:

> We should think of the many different kinds of relationship which we can have with other people—as sharers of a common interest, as members of the same family, as colleagues, as

friends, as lovers, as chance parties to an enormous range of transactions and encounters. Then we should think, in each of these connections in turn and in others, of the kind of importance we attach to the attitudes and intentions towards us of those who stand in these relationships to us, and of the kinds of reactive attitudes to which we ourselves are prone. (p. 6)

What I want to contrast is the attitude (or range of attitudes) of involvement or participation, on the one hand, and what might be called the objective attitude (or range of attitudes) to another human being, on the other. Even in the same situation, I must add, they are not exclusive of each other; but they are, profoundly, opposed to each other. (p. 9)

Exceptionally, I have said, we can have direct dealings with other human beings without any degree of personal involvement, treating them simply as creatures to be handled in our own interests, or our side's, or society's—or even theirs. In the extreme case of the mentally deranged, it is easy to see the connection between the possibility of a wholly objective attitude and the impossibility of what we understand by ordinary interpersonal relationships. (p. 12)

Notice that reactive attitudes are responsive to the intentions and attitudes of others as beings to whom we relate intersubjectively and that objective attitudes do not exclude them but are 'opposed' to them in a morally relevant way in that the objective stance treats others 'simply as creatures to be handled in our own interests . . . or even theirs'. Psychiatric patients present a third possibility: neither thing nor 'real person' but *abject*, unsettling, frightening, threatening the boundaries of our being, and to be avoided at all costs.

Reactive attitudes engage one in a certain kind of reciprocity with the other whereby the other person has a complex role: she serves both as a proper object of reactive attitudes, as a source for validation of one's own attitudes, and as part of the mirror held up to oneself by others. Objective attitudes, by contrast, detach one from the other person so that it is not an intersubjective relationship but she is rather a phenomenon for 'observation and assessment' so that she cannot legitimately affect one and one is entitled to have an attitude of control (It's for the best). A caring person working in this liminal zone may slip in and out of the two stances in a quasi-stable and subtle interplay of personae or register that she or he is in the presence of something incomprehensible that threatens the categories of human existence, something abject, who traps one in false actions where misconception is evident.

Karl Jaspers (1913/1974) distinguishes what is learned within 'empathic experience' from 'evidence based on the principle of causality' (p. 84): 'objective psychology . . . is capable of reaching extraordinarily exact results, but by the same token, by its very nature, it never can give an answer to the question of phenomenology and of the psychology of meaning' (pp. 83–84). Understanding a person and her intentions, framed by a genuine appreciation of what means something to her, is coeval with respect, intersubjective appreciation, and understanding rather than an objective stance associated with categorization and control. The abject slips away from both forms of 'capture' frustrating the observer and fellow-traveller, making them mad.

The tension between these modes of appreciation is evident in their epistemology. Reactive attitudes rest on a principle of charity or recognition of others as persons that tries to make sense of another person's behaviour, assuming that people aim to believe what is true and want what is good (Davidson, 1984) The charitable stance allows communication and fosters interpersonal reciprocity or understanding 'from the inside', and when all stances fail, we are confronted by the indigestible abject who leaves us stranded (and can, epistemically, pull us apart).

'Stop here! This is where I get off.'

'But you can't get off, we're in an aeroplane.'

'Are you crazy? I'm hitchhiking and I don't want to go any further!'

'Look, I think I'd better call the hostess.'

Or the following:

'I want that rock to eat.'

'You what?'

'I want that to eat with tomato sauce'

'But it's a rock'

'I know; that's why I'm not having cream with it.'

In neither case can we make sense of what is said because the perspectives of the subjects involved are inaccessible. Their intentions and desires are so unlike anything we could imagine in ourselves that our empathy fails, not because of pure illogicality but because of failure of human congruence:

> We see the agent . . . as one whose picture of the world is an insane delusion; . . . whose behaviour . . . is unintelligible to us, perhaps even to him, in terms of conscious purposes, and intelligible only in terms of unconscious purposes; or even perhaps, as one wholly impervious to the self-reactive attitudes I spoke of. Seeing an agent in such a light as this tends . . . to inhibit ordinary interpersonal attitudes in general, and the kind of demand and expectation which those attitudes involve, and tends to promote instead the purely objective view of the agent as one posing problems simply of intellectual understanding, management, treatment, and control.
>
> (Strawson, 1974, p. 16)

Suspending the principle of charity and the reciprocity that flows from it casts us adrift into an alien or uncharted sea where our ordinary maps do not work. Thus, praise or blame (or other forensic practices) become insecure and an interpersonal mode of interaction is jeopardized. But the presence of the person who embodies insanity also defeats the objective stance and pulls us into an abject and schizoid place of *non-empathy* and *non-explanation*.

Our reactive attitudes are based on the perceived beliefs, desires, intentions, and attitudes of others whereby we recognize our affinity with and develop relationships to them. When someone's discursive moves are 'alien', we are on unfamiliar turf and lose our grip on the fundamental ground not only for dealing with others but also for understanding oneself as a thinking subject. The ground of my being (or belonging) is where I feel understood and have encountered care and recognition; on that ground, I can rely on certain moral constraints regulating the exchanges between self and others, whereas outside of it, excluded from reactive discourse, the world is a scary place where even 'good' words can take on sinister overtones.

> Shock treatment! It had a very bad ring to it. Especially the word 'treatment'. When they biffed you it was pretty bad, but at least you knew they were doing something they shouldn't be doing. They knew it too . . . But 'treatment' was different . . . They could do it with a clean conscience because they were just trying to help you.

> (Kocan, 1980, p. 9)

The 'help' here is often based on the objective model in which malfunctioning entities are dealt with, not subjective beings with hopes, fears, feelings, intentions, and projects but otherwise. The 'help' abandons empathy with the patient and detaches their treatment from the moral constraints linked to empathic appreciation. Laing (1994) talks of the objectifying milieu surrounding the doctor in many psychiatric hospitals of the 1950s: 'He administered drugs, he gave electric shocks, he induced comas and epileptic fits through the injection of insulin. Straitjackets and padded cells were integral to psychiatric practice at the time. Doctors were not expected to speak to psychiatric patients.'

However, objective attitudes operate in two directions, affecting both their targets and those adopting them so that the professionals find themselves acting in ways that they would never do towards 'normal people' because reactive attitudes are not only central in adult relationships but are also important in the development of self. Just as I appreciate others as persons through empathic experience so I learn what-it-is-like-to-be-a-person (i.e. how to structure my own experience according to the concepts they teach me): for instance, I learn what counts as being hurt, and how to articulate what is happening to me and others by using the concept (and related concepts). *Hurt*, in fact, bridges between descriptive psychological concepts and moral concepts, both of which are explanatory, communicative, and formative in a thinker's mental life as they are taught and learnt in interpersonal exchanges in which we do things to each other by using words and allied discursive tools and so develop reactive attitudes as part of that subjective context. Hurt, joy, concern, fear, anticipation, disappointment, and concepts such as them draw us into engagement with one another and help articulate that engagement, but the abject world of the unreasonable (borderline or marginal souls) disrupts the articulations between such concepts so that the discursive context of the treatment of aliens (the abject, excluded) grossly distorts the self-constructions of those who inhabit it.

Empathic experiences of others also provide me with techniques of self-reflection and self-mastery. For example, if I ask my father why he shouted at my mother, he could respond with resentment and rejection or, alternatively, take my question as an opportunity to explain his own reactions (implicitly modelling the discursive skills of self-reflection). The latter response conveys to me that my thoughts matter to him and includes me in that intersubjective moment in my (and his) narrative. On the other hand, if he always reacts defensively ('Mind your own business!' or 'So you're on her side as well!'), I myself may never learn the reflective skills I need to deal with my emotions. Even if I do not feel as he thinks I do, his responses connect (perhaps inchoately or subconsciously) questioning behaviour and hostile attitudes that can crush the 'spring growth' (Janet Frame) of a youthful and searching mind, putting in its place congealed patterns of latent hostility and insecurity.

Openness to the lessons of experience and the perspectives of others may be stunted by fixing modes of responding and personality structures designed to guard against anxiety (or perceived threats to the self) and crystallize modes of discourse hiding ignored, and unexplored (therefore unmoderated—by argument) feelings. The 'repressed' aspects of the psyche, lacking articulation, are not engaged with one's self-narrative skills so as to equip one to examine them, limn their contours, and expand the skills that adapt one to being-in-the-world-with-others into which one fits as if one were made for it—just as a hand fits a glove. The alternative is to be unfitting, out of place, abject, neither this nor that.

Neurath pictured a boat being rebuilt as it stays afloat (and likened it to our knowledge of the world), and personality theory can make use of the metaphor. The obvious application to the psyche implies that even if aspects of oneself are maladaptive, one can, as a result of experience, reform and modify them bit by bit. One's psyche, as we shall see, can be and is modified by reflection inspired by the modelling and responses of other One's subjective-being-in-the-world-with-others emerges from the discursive moments in the psychic narrative in which one feels the influence of others, responds to their demands, takes account of their reactions and feelings, and adjusts oneself to be a good-enough person.

3.2 **Normative influences, social context, and mental life**

Mental self-ascriptions have distinctive normative properties related to the 'oughts' that I should heed rather than those that I am bound to comply with, and all my self-knowledge works within that framework of normativity that fits me for the world of others.

> I may infer from signs and behavioural indications what my past beliefs were—'I must have believed him'—as I may infer the present beliefs of another. But one cannot infer what one's beliefs are to be, starting from now. Either one already knows or one has to answer a normative question to form a belief on the evidences of truth, as one takes them to be.
>
> Similarly with the two-faced concept of desire: While I make up my mind what I now want, there are no knowable facts to be expressed in the words 'I want to do so-and-so.' If I infer that I must already want so-and-so or that I must already have such-and-such an unconscious desire, it is still an open question whether I dissociate myself from this desire, now brought to consciousness . . . Do I want to get rid of this desire, if I can, or do I now endorse it? Does it now persist as a conscious desire? . . . In this uncertainty, there is room for deliberation: that is, for determining what is to be true of me.

> (Hampshire, 1969/1979, p. 37)

Hampshire argues that any uncertainty about what I think or want is not settled by further gathering of facts about my present state but by my shaping myself in accordance with what I think I ought to believe or desire. This 'ought' is something like 'best—all things considered' (not a moral ought), and a subject evaluates herself or himself in the light of what is warranted or 'right' around here in terms of shared projects, moral and emotional commitments, and so on. One's psychic life is therefore a 'montage' (Lacan, 1979, p. 169) or montages pervaded by evaluative judgments about what one ought to do or think and not merely reflecting primitive givens; it is therefore surreal rather than real and its surreality can become exaggerated into abjection.

A thinker does or can reflect upon and evaluate her or his own thoughts and judgements, a basic normative feature of thought that emerges from the myriad reactions of others to that person, and is continuous with the reactive attitudes or judgements about the person as a being-among-others that are part of all interpersonal relations. The close connection between usable, integrated mental content and one's relationships can be a powerful tool (transference) working on the side of the therapist attempting to assist a disturbed patient. The ability to reintegrate a fragmented and unsettled self-narrative is, one might say, dependent upon non-threatening, empathic, communications about one's experience and one's being-among-others.

Laing notices the effect of humanizing and re-engaging patients as persons in his own psychiatric unit:

> The patients lost many of the features of chronic psychoses; they were less violent to each other and to the staff, they were less dishevelled, and their language ceased to be obscene. The nurses came to know the patients well, and spoke warmly of them . . . And the most important thing about the nurses and other people in the environment is how they feel towards their patients.

> (Cameron *et al.*, 1955)

The effects of understanding and respect are also seen in the treatment of *bulimia nervosa*, the eating disorder marked by binges of overeating and vomiting: 'bulimia tends to start in women in late adolescence or early adulthood'; there is a 'high prevalence of depressive symptoms . . . attempted suicide . . . self-mutilating behaviour, alcohol and drug abuse, and low self-esteem' (Freeman *et al.*, 1988). Recent studies suggest that 'interpersonal therapy' is superior to or at least as effective as other types of therapy both in terms of objective indicators and in terms of patient self-esteem and relationships (McCarthy & Thomson, 1996; Orbach, 1993; Zerbe, 1996). A similar trend is seen in the growth of self-help, self-worth, and family-based therapies in which intrapersonal conflict is addressed within an engaged and reactive milieu and the sufferers enabled to renegotiate the norms they live by so that they are no longer destructive. It therefore seems that reflective control of maladaptive and unconsciously driven behaviour (associated with disruptions of self-esteem and personal relationships) can occur through interpersonal contact and participation in situations in which people react to one another and incorporate the evaluations and reactions of sympathetic others so as to refashion their life narratives[1]. Recognition (as someone who is *somebody*) is important in recovery from a mental disorder, in which emotional, internal, and often subconscious influences have distorted a patient's

---

[1] See Chapter 11.

behaviour—it reverses abjection and welcomes a person home. When the subject is recognized as one of us, she or he is treated as having a valid perspective of her or his own and as having an autobiographical role in the formation of self, but complications arise when these attitudes are suspended and we move into an objective (or worse, abjective) mode (especially in a person already psychologically disturbed).

3.3 'Loonies'

> Janet Frame, as I have noted, hoped for a glimpse of the 'loonies', whom she would recognise because of 'the funny look in their eye' or perhaps because of something even more spectacular as her train passed Seacliff, the mental hospital to which (ironically) she herself would later be sent and have her brush with frontal leucotomy.
>
> (Frame, 1989, p. 150)

So Janet Frame reports her reactions on passing Seacliff, the mental hospital to which she would be sent. I have noted that, similar to all such places, it was sited at the margins of normal life. The term 'loonies' demarcates the inmates of Seacliff as 'different', with thoughts that are opaque to us, lacking sense, crazy, and abject. As other, they are marginalized, not only geographically but also in folk representations (Jodelet, 1991); as aliens,[2] they do not speak to us as normal folk do.

(i) Their opinions are negated or devalued. 'No one thought to ask me why I had screamed at my mother, no one asked me what my plans were for the future. I became an instant third person, or even personless. . . I was taken (third-person people are thrust into the passive mood) to Seacliff.' (Frame, 1989, p. 191) The patient is outside comprehension and reason, abject in a world of interpersonal communication.

(ii) Because the patient does not warrant reciprocity and openness, the therapeutic relationship can slide into a duplicity of 'hidden agendas'.

> My consolation was my talks with [J.F.], as he was my link with the world I had known, and because I wanted these talks to continue, I built up a formidable schizophrenic repertoire: I'd lie on the couch, while the handsome [J.F.], glistening with newly applied Freud, took note of what I said and did, and suddenly I'd put a glazed look in my eye and begin to relate a fantasy as if I experienced it as a reality.
>
> (Frame, 1989, p. 201)

There is, indeed, a fine line between acting as if you are mad and being mad (indeed, one of my professors said 'If you're mad enough to act mad, you are mad') especially when we consider the mirror of social representation and the interactive nature of what we say and do.

(iii) The patient is condescended to, treated as a proprietary item, subhuman or non-human presence, or infantilized rather than being seen and responded to as a locus of adult thoughts and attitudes: 'My shyness and self-consciousness, arising

---

2 See Appendix D on Varieties of Alienation.

from my feelings of being nowhere, increased when my sister's friends asked, 'How is she?' 'Does she like being in Auckland?' I had become a third person, at home in Willowglen and now here in Auckland.' (Frame, 1989, p. 215) This person who is not present is abject, not here and yet here, a topic of conversation not its target or source.

(iv) A range of barbaric, unproven, and terrible (or terror-full) treatments have been applied to psychiatric patients, allegedly in their own best interests.

> I was discharged from hospital on probation. After having received over two hundred applications of unmodified ECT, each the equivalent, in degree of fear, to an execution, and in the process having my memory shredded and after having been subjected to proposals to have myself changed, by a physical operation into a more acceptable, amenable, normal person, I arrived home at Willowglen, outwardly smiling and calm, but inwardly with all confidence gone, with the conviction at last that I was officially a non-person.

> (Frame, 1989, p. 224)

The moment of abjection is internalized by the non-person. It was eventually concluded that 'there had been an awful mistake even in my first admission to hospital and from then on a continued misinterpretation of my plight' (Frame, 1989, p. 277) signalling, or better licensing, the return home.

Once started, the process of being discounted as a person is hard to stop, as witnessed by the famous study of the psychiatric admission of normal individuals (Rosenham, 1973). Peter Kocan (1980) describes the case of Con Pappas who, during his psychiatric admission, tries to change from the chronic psychiatric 'habitus' that many patients develop from years of marginalization. He combs his hair, grows a trim moustache, and 'spends all his spare time trying to socialize with women inmates.' (p. 229) This begins a process—'the Snowball':

> It builds gradually, with Blue making remarks about the 'two-bit Casanova.'

Con Pappas is singled out from a group of patients listening to a radio behind a partition in the dayroom.

> There are half a dozen patients behind the partition, but the screw has Con Pappas firmly in his mind.

> 'I told you before to come outta there!'

> Con Pappas comes out, half-grinning.

> Do you reckon it's a bloody joke?' snaps the screw. 'Alright then, you can get to bed!'

From here things progress, an apparent hesitation and the attendant grabs Con Pappas to frog march him away.

> 'Con Pappas puts up his arm in surprise. The attendant bends his arm up his back and forces him out of the room.

> Then he goes to write it all up in his report book:

>> Sexually molesting a female patient

> Disruptive behaviour
>
> Abuse of ward property
>
> Disobedience

Attempted assault of staff member

By now the process is well under way.

> The Snowball—It begins with something trivial and gathers its own momentum . . . .
> Some female patients have realized how much better Blue treats them if they can report
> being 'bothered' by Con Pappas . . . 'I saw him interfering with Denise Williams . . .'
>
> 'Is this true, Denise?' Blue demands.
>
> Denise Williams looks vague.
>
> 'Did you agree to go to the canteen with him?'
>
> 'No.'
>
> 'So he forced himself on you?'
>
> 'I went by myself.'
>
> 'Did you or did you not encourage him, Denise?'
>
> Blue turns to Con Pappas. 'Well, what have you got to say for yourself?'
>
> 'I do nothing wrong. I just go for walk.'
>
> 'We all know what kind of walks you go for!'

Here, the Snowball begins when a patient tries to humanize himself and fraternize with woman as is normal in the outside world. It ends with him being overmedicated, less involved in normal ward activities, losing any sense of personal worth, 'depressed' behaviour, ECT, and a return to his dishevelled state. Psychomotor retardation caused by his ECT and medication makes him clumsy so he spills his medication and is bullied by an attendant.

> Con Pappas stares vaguely back at him. Bull is fully stirred now. He pushes Con Pappas
> harder so that he falls against the servery and a Dixie of custard crashes to the floor. Bull
> wrestles a headlock on to Con Pappas and the two of them lurch and slide together in the
> spilt custard . . . It will all go in the report book.
>
> > Refusing medication
> >
> > Running amok in the dining room
> >
> > Attempted assault of a staff member
>
> The Snowball has begun again for Con Pappas. (Kocan, 1980, pp. 229–235)

Kocan chillingly details a process that constructs the patient according to a powerful institutional discourse so that everything he does, every word he says, and the expressions on his face take on an-'other' significance. This process dehumanizes the person and deprives him of the interpersonal contact essential to repairing his broken story; 'the powerlessness, depersonalization, segregation, mortification, and self-labelling seem undoubtedly counter-therapeutic' (Rosenham, 1973). The patient loses a sense of 'I' as a being-among-others so that he is no longer 'in-the-world': he is alienated by the transforming 'gaze' (to use Foucault's term) of the institution leeching meaning (and therefore its life) from the psyche of someone for whom the reconstruction of meaning and identity is vital. The 'gaze' informs the institutional report, or 'the constitution of the individual as a describable analysable object' (Foucault, 1984, p. 202), a record that may bear little relation to the subjectivity or narrative of the person it concerns.

The tendency to infantilize, objectify, and dehumanize or make abject are, such as other tendencies in contemporary biomedicine, exaggerated by commercial influences—predicating treatments on a medical (or even market) model, differentially rewarding research focused on medication, pressuring inpatient and outpatient clinic times, and overbiologizing psychiatry ('Is there any other kind?')—results in a neglect of the lived experience of a disturbed subjectivity and the narrative fracture induced by mental disorder is worsened in ways we ought to resist (Chodoff, 1987).

First, the disorder affects the psyche (or soul)—'the present correlative of a certain technology of power over the body' (Foucault, 1984, p. 176). Soul damage has, at least, two aspects: (i) an ongoing cause of mental disarray whether biochemical, cognitive, or social and cultural; and (ii) a broken story (Freud). Therefore, even where the cause of a mental disorder is biological, neglecting a person's need for recognition, understanding, and help in the task of narrative reconstruction can perpetuate the damage. A saving factor in the face of a devaluation of such discursive work is our tendency to relate to other human beings in reactive and interpersonal ways so that everyday human contact has a normalizing and therapeutic influence (that can be effaced by seeing others as aliens). We ought however to be alert to the fact that certain kinds of contact are harmful, or even, arguably, causal in soul sickness (as in some of the more radical claims of the anti-psychiatrists) even though recognition and a witness to one's ordeal are essential to the reconstruction of personality and a sense of being somebody.

Second, the reconstructive work is interpersonal—it involves restoring relational skills that may be profoundly disturbed by the person's past dealings with others. Jung argued that for human beings 'optimum development tends towards a goal called 'wholeness' or 'integration': a condition in which the different elements of the psyche, both conscious and unconscious, are welded together indissolubly' (Storr, 1987, p. 159). A person has a unique narrative position and a constituted <self> cumulatively defined and refined in ongoing interactions (Gillett, 2008; Schechtman, 1996), but the self so constituted may be driven by conflict and disharmony and so destructive or even self-destructive in ways the person themselves may not understand.

Sartre argues that by acting in the world, one becomes somebody and defines oneself as a distinct being-in-the-world-with-others, in stark contrast to what is found in many psychiatric settings.

> I grew to know and like my fellow patients. I was impressed and saddened by their—our—capacity to learn and adhere to and often relish the spoken and unspoken rules of institutional life, by the pride in the daily routine, shown by patients who had been in hospital for many years. There was a personal, geographical, even linguistic exclusiveness in this community of the insane, who had no legal or personal external identity—no

clothes of their own to wear, no handbags, purses, no possessions but a temporary bed to sleep in with a locker beside it, and a room to sit in and stare called the dayroom.

(Frame, 1989, p. 193)

The same alienation from the possibility of autobiography is seen in *A Day in the Life of Ivan Denisovich* (Alexandr Solzehnitsyn) and is a heart-rending and melancholy feature of many other testimonies of the incarcerated and institutionalized.

Aimlessness and a loss of subjective identity or purpose (*anomie*) is a dominant theme in the narrative of many who suffer mental disorders (or cognitive decline). An uninspiring mental life and the discounting of self as agent undermines the patient as a person in his or her own right, and objective attitudes endorse and reinforce this sense of inertia or passivity creating the institutional habitus. Reactive attitudes treat the other as a locus of mental life with his or her own attitudes, beliefs, intentions, and emotional stances and thereby constitute the other as worth participating with in a shared human life-world, a locus of initiative, inscribed on the body of the patient as a certain vivacity and engagement with others. Abjection expels the person, perhaps fuelled by their disturbing likeness to oneself and the gaze of the (inhuman) human being that they direct at one. The abject make the world uncomfortable and bear silent witness to our lack of care for one another, which can cause a person to react even more violently so that they become, unquestionably, other—not a real part of our intersubjective world at all; the alternative is too painful.

3.4 **Reactive attitudes and genealogy**

Social and personal factors, through the perceived or subjective contingencies in an environment, can distort the normal process of personality formation and rewrite the (cerebral and other) inscriptions that form the soul. I have argued that disorder arises, in part, because a person is not treated as a moral individual who is taken seriously. In the eating disorders we see, perhaps more clearly than anywhere else, the visible inscription of such a disorder. The anorexic body is inscribed by and exhibits the psyche both subjectively and objectively, and the relevant inscription or informing is seen in the brain scans of children raised in an adverse environment (Bremner *et al.*, 1997; Stein *et al.*, 1997).

Brain processing networks realize the cumulative effects of experience so that personal, reactive, interactions 'shape' the body and the brain (in complementary ways). The disorders are therefore just as real as and perhaps even more enduring than any biological influence. The extent to which such effects can be changed depends on the way one is helped to bear the weight of 'future years' accumulating upon them and fixing them in place (Frame). That such effects can be implicated in the genesis of a mental disorder is suggested when interpersonal therapy of some type ameliorates it but, whatever the cause of an aberrant mode of being, one would expect that rehabilitation through new ways of dealing with challenges is enhanced by interactions in which the patient finds supportive and normalizing reactive attitudes and learns skills that can be used in the reconstruction of mental life and identity.

In many situations, the production of an individual as a psychiatric object or thing seems to be a cumulative process in which small problems are amplified and concretized by the significations surrounding the person. In that problematic space, human life is framed accusatively—we who should care are accused for our normality and they whom we should care for silently reproach us for their suffering. As we all seek to live our stories from the moral positions in which we find ourselves, we encounter confusing and disfiguring texts, some of which are acted out as the worst scenarios envisaged by Laing. The abject are disempowered and depersonalized in ways that they lack the discursive techniques to resist, especially when fixed in the objectifying psychiatric gaze, and their caregivers can react in kind, horrified into willful ignorance by the suffering in the midst of which they find themselves. Fortunately, psychiatry is actively transforming itself and many have taken to heart the lessons of past abuses.

The loss of a context of reactive and empathic attitudes is particularly evident in some of the more brutal facets of psychiatric history.

3.5 **Psychiatric interventions**

> As Dave goes past, you turn your eyes away, as though there's something terribly interesting on the far side of the lake. Dave and the doctor and Arthur go into a small room after the screw. There is silence for a couple of minutes and then you hear Dave yelling: 'I don't want it! Please! I'm all right! Oh please don't! Oh please! Oh please!' There is a sound of struggling. You hear screws' voices: 'Don't be such a bloody kid, Dave!' and 'The doctor knows what's best!' and 'Hold his arms!' and other things. Then there's a sudden buzzing sound and a choking and gargling, then silence. Your stomach is watery and you're shaking.

(Kocan, 1980, p. 21)

ECT and psychosurgery are quite unlike psychotherapy: (in the broad sense) they are objective interventions that 'readjust the machinery of the mind'. A simple surgeon such as myself can relate to patients as persons when I meet them and discuss their problems, but treat them as objects in an operating theatre using different tools and techniques. A psychotherapist has no such clear separation in much of what she does. She uses discourse both to correct the deficiencies of thought and action she discloses and as the medium of her contact with the patient as a person (Some surgeons even notice that puzzling as it is, sometimes their words, as much as their use of cold steel, are vital in the recovery of their patients.)

In both reactive and instrumental uses of discourse, a therapist aims at the well-being of the patient as a person—a rational, social being with his or her own attitudes and initiatives and an important perspective on life events. But this stance cannot be assumed from the start in the treatment of mental disorder because there is often something profoundly wrong with the functions enabling the reciprocal interaction. One of the areas where the well-being of the patient as a person and psychiatric treatment most obviously seem to come into conflict is in relation to physical interventions. ECT and psychosurgery are feared beyond all others for reasons that have little to do with any scientific evidence for and against their efficacy (Stek *et al.*, 2003). First, the treatments are violent and apparently irrational. Second, the changes induced by psychosurgery in particular seem to damage a person at the centre of their being. Third, ECT and psychosurgery seem like punishments of a particularly unpleasant kind—electric shocks on the one hand and a physical wounding of the brain on the other. And fourth, none of us can ever imagine wanting such a thing done to ourselves.

The formal credentials of ECT as a treatment belie its fearsome reputation in that, when used wisely, it is a very useful adjunct to other modes of treatment (APA, 1978; Harris, 2006). Its best use seems to be for serious and severe depression unresponsive to other forms of treatment. Indeed, the desperate nature of that state and its association with suicide seems to justify extreme measures despite their 'bad press': 'Such political activity over a highly successful treatment owes little to knowledge of clinical practice and is also an interference with a patient's free choice of treatment' (Merskey, 1999, p. 280).

Recent subjective reports from New Zealand suggest that its negative features have, in the past, occasioned its use as a punishment inflicted (contingently or capriciously) on patients including children with conduct disorders and poor psychosocial backgrounds (Radio NZ, 1997).

> They demoralized me, they shocked me, they jabbed me with injections, they stripped me. That teenage kid that was in that hospital was never allowed to live.

Clearly, its use for punitive rather than therapeutic indications is a particularly barbaric form of the treatment of aliens.

Prefrontal leucotomy and psychosurgery in general seems qualitatively different from ECT in that the organ being damaged is the basis for successful social adaptation and therefore essential for recovery and rehabilitation from a psychiatric disorder. Merskey (1999) is, once again, sanguine, but the arguments seem quite disturbing:

> What from one point of view seemed to indicate a positive result (the removal of unwanted symptoms), from another point of view could be seen as a deterioration in condition (because of side effects). How should success be measured? How should risk–benefit ratios be calculated? And by whom?
>
> (Kleinig, 1985, p. 13)

Kleinig notes that making a patient more tractable and compliant may also destroy some of the spirit, verve, or individuality of a person; indeed it does if we believe anecdotal reports from psychiatric survivors such as Janet Frame and clinicians who have used the treatment: 'She is my daughter but yet a different person,' 'She is with me in body but her soul is in some way lost,' or 'His soul appears to be destroyed' (Pressman, 1998, p. 328). Here is abjection.

> After her operation, Louise became more docile, less inclined to fly into a rage if people refused to hear her 'story'; she wet her pants and giggled delightedly, and yet began to take a pride in her appearance.
>
> She was given every attention and plied with curious morbid questions by the nurses who shuddered when they looked at her and at the others with their bald heads and said, amongst themselves, 'I'm glad it's not me. It gives you the creeps.'
>
> Louise improved. The doctor came to see her twice in one week! And then, as she stayed day after day in Lawn Lodge, and the novelty of the operation wore off, and the doctor had no more time to see her twice a week, although still docile, she grew more careless about her appearance, she did not mind wetting her pants, and the nurses, feeling cheated, as

people do when change refuses to adopt the dramatic forms expected of it, at the sight of the 'old' Louise still settled comfortably under the 'new', gave up trying to re-educate her, and very soon she was again just one of the hopping, screaming people in the dayroom.

(Frame, 1961/1980, p. 111)

These passages highlight the problematic nature of assessments of efficacy in psychiatry (and indeed in medicine in general). In many cases, it is impossible to say what psychosurgery achieves and the procedure has undergone many changes in indication, method, and even site of operation since its simple beginnings with Egas Moniz. This dynamic and changing spectrum of relations between indications, procedure, and outcome measures explains what one commentator calls 'collective uncertainty which should not be eliminated from judgements of psychosurgical efficacy' (Kleinig, 1985, p. 110). The major ethical issue in relation to psychosurgery is that we seem to lack good evidence of sufficient benefit to the patient to make it defensible or indicated, although the progressive reduction of collateral damage to significant (but often subtle) neurological function has greatly reduced the associated harms (Kim *et al.*, 2002; Manshour *et al.*, 2005; Merskey, 1999). Lacking good empirical studies of effectiveness, we must, at best, consider psychosurgery as a treatment of last resort, and at worst, as an unjustified and potentially damaging interference with the integrity of the person.

A further problem hinges on 'old unacceptable personalities' (Frame, 1961, p. 111). The problem is evident in Phineas Gage, who was impaled by a tamping iron that destroyed a significant part of both frontal lobes when it was blasted into his head. After the accident, he was completely changed in that his former civilized and responsible demeanour gave way to a profane and feckless attitude towards life in general and an inability to hold down any position requiring application and reasonable continence (of habits and temper). There is no question that Gage survived his horrendous accident, but as whom did he survive? What happens to the personality and identity of the individual who has a frontal leucotomy. The popular image is that it makes people into 'zombies'; 'Her soul is in some way lost' (Pressman, 1998) and, if so, we should surely not allow it because the risk of injury and alterations of the self cannot be accepted unless there is such compelling evidence of benefit that it would be unethical not to offer a patient the 'last resort' (Pressman).

3.6 Reactive attitudes, the law, and psychiatric care

Our aim in psychiatry is to restore the patient to proper functioning as a person so that an objective attitude should be a provisional and temporary stance and the patient should be encouraged to assume responsibility where she or he is able, an orientation that Janet Frame found reassuring when she came to London. 'Her only stated criticism of her years in hospital is 'No-one listened to me' (Bragan, 1987, p. 73), not a good basis on which the person damaged by a psychological disorder can be recognized and nurtured back into health. Decisions about psychiatric patients may initially disempower the patient because of his or her mental disorder (a benign paternalism in line with a duty of care), but the patient in partnership with the therapist must resume a kind of 'good-as-it-gets' autonomy (that, even in 'normal' people, is not as clear as some ethicists seem to suggest). The whole panoply of truth-telling, informed consent, and confidentiality then goes in step with that restoration.

Many psychiatric patients cannot make well-grounded choices in line with their own best interests quite beyond the fact that many people have inchoate and often poorly formulated life-goals and value structures and a poorly integrated life story. That characteristic of our thinking often makes a demand on doctors and health-care workers as persons and not as objective observers and therapists. Patients look to health-care professionals for expertise but also for respect, guidance, and care so there needs to be a mix of expertise and engagement that helps the patient to overcome his problems while recognizing him or her as a person.

A persistent problem in clinical practice is the formation of habits of thought and reaction that can trap a person in a web of dealings where she or he is regarded as an object, different from the rest of us, and able to be treated in ways that we would never treat each other. But, it is also found more widely in social constructions of insanity, which are inherently alienating even where patients live in the community among 'normal' people, as we have seen.

> They are people you can't put together with others. They're ill after all. They can't live with us or eat with us or anything like that.
>
> (Jodelet, 1991, p. 127)

> No they're not like the rest of us. They've all got something, all of them. All of them are abnormal. (p. 155)

This attitude is also evident in cases of institutional abuse and maltreatment that have marred the history of psychiatry.

Lakeside and Aradale

Two reports from Australia tend to undercut attempts to create historical distance between ourselves and the abuses that mark the treatment of aliens. A psychiatric institution called the Lakeside Hospital at Ballarat (Health Department Victoria, 1990) was investigated after the death of a patient from acute alcohol and amphetamine poisoning and it revealed widespread failures of proper medical treatment and the management of patients' personal funds and ward activities in the chronic psychiatric ward. The report concluded that the actions of those looking after patients 'were subtly influenced by the low esteem of Lakeside Hospital' resulting in neglect of the most appropriate treatment for health problems and 'a need to protect the professional reputation of Lakeside and its staff' (p. 34). Thus, the patients' well-being and even their lives were considered secondary to other staff concerns. The Board of Investigation found that the death was symptomatic of a more general problem, evident on a controversial outing to a local hotel where the staff ate their meals separate from the patients but used patients' personal funds to pay for their food and beverages (p. 52).

> In appearing before the Board, staff made frequent reference to and implied that they understood principles such as least-restrictive care options, the notion that the needs of individuals are best served in environments which reflect the norms of society, and the

rights of people who are mentally ill to access standards of care and treatment which are at least equal to those provided for people with other forms of illness.

Although these beliefs and service objectives appear to have been assumed by Lakeside staff, the Board found little evidence to demonstrate that these concepts have been operationalized in a manner consistent with their philosophical thrust. (pp. 59–60)

Similar conclusions arose from an investigation at Aradale Hospital where patients were poorly fed, poorly occupied, reduced to vegetative roles, custodially confined for the sake of advantageous staff rosters, and exploited to provide jobs for the local community as caregivers (Investigative Task Force, 1991). For instance, the staff deprived the patients of food bought for them and sold it on a thriving black market. The Task Force concluded, 'Resources have been utilized not only without regard to improving conditions for clients but at a direct cost to client independence' (p. 10). The Human Rights Commissioner 'posed the question as to "whether union rights and industrial rights take precedence over human rights"'and reluctantly concluded, 'At Aradale, they appear to have.' (p. 11)

In both cases, psychiatric patients were treated worse, in certain respects, than vulnerable and suffering animals as a result of dehumanizing and degrading practices adopted by caregivers. The objective attitudes in evidence not only caused the human needs of patients to be neglected but also their basic needs to be ignored and actively denied despite official policies mandating otherwise. This alienation (the treatment of psychiatric patients as 'other', not like us, abnormal, threatening, disruptive as if they are a contagion in normal society, abject) is insidiously objectifying and/or abjectifying in ways that pose a deep moral and personal challenge to all dealing with injured and damaged human souls.

3.7 **Forensic confusions**

The confusion between normal reactive judgements about individuals and objective or impersonal judgments also arises where criminal actions fall outside the bounds of comprehensible human action but the person concerned presents as one of us and reminds us of 'the stranger within'.

The David Bain case

On the 20th of June 1994, a young man, 22 years of age, finished his morning paper round (at least somebody did his round that morning) and went home at about 7 a.m. He went and got the .22 calibre rifle that he had been practicing with all week, fitted a silencer to it, and proceeded to stalk through his home and kill his mother, two sisters, and younger brother. He then went into the sitting room, where his father was, having come in from the caravan in the back garden which served as his bedroom, and also shot him. Shortly after this, he rang the police and said that an awful tragedy had happened, which he had discovered on returning home from his paper run. He was arrested for the murders four days later but protested his innocence. He was tried and found guilty and, although he did not enter a plea of insanity, an examining psychiatrist determined that he was not insane. He is currently serving sentence for murdering five members of his family.

One asks, 'How could one do such a thing and not be insane?' An answer (of sorts) is found in the insanity plea and attempts to codify the nature of insanity and its relevance to forensic responsibility, as in the so-called 'McNaghten rules' drawn up by the House of Lords.

> To establish a defence on the grounds of insanity, it must be clearly proved that, at the time of committing the act, the party accused was labouring under such a defect of reason, from a disease of mind, as not to know the nature and quality of the act he was doing or, if he did know it, that he did not know that what he was doing was wrong.
>
> (Gelder *et al.*, 1983, p. 727)

The two criteria for a successful plea of not-guilty on the grounds of insanity can be illustrated by contrasting two (imaginary) cases.

> 1. Anton wakes one night to see his mother walking through the house. He is struck by the thought that she is a witch-demon in his mother's guise, a spirit creature haunting his mother and the rest of his family. He therefore knocks her to the ground and kills her and goes to wake his mother and father to tell them that he has delivered the family from this evil. To his horror, he finds his mother is not there; but after initially believing that she had been taken away, he realizes that he has killed his mother, and breaks down in tears of remorse. Anton's action satisfies the first aspect of the insanity plea in that he was delusionally mistaken about 'the nature and quality of his act' while he believed himself to be destroying a demon-spirit when he was actually killing his mother.

> 2. Beth believes that her brother is a vampire and that he will only have rest from his awful fate if she drives a stake through his heart and says a prayer over him while holding a silver cross. Now she may know that she is attempting to kill her brother and that he will die if she succeeds and yet genuinely believe she is doing good because it is the only way to save his own soul, and the souls of any victims he might prey on, from eternal damnation. Now Beth knows the nature and quality of her act but is genuinely mistaken about its moral qualities in regarding it as a loving act when it is actually homicide.

The McNaghten rules reveal the basis for judging an act to be exempt from the reactive or moral implications that would otherwise follow. They were temporarily displaced by the Durham standard, whereby the disease had to be causally implicated in the act. The exact test is, however, unclear. To conclude that the state of mind of an offender is sufficiently disordered to constitute an excusing condition (on the ground of insanity) according to the McNaghten rules, relies on a judgement that an agent who thought things were as the disordered state of mind pictured them, the action would be permitted (McMillan, 1982, p. 30). But that is not a matter for scientific determination; it rests on the view that 'people, as rational beings, made free choices informed by conscious consideration' (Bazelon, 1974, p. 20), a view criticized by those who argue that a clinician can only give an expert opinion on the kinds of behaviour to which a disorder is likely to give rise and not on the moral qualities of the defendant (the basis of the Durham test).

The Durham test—whether the unlawful act is 'the product of mental disease or mental defect'—rests on a problematic conception. It is clear, for instance, what is meant if the patient were an epileptic and the convulsive movements cause him to strike somebody so that they die. We could also imagine an omission to perform one's proper duty being caused by an absence attack or a hallucinatory disorder. But acts such as those of Anton, Beth, or David Bain are not of that kind but proceed from a plan or set of intentions conceived and enacted by the individual. These are not mere manifestations of some altered psychic state. They may be understandable were things to be as the psychic state in question led the person to think they were; we still have to judge whether a well-intentioned person would do what was in fact done in the situation they believed themselves to be in and that is an interpersonal or reactive judgement. There is one further mitigating condition, aside from ignorance of the nature of the act or its moral significance, when a disorder excuses an otherwise criminal act because it creates an irresistible impulse (Elliot, 1991).

A state of mind giving rise to an irresistible impulse mitigates guilt as in a case involving second-degree murder (the defendant is Brawner).

> A person is not responsible for criminal conduct if, at the time of such conduct, as a result of mental disease or defect he lacks substantial capacity to appreciate the wrongfulness of his conduct or conform his conduct to the requirements of the law.
>
> (Bazelon, 1974, p. 23)

The decision rehearses the knowledge component (as in the McNaghten rules) but adds an impairment of volition (or self-control), as in kleptomania.

A. Recurrent failure to resist impulses to steal objects that are not needed for personal use or for their monetary value

B. Increasing sense of tension before the theft

C. Pleasure, gratification, or relief at the time of committing the theft (DSM IV [APA, 1994a, p. 613])

Acting is such a way is odd or alien; Elliot (1991) likens it to being under duress from a strong and irrational impulse arising from an illness.

> As in more typical cases of duress, the volitionally disordered person would often strongly prefer not to be faced with the choice he must make. He has desires which he wishes he did not have, and he is in a situation in which he would prefer not to be. Yet he must choose whether to act on his desire or resist. (p. 51)

Elliot argues that we feel sympathy for the sufferer because of his or her obvious psychological distress and our intuition that they are not 'an expression of the personality [such that] the person who has them is somehow responsible for their existence' (p. 53). He argues that the compulsive nature of the desires concerned serves as an excusing condition (along with their alien nature with respect to the person's character).

A commonsensical version of the intuition concerned is captured by the 'policeman at the elbow' test: 'Would the person have acted as he or she did if there had been a policeman standing at their elbow?' An action meeting this test is said to result when the psyche 'deprives the person of the power of choice or volition' (Dresser, 1997, p. 10), but notice that the test appeals to commonsense or lay knowledge of persons rather than scientific evidence *per se*, even though expert opinion may be needed to assess the effects of a given condition on the individuals who suffer from it.

Impulse disorders clarify the respective roles of scientific opinion and the human judgement that humans develop and practice in understanding people and developing reactive attitudes (of praise and blame and so forth) towards them. In fact, as I have noted, our understanding of people draws heavily on the situations in which language is learnt (Gillett, 1993d). That context is, of course, interpersonal in that we are influenced by those around us, their evaluations of us, and the expectations they convey as they nurture and train us (Lacan, 1977; Morris, 1992). Thus, the framework of our thought and knowledge about the world is a milieu incorporating reactive attitudes embedding values so that the psyche is not a domain of explanatory states and events (whether real or notional) but a relational aspect of our being through which we engage with others and (through them) the world around us (Gillett, 1992; Gillett, 2008; Harre & Gillett, 1994).

Thus, the reactive or interpersonal side of our nature, evident in assessments of responsibility, is fundamental and prior to any theorizing about the mechanisms governing human behaviour, and it (generally) yields reliable knowledge about people and the moral qualities of their actions. Problems arise when we shift to thinking of human beings according to a scientific framework (we see ourselves as mechanisms of a complex sort obeying laws of nature) with no place for the reactive attitudes (intrinsic to dealing with each other). Kant's remark that human beings not only obey laws but also obey their conceptions of laws—what they think they *ought* to do—underpins the claim that human agents are responsible for their actions (Gillett, 1993b). Psychiatrists wedded to the scientific attitude therefore find traditional legal or jurisprudential models of human agency problematic, as when the Durham rule tries to characterize some behaviour as being caused by a mental disease. The *International Classification of Diseases-9* (ICD 9) has 'deeply ingrained maladaptive patterns of behaviour' (Elliot, 1994), a description that recognizes, as Aristotle did, the tension between free and reasoned action in a particular situation and those habits and weaknesses of character eroding it.

The 'full-blooded' sense of *ought* is diminished by defects of character, but a dispositional bias towards violence and hostility can be distinguished from mental disorder as the basis for an insanity plea in that it blurs the distinction between inability and inclination.

> There is no mental disorder. Paul has had an inadequate parenting. He was sexually abused as a child. He is well above average in intelligence. He is easily slighted, bears a grudge, tends to keep it to himself, and . . . according to records, he is . . .able to build up a homicidal image which he can carry out in a very violent way. He showed that these homicidal acts have no emotional value. He showed no remorse or sorrow. Because of these findings, we feel that Mr. J could easily kill again if he was not maintained in conditions of maximum security.
>
> (Mental Health Review Tribunal, 1993, p. 5)

In this judgement, a summary of the mental state gives rise to a moral assessment, but not according to a scientific train of 'proof' or reasoning (such as disease or disorder-based causal reasoning in psychiatry), rather in terms that a relatively astute observer of the human condition, familiar with the failures of reason found in everyday life, could clearly appreciate. It is in such terms that we understand weakness of the will and self-deception and recognize Aristotle's diagnosis of the need for training in the skills of self-control to overcome such problems. We struggle however, with psychiatric disorders because the cases we find there are alien to our commonsensical notions of action and responsibility, and the failures of reason and self-control often seem quite incomprehensible (Fulford, 1990).

The boundary between 'normal behaviour' and 'personality disorder' (similar to most in the social sciences) is fuzzy. Elliot remarks that the inner defect in a personality disorder is not separable from the identity (in some all-in sense) of the person involved, but unlike our everyday assessments of personality and character, it is dressed in the finery of a scientifically characterized disorder. Elliot suggests that we need the full resources of our reactive attitudes (of praise, blame, excuse, and so on) to cope with forensic judgements in such 'disorders' so that we need good reasons, according to our human understanding of others and their situations, to conclude that the individual concerned is less responsible than a normal person would be to justify disorder type excuses. Thus, we need good phenomenological knowledge of the disorder and the experiences of the person suffering from it so that we can make up our minds on the moral issues of culpability and responsibility on the basis of our interpersonal or reactive knowledge. This puts the language of mechanism where it should be; it should be invoked only when we conclude that, for the purposes of the events under question, our commonsensical judgement is that the person acted less-than-freely and was influenced in a way that would make it unreasonable to praise or blame him or her for the action. That may be the case (as I have already suggested) in kleptomania, in which the deep irrationality of the act defeats our normal understanding of intention and action; in other cases, the excuse of disorder is less clear-cut.

The tribunal's judgement in the matter of Mr. J was that a difficult life history is not enough to explain away (or excuse) a range of vicious and harmful actions; one needs also to argue that the person could not be expected to take the kind of control over their behaviour and personality that most people manage to achieve. Aristotle argues that the vices of weakness and lack of training are not excuses but character defects (whatever their origin) and should be treated as such. Persons who act badly out of a weak or morally deficient character disposed to do immoral and antisocial things are, despite their failings, not incapacitated by a defect of reason, nor are they rendered incapable of pursuing a purposive course of action by an affliction of the soul disabling their self–control; therefore, they deserve to suffer the consequences of their criminal act, a conclusion that bears closely on the problem of psychopathy (or antisocial personality disorder).

Therefore, we must, it seems, make commonsensical judgements, based on our critical but intuitive command of the complex (and often culturally specific) relations between personal skills, character, personality, reactive attitudes, and their conditions of application in a particular set of circumstances, in many psychiatric settings. We should trust our moral judgements provided only that we understand the subjectivities, positions, and discursive options open to the individuals concerned and suspend them when we find that the alienation outstrips our making sense of what has happened without recourse to an illness model (for instance, when we d iagnose a disorder or malfunction that may imply that the person concerned should be treated by, for instance, drugs rather than be judged as being fully responsible for their acts). In some cases, 'treatment' might involve human relationships and skilful discourse to try and help the offender mature and develop the relevant personality skills; in others, the person concerned might receive more objective treatment (such as drugs and behaviour modification) before any interpersonal techniques can usefully get underway.

David Bain revisited

I have couched the forensic questions about insanity in terms of actions attributable to a mental disorder, irresistible impulses, and serious disorders of thought impairing a person's ability to assess or understand the nature and moral properties of their own actions. None of these are present in the Bain murders where we meet a killer who seems very similar to anyone else but where our intuitions falter because of the incomprehensibility of his actions.

David Bain did not seem to be acting out the effects of a disease state but rather executing a premeditated course of action with lethal consequences for his family.

David Bain was not suffering from irrational impulses as in a condition such as kleptomania but was enacting a conscious, albeit highly aberrant, set of intentions.

David Bain was not disordered in his thinking to the point where he did not understand he was killing his family or that killing them was wrong.

The last finding is clear from the actions he took, on the morning of the deaths, to deflect suspicion from himself and then his sustained attempt to defend himself against the charge of murder. One can only imagine the kind of emotional and mental contortions that must have produced his deadly intentions and focused such destructive forces on those close to him; but, once the psychological background is filled in, perhaps those actions make an alien kind of sense. The symbolism, the unusual patterns of family interaction, and the hidden conflicts and tensions within a growing young man can be woven into a plausible story (McNeish, 1997) even though that story is bizarre and the actions extreme. The story does not require a descent into brute mechanism or the loss of a recognizably human narrative to explain the events appearing in it so that our interpersonal, reactive judgements do find purchase and not laws of nature undermining the reason of an admittedly disturbed young person and discrediting the significance of his subjective narrative.

Elliot raises important points about the boundary between our understanding of human beings as persons to whom we relate and individuals who present to us for professional help, highlighting the fact that psychiatry can easily become a hunting ground for poorly formulated theories about the psychic determinants of human behaviour. When it does, it threatens to undermine our reasonable and well-established practices in which we understand each other as subjects weaving inclusive narratives out of the events that we are caught up in. If we can avoid this mistake tied to the abject, unfitting nature of maladies of the soul, we will gain much in our proper study (humankind), the source of our insights into ourselves as agents and personalities.

3.8 **Concluding philosophical arguments**

The philosophical problems fuelling this chapter concern the role of reactive and objective attitudes as sources of knowledge about others. Reactive attitudes lead to discursive knowledge potentiating empathic understanding. This, in turn, allows one to appreciate the position of the other and his or her attempts to cope with the relationships of power structuring his or her experience of the world. Reactive attitudes are set aside when psychiatric patients are treated as aliens and, as a result, they become not only alienated from themselves but also alienated from those who should care for and about them. The contemporary importance of psychiatric abuses of the past is the possibility of alienation from self and others as an inherent feature of mental disorder that leads to uncertainty, frustration, exclusion, and anger, potentiating diverse kinds of violence towards the psychiatric patient.

The existence of two types of attitudes reveals a flaw, as Peter Strawson noted, in the following argument.

The argument for scientific objectivity in psychiatry

(1) Knowledge can be reactive and morally loaded or objective and scientific.

(2) The most reliable and productive knowledge about any natural phenomenon is objective scientific knowledge.

(3) Persons are natural phenomena.

(4) The most reliable and productive knowledge about persons is objective scientific knowledge.

(5) Reactive and moral knowledge of persons ought not to figure prominently in psychology and psychiatry.

But 3 is only a partial truth and should be amplified to read as follows:

(3a) Persons are natural and discursive phenomena.

Thus 4 should read as follows:

(4a) Not all facts about persons can be reliably ascertained by the methods of natural science.

4a undermines 5 and is more congenial with the claims (expressed in 5a and 6) that follow:

(5a) Certain interventions potentiated by scientific and objective knowledge are important in psychiatry.

(6) Certain modes of relationship have reactive and moral aspects and are universally important in healing professions such as psychiatry.

These two claims jointly overturn 5 and deconstruct totalizing alienation (that devalues individuals because they are 'other').

Psychiatric disorders force us to confront the tension in our attitudes to one another more clearly than many other areas of human life and highlight the fragility of the reactive attitudes recognizing, constituting, and affirming us as loci of self-conscious thoughts and considered actions. When we recognize and respect each other's hopes, fears, insights, needs, and intentions, we enter participant roles that are the norm of interpersonal discourse in intelligent communities. Janet Frame (1989) descended into the 'land of shades' where she 'became' alienated, less than a person:

> I remember one instance of a letter written to my sister June where I was actually quoting from Virginia Woolf, in describing the gorse as having a 'peanut buttery smell'. This description was questioned by the doctor who read the letters, and judged to be an example of my 'schizophrenia', although I had had no conversation with the doctors, or tests. I had woven myself into a trap, remembering that a trap is also a refuge. (p. 213)

Bragan (1987) remarks, 'Her self was not recognized or understood, and whereas that failure may have been largely the result of the limitation of time that could be given to each patient, lack of an adequate conceptual framework for understanding her type of illness may have been a significant factor too' (p. 71). Janet Frame entered the abject world of living as an inhuman or subhuman human being and came back to tell the story. The discursive and reactive conceptual framework pervades the present work. The world of letters is richer and Janet Frame (1989) herself is fortunate that she was reinstated from her trap and/or refuge to the world of normal discourse to become one of the foremost female writers that New Zealand has ever seen.

> I joined the new town library and discovered William Faulkner and Franz Kafka, and I rediscovered the few books left on my own bookshelf. I began to write stories and poems and to think of a future without being overcome by fear that I would be seized and 'treated' without being able to escape. (p. 225)

Chapter 4

The depths of the self

> How then is the child's consciousness to be determined?
> It is actually quite indeterminate, which can also be
> expressed by saying that it is immediate. *Immediacy* is
> precisely *indeterminacy*. In immediacy, there is no
> relation, for as soon as there is a relation, immediacy is
> annulled. *Immediately therefore everything is true*; but this
> truth is at the next moment untruth, for *in immediacy,
> everything is untrue*. If consciousness can remain in
> immediacy, then the question of truth is annulled.
> *(Kierkegaard, 1843/2001, p. 78)*

An account of consciousness and the unconscious allows further exploration of the
apparent dichotomy between physiological and biologically inspired accounts of brain
function through the work of Thomas Metzinger and Jacques Lacan. That path reveals
a strange hinterland between consciousness and intentionality inhabited by *meconnaissance* in a way that gives rise to a host of misleading philosophical (and
neurophilosophical) dogmata

4.1 Mental and physical: antireductive thoughts

The biological basis of certain conditions (such as acute schizophrenia and
Manic-Depressive Psychosis, and possibly, obsessive-compulsive disorder, depression,
and certain agitated mood disorders) is so evident that to deny the connection is
foolish. But the system in which the biological changes act—a set of biochemically
mediated structural–functional complexes or a 'wet-wired' processing network—is
designed to interact with and be changed by its environment—the human life-
world—as a result of experience. The causes of change in this network therefore
include both biochemical agents that affect transmission of excitation in the system
and information-preserving configurations of the patterns of connectivity realized by
the system. The biology entails that a model of the system dealing only with its
physiological features (not, I have argued, amenable to symbolic information-processing
terms, and including neurohumoral or biochemical factors influencing excitation
patterns) omits the role of social and cultural context so that explanations of neural

function in biological terms are inevitably incomplete because of discursive influences and their explanatory role in psychology and psychiatry.

The human organism is exquisitely sensitive to the way that environmental conditions are marked by conspecifics so that the cognitive 'significance' (or sense) of information received is determined not only by its physical or causal characteristics but also by the way it figures in the behaviour of other human beings who interact with a human subject (in emotively relevant ways). Other human beings, through their own responses, pick out items and features of the environment, and a developing thinker responds so as to incorporate those items, according to the discourse in play, into the control structures of his or her behavioural repertoire.

Consider, for instance, a stone lying on the ground unnoticed until one of the human beings present picks it up and uses it in some way thereby constituting the item as a thing worth noting rather than merely part of the background. The brain records the experience (and others similar to it), giving rise to cumulative abilities to adapt to the many contingencies and possibilities of situations as they figure in our language games and human forms of life. Something similar to a representation of the stone— a node or focus of processing activity linked, on the one hand, to the stone (as a 'trackable' thing out there) and other objects similar to it and, on the other, to the human behaviour (including linguistic behaviour exhibited)—then arises in the subject (or in the brain). Thus, the stone, fixed (in cognitive space) by a set of (linguistically informed) human responses to it (manifest in practices in which human beings repeatedly or customarily react thus and so to things about them), appears with a determinate profile (in our human network or structure of adaptive responses and associated discourse).

Words operate in shared practices (and therefore, as I have argued, link the responses of one person to those of others in normative ways). Where they focus on interpersonal exchanges and our reactions to one another, they touch chords strung early in our development as (uncoordinated and prematurely born; Lacan) subjects. Many of our basic reactions and modes of responding are therefore formed in close, indeed intense, relationships where personal needs have either been recognized or ignored and met or unmet by those who care for us (a domain of imperatives and appeals; Lacan). Thus, words and propositional attitudes (PAs) involving mental ascriptions and self-ascriptions such as <he-is or I-am in distress> introduce content preformed within close relationships in one's personal history. The matter of these significations has more than one face, only one of which is a fully explicit conscious signification for the subject. But what is involved in material that is not conscious and what aspects of behaviour does it explain? Answering these troubled philosophical questions yields an idea of the relation between conscious and unconscious mental content and the role of language and communication in self-knowledge (Gillett, 1988, 1992, 1997b).

Human beings are active perceivers exhibiting a holistic interplay between conative (affect-related) and cognitive (enquiry-related) intentionality. Thus, we constantly think about and evaluate situations on the basis of a two-way dynamic interaction between mental acts weighted more heavily towards one or other pole on the informative-evaluative continuum. This activity (comprising one's experiential or mental life) is 'inscribed', in the sense already discussed, on the brain and body with the resulting thoughts and attitudes reverberating in a brain network that realizes the accumulated weight of experience in the shared, discursively structured, human life-world.

The brain, as an interconnected network of neuronal activity, does not show step-by-step chains of discrete causal state or event transitions but rather patterns of excitation forming a stream linking the markers of one's mental economy into a dynamic, integrated, ramified, and complex whole that may surprize us by the experiential links it reveals. The unfolding subjective reality follows a narrative rather than rational path of articulation, constantly linking new stimuli to old in ways that both open and close off possibilities for connection (and therefore, meaning). Because humans depend greatly on shared practices in their adaptations to their environment, the structure into which the units of such a system dispose themselves is heavily influenced by language. The milieu in which linguistic expressions derive meaning from their uses (Vygotsky, 1929/1962; Wittgenstein, 1953) is an intersubjective context enabling a synthesis of biological and meaningful aspects of being-in-the-world-with-others and grounding cognitive and/or dynamic and biological approaches to abnormal human behaviour in a way that implies an overall antireductive orientation.

We need, at this point, to tighten up the loose account of stimuli being linked to others through their processing by similar pathways and carrying significance grounded in the experiences where they are encountered. Imagine a subject confronted by a certain kind of object or event: for instance, an eleven-year-old boy who sees his mother making love (e.g. in the front seat of a car) with someone other than his father. The significance of the situation depends on brain pathways registering the object *mother* and linking the presentation <this man before me> with the patterns caused by *father* (a structurally related significant object). Social and evaluative colourings tied up with those significations alter the emotional tone of the encounter and its cognitive effects and explain why it reverberates through the boy's neuronal networks because he is situated in a discursive milieu involving his mother, his father, the concepts of marriage and family, taboos relating to those significations, and so on. The subject, *qua* discursively located subject, is therefore part of the explanation of his brain activity in terms of its social-discursive descriptions and connections. Biology is not sidelined but incorporated into a complex of meaning and structures of signification that are articulated elsewhere even though he does not, as a conscious intentional agent, choose what happens to his brain activity (or, as we shall see, to his psyche). The impact of events, whether conscious or unconscious, can only be understood by reference to the discursive (as well as the biological) realities (mediately) determining them. Enter Lacan, and Dennett, in pursuit of this insight.

4.2 Mind and brain: worlds apart

Dennett's (1991) model of the relationship between mind and brain undercuts naive attempts to correlate mental phenomena and brain events and states, and gives us a useful approach to the idea of the unconscious as that which is immediate and determined by narrative and meaning.

An event of which one is conscious can, as it were, be cognitively examined using a number of different analytic and conceptual resources so that various features of it emerge for reflection. We should also notice that the fact that there are neural or cognitive 'goings-on' beneath consciousness does not imply that they can properly be said to have psychic content apt to contribute to intentional explanations of an individual's behaviour.

Consider the phenomenon of blindsight (Weiskrantz, 1986) in which a subject has residual visual abilities in a scotoma after a brain injury or stroke. The abilities include 'detection of location, movement, stimulus intensity, along with some crude detection of form and colour' (Parkin, 1996, p. 37), all relatively undeveloped and unable to be elaborated in terms of any detailed or explicit knowledge of what is going on. In fact, my patients of this type normally report that they are uncertain whether what they can 'see' is real or a fleeting visual aberration and it takes something similar to a signal detection task to reveal the residual function. Tasks involving dichotic listening are also used to investigate stimuli not available for detailed cognitive work (Gleitman, 1991, p. 228; Holender, 1986), showing that some features of the suppressed or neglected message are implicitly detected (Moray, 1987), including its emotional significance, relevance to the current task, and convergence with attended material (all relatively higher-order features suggesting that mental or semantic content is in play).

Cognitive incubation effects, such as the observation that subjects can solve an 'insoluble' (for them) problem if they are retested after a delay in which they are given distracting but cognitively demanding tasks to do, are also relevant to the concept of a subconscious mind (Smith & Blankenship, 1991). What is more, the effects of such a delay can be enhanced if the subjects are primed with relevant but ultimately misleading stimulus items, suggesting that the subconscious mind is a repository of highly meaningful information that can be manipulated even if the conscious mind is caught up in a different task.

Implicit learning and perceptual processing of degraded stimuli are all tasks in which reasoning and inference (by hypothesis testing and other means) are at work although the subject is not doing such things consciously (Baars, 1988) so that, again, we seem to be dealing with contentful and relatively sophisticated mental operations outside the field of consciousness.

Semantic priming usually involves a task in which the semantic relatedness of word stimuli enhances lexical decision-making or retrieval performance even though the subject may not actually report the stimulus words or consciously recall the words used to prime the present response (Blank & Foss, 1978; Meyer & Schvanenveldt, 1971; Spitzer, 1992), a further fact taken to suggest that some sorting of words on the basis of semantic features goes on at an unconscious level (in the network of signifiers) and helps to structure cognition.

On the basis of such findings, a number of theories about consciousness and the unconscious mind are current in the literature. Block (1995) makes a fundamental distinction between access and phenomenal consciousness and argues, with others such as Chalmers (1996), that there is an unbridgeable, even metaphysical gap between the functions associated with cognitive access and the raw feels or *qualia* of phenomenal consciousness[1]. Weiskrantz (1987) elaborates a *central monitor theory of consciousness*, commenting on patients with disordered consciousness due to brain damage as follows: 'What I think has become disconnected is a monitoring system,

---

[1] I shall discuss this in Appendix C.

one that is not part of the serial information-processing chain itself but which can monitor what is going on' (p. 316). This is a 'second-order' theory as in the phenomenological analysis of consciousness (that distinguishes being conscious of 'X' from being conscious of being-conscious-of-X) interpreting that phenomenon in terms of internal monitoring of the system's function. *The public relations theory* is a simplified version of a view attributed to Dennett (1981) on the basis of his early stress on semantic intentions (p. 171). It is a functionalist analysis of consciousness in terms of access to (or control of) the speech (or expressive language) mechanisms in the brain. However, it seems to ignore the fact that many active intentions and conscious projects are not verbal and seem primarily to involve skilled movement, graphic art, or music (perhaps learned as language-related activities).

Dennett's (1991) later *'cerebral celebrity'* view of consciousness moves beyond a linguistic view to embrace widespread effects on the ongoing stream of neurocognitive processes:

> According to our sketch, there is a competition among many concurrent contentful events in the brain, and a select subset of such events 'win'. That is, they manage to spawn continuing effects of various sorts. Some, uniting with language demons, contribute to subsequent sayings, both sayings-aloud to others and silent (and out-loud) saying to oneself. Some lend their content to other forms of subsequent self-stimulation, such as diagramming to oneself. The rest die out almost immediately, leaving only faint traces—circumstantial evidence—that they ever occurred at all. (p. 275)

The emphasis on dissemination of neural activity within dynamic systems is also central in the *patterned process* view of consciousness in which 'spatiotemporal transitions of states defined by particular forms, shapes, or configurations unfolding in an orderly fashion' are considered to be what differentiates conscious mental events (Diaz, 1997). There is, however, a great deal of ambiguity about the exact way in which such features of physical states actually yield the properties we would associate with consciousness and something similar to the *global workspace access theory* is far more intuitively appealing (Baars, 1988). This theory, similar to Dennett's, focuses on the cognitive connectedness of material that becomes conscious and, to some extent, incorporates phenomenological intuitions about conceptual exploration. O'Brien and Opie (1997, p. 271) point out certain difficulties in specifying just which content items one might include in the range of states that are to count as conscious and offer a cognitive theory in terms of explicit representational content.

They describe their own approach as a *vehicle theory* (O'Brien & Opie, 1997) such that

> All phenomenal experience is the result of the tokening of explicit representations in the brain's representational media, and that whenever such a representation is tokened, its content is phenomenally experienced. (p. 280)

Koch (2004) uses explicit content in seeking the neural basis of consciousness but begs serious questions about mental realism and takes the idea of 'encoding' somewhat further than cautious commentators such as Bolton and Hill (1996).

The present anti-realist reading of mental activity is compatible with the *discursive integration theory* of consciousness implicitly supported by Searle (1992) and Worley (1997), both of whom argue that explicit propositional content is problematic in a way that undermines attributions of mental states not subject to the array of discursive skills people use to frame and give an account of their thoughts, attitudes, and actions. The present view argues that the life of the psyche is the life of an engaged subjective being among others structured, owned, and enacted by using discursive skills and modes of interaction.

In fleshing out a discursive theory of consciousness and the subconscious mind, we can pursue Dennett's thesis that consciousness is a narrative composed in 'Multiple Drafts' (p. 111).

> According to the Multiple Drafts model, all varieties of perception—indeed, all varieties of thought or mental activity—are accomplished in the brain by parallel, multitrack processes of interpretation and elaboration of sensory inputs. Information entering the nervous system is under continuous 'editorial revision.' (p. 111)

In order to formulate a clear and distinct idea of what is being said here, we can substitute information-processing terms for 'interpretation', and 'editorial revision' as follows:

> The patterns of neural excitation do not firmly fall into well-developed processing pathways on initial registration but rather excite a number of possible pathways, the relative strengths of activity in which change relative to each other as each new bit of information arrives.

The resulting theory meshes well with a narrative or autobiographical theory of the self:

> Probing this stream at different places and times produces different effects, precipitates different narratives from the subject . . . Most important, the Multiple Drafts model avoids the tempting mistake of supposing that there must be a single narrative (the 'final' or 'published' draft, you might say) that is canonical—that is the actual stream of consciousness of the subject, whether or not the experimenter (or even the subject) can gain access to it. (p. 113)

The last point is crucial. It is clarified by one of Dennett's experimental examples: Kolers' *colour phi phenomenon* (Kolers & Grunau, 1976) in which subjects are exposed to a red spot of light and then a green spot of light 200 msec later and a short but significant distance away. In this situation, the subject reports a coloured spot that moves and changes colour in going from one position to the next. Now, it is clear that the consciously experienced phenomenon is not what physically happens (out there in the world) and stimulates the brain. Dennett (1991) remarks:

> So somehow the information from the second spot (about its colour and location) has to be used by the brain to create the 'edited' version that the subjects report. (p. 120)

It seems that the subject actually 'fills in' the non-existent trajectory during which they report the spot moving and changing colour and that 'the temporal order of discriminations cannot be what fixes the subjective order in experience' (p. 119). Conscious experience therefore is a 'best guess' (and, in an ecological setting, usually a very good guess) about what (in the world) has caused the pattern of excitations in the brain.

Such an ecologically situated 'best guess' takes into account the kinds of thing that normally happen in the world in which the subject is situated. The model has the following implication about brain activity and conscious experience:

> If one wants to settle on some moment in the brain as the moment of consciousness, this has to be arbitrary. One can always 'draw a line' in the stream of processing in the brain, but there are no functional differences that could motivate declaring all prior stages and revisions to be unconscious or preconscious adjustments, and all subsequent emendations to the content (as revealed by recollection) to be post-experiential memory contamination. (p. 126)

This implies that there is no story about the events of consciousness picked out by pointing at some feature of those brain events that are conscious and driven from the bottom up; rather, there is a narrative supplied by the subject that signifies or selects from what is happening to him or her those things to be given a certain prominence (in the light of learnt significance). This narrative has its moments or events as elements in a signified narrative, not a report of internal states, and it is subject, as are all narratives, to socially productive effects. Once composed, the narrative structures one's experiences (but not totally) and it is not ever (nor could it be) a description of brain events; it is rather a commentary on or signification of the impingement of a situation and its component conditions upon the discursive subject.

This account stresses the discursive and narrative nature of conscious experience in a way that becomes important when we begin to discuss pathologies of identity, but it also makes visible the fact (noted by Bolton and Hill) that the subject is situated in a world to which he or she must adapt. The world contains natural contingencies and social contingencies and the techniques of adaptation combine natural responses and cultural techniques inextricably bound together. Thus, the myth of the noble savage in tune with nature and constrained by society is just that—a myth. We are all constituted as social products, consciousness is a social product, and the skills producing the contents of consciousness are social techniques. But that does not imply there is anything more false and flimsy to consciousness than the very real experience of feeling a brick hit my foot or my foot step on the rung of a ladder given that I am constantly working with my very real engagement with the world around me[2].

In summary, there are two worlds in which each of us is situated, narratively constructed with their own metaphors, models, signifiable events or moments, and their own timescales and relationships. (In fact, the events and relations can only be identified by using significations available in a particular narrative context.) There is a world of events described by neuroscience and the other natural sciences (with its spatiotemporal relations and notions of causality according to scientific description and laws of nature), but there is also a world of mental phenomena appearing within a narrative that is rooted in the evaluative, interpersonal, and historical context of human discourse. Each set of descriptions or significations is in part constituted by rules, and the rules of each cannot be mapped onto the rules of the other so that mind-brain identity theories are ill-conceived and metaphysically naive.

---

[2] Again, this is discussed in Appendix C.

Those philosophical preliminaries lay the groundwork for an informed theory of the unconscious reminiscent, in certain respects, of Freud's (1986) own theory. Consciousness, he remarks, 'is only a quality or attribute of what is psychical, and moreover, an inconstant one' (p. 188). It 'can only offer us an incomplete and broken chain of phenomena' (p. 189). Consciousness, we might say, is a selection from events inscribed on the body (including the brain) through experience as they appear in a world of intersubjective and relational beings.

4.3 Consciousness and the unconscious

Freud

Freud (1986) revolutionized psychology and psychiatry by arguing that there were unconscious mechanisms underlying conscious behaviour and thereby severing the conceptual connection between introspectability and mental contents. He drew on the following phenomena:

(i) The gaps in psychological explanation evident when one is limited to conscious phenomena;

(ii) The nature of post-hypnotic suggestion; and

(iii) The coherence and meaningfulness of dream interpretations (p. 135ff).

The gaps in explanation are filled by two different types of psychic contents: those not present to consciousness at a given point in time and those later characterized as repressed. Such contents are uncontentious when we consider memories or beliefs not currently the focus of attention, but Freud (1986) also invokes unconscious contents to explain slips of the tongue, irrational behaviour, and other 'ideas keeping apart from consciousness in spite of their intensity and activity' (p. 137), such things as wishes and thoughts with an attached cathexis or meaningful and/or emotional loading and psychical effects.

The dynamic thesis whereby unconscious contents have psychic content that explains what people do and the attitudes they adopt is not merely the idea that there are unconscious informational processes explaining our cognitive performance in solving problems or in relation to thought in general. Dennett's theory of consciousness, Metzinger's no-self theory, and Lacan's *meconnaissance* or *me-connaissance* can all be seen as elaborations of the idea that the unconscious is the core of the psyche in ways that illuminate the dynamic and interpersonal aspects of disorders such as Multiple Personality Disorder, Hysteria, and anorexia.

Freud appeals to the fact that we rationalize and minimize the significance of phenomena such as 'slips of the tongue' or laugh at a slightly 'off' joke (with respect to the discursively constructed self we present to the world) but that they are deeply revealing. He also discusses post-hypnotic suggestion and the feeble rationalizations to which it gives rise as evidence that the unconscious can affect conscious behaviour. Freud (1986) mentions, *inter alia*, a patient who, under the influence of post-hypnotic suggestion, picks up a doctor's umbrella and holds it over the doctor's head to ward off the rain when the doctor comes to his ward. When challenged, the patient makes 'some lame remark' about why he is doing that (p. 188). Freud claims that such evidence indicates that contents in the psyche have behavioural effects without being accessible to the conscious awareness of the patient.

Another well-known Freudian phenomenon is the interpretation of dreams whereby he brings out their 'latent thought content' and locates them in relation to a patient's conscious mental life and, in particular, unspoken wishes and fantasies. Dream analysis illustrates the general structure of psychoanalytic theory as it fills in gaps in conscious self-understanding by positing subconscious contents completing otherwise deficient chains of intentional explanation (in terms of quasi-desires and quasi-beliefs in a mind-like 'zone' beneath conscious thought).

Freud (1940) formulates a threefold structure for the mind consisting of *id*, *ego*, and *superego*.

> The *id* 'contains everything that is inherited . . . above all . . . the instincts which originate from the somatic organization and which find a first psychical expression here [in the id] in forms unknown to us.' (p. 28)

The *ego* 'acts as an intermediary between the id and the external world' (p. 28) through consciousness and the voluntary control of behaviour so that it is the seat of intentions (whereas the deeper motives and attitudes affecting behaviour are found in the id). Freud (1940) believes that conscious intentions and attitudes are constructed by striking a balance between the urges and instinctive dispositions of the id and the moulding influence of the world in producing personal strategies for public self-presentation and a significant factor in that process is a further division of the psyche—the *superego*.

> The long period of childhood in which the growing human being lives in dependence on his parents leaves behind it as a precipitate the formation in his ego of a special agency in which this parental influence is prolonged. It has received the name of *superego*. (p. 29)
>
> The superego does not merely serve as a representative of the parents but is a precipitate of 'not only the personalities of the actual parents but also the family, racial, and national traditions handed on through them, as well as the demands of the immediate social milieu which they represent.' (p. 29)
>
> *Ex hypothesi*, problems arise when the ego cannot strike a balance between the conflicting demands of the id, the ego, and the superego so that 'normal and abnormal manifestations' arise that 'need to be described from the point of view of their dynamics and economics (in our case, from the point of view of the quantitative distribution of the libido).' (p. 39)

Freud (1940) claims that we need to understand what shapes the conscious field to make sense of what is going on in experience and that three different types of psychic processes—'conscious, preconscious, and unconscious'—are involved (p. 44). All are 'folk-psychological' (in the contemporary sense), 'the same as the consciousness of philosophers and of everyday opinion' (p. 43). Preconscious material is 'capable of becoming conscious' whereas 'other psychical processes and psychical material . . . have no such easy access to consciousness' and 'for such material we reserve the name of the unconscious proper' (p. 44). Each set of processes forms a system in which an idea can be located in relation to other ideas and the objects (or 'things' which have given rise to them). Ideational complexes move between the Ucs, Pcs, and Cs systems, and their 'psychical topography' in different 'regions of the mental apparatus' (1986, p. 150) reflects the way they are presented to and operate on the psyche.

Psychic resistance prevents unconscious material from becoming conscious and is caused by the difficulty in accepting into consciousness certain highly significant material with profound (and disruptive) significance to the subject. Freud sees the transition from Ucs or Pcs to the conscious level of recognition as having two phases.

(i) The transition from Ucs to Pcs, linked to the developmental history of the individual;

> In the course of this slow development, certain of the contents of the id were transformed into the preconscious state and so taken into the ego; others of its contents remained in the id unchanged, as its scarcely accessible nucleus. (1940, p. 47)

This first transition is affected by psychic trauma resulting in repression so that certain contents remain as unconscious influences on the thinking and behaviour of the subject. The ideas confined to Ucs exist in an inchoate form with variable effects creating pressure on the Pcs even though any of their cathexes (emotional accompaniments) exists as 'a potential beginning . . . prevented from developing' (1986, p. 153). This lack of development (articulation or determination) is important in a discursive and particularly in a post-Lacanian account.

(ii) The second transition from Pcs into full consciousness, which is intimately involved with speech;

> This is the work of the function of speech, which brings material in the ego into a firm connection with mnemonic residues of visual but more particularly of auditory perceptions. (1940, p. 46)

Freud sees the passage of preconscious material into the ego as effected by mechanisms tied to language and the meanings available to the patient such that traumatic associations of an idea *qua* idea can prevent it becoming explicitly formulated in terms acceptable to the ego. If the ego is too weak or 'young and feeble' to accept the material and render it in a consciously articulate form, the material is returned to Pcs or even Ucs (p. 47). Ideas in Ucs are associated with cathexes (associations and images linked to gratification and threat or harm). These cathexes are mobile and can be displaced from one idea to another or even condensed with the cathexis of another idea, perhaps in response to drives or wishes or perhaps for some apparently incidental contingency such as an auditory resemblance in the words used to express the idea (Cavell, 1993, p. 162). Unconscious ideas are also unlike conscious material in that they are not clearly located in time and carry no essential reference to a particular event or episode. Finally, the processes in Ucs do not track nor become firmly linked to reality as revealed by perception of and conscious thoughts about the world. Ucs is not interested in what is out there and validated by others but concerns itself with the psychic moments of an individual subjectivity. This mode of thought is characteristic of the 'primary process' so called because it is primitive in the development of mind and precedes the development of language with its implicit discursive norms. Anna Freud (1986) describes the primary process as follows:

> We are dealing here with modes of expression that are closer to hallucination than they are to thinking in words: opposites become one and the same thing, temporal relationships and sequences are disregarded, logical thinking and consequential cause–effect connections

are missing, emotions are easily displaced from the real object to another, mixed figures are formed as the result of the condensation of several single figures. Altogether, this mode of thinking characteristic of the unconscious strikes one as extraordinarily primitive; it is not different from what we assume to prevail in the infant before the acquisition of language. (p. 132)

We will later see that the promiscuity of association (or indeterminacy) indicated here is what one might expect where cognitive operations are not configured by and subject to the rules of discourse. Discourse moderates the immediacy of *le jouissance* (Lacan) so that the encounter with the real is constrained and transformed through its link with a signifier and the material that results is a semi-organized hybrid of indeterminate meaning and raw engagement. The 'subconscious', psychic material that is not clearly conscious rather than physiological processes or presumed cognitive mechanisms (Jaspers' 'extraconscious' processes) is, in what follows, that which is significant to the subject even though it may be inchoate.

Thus far, Freud's claims are more or less common to all types of psychoanalytic theory and his basic divisions in the psyche correspond to theoretical structures often invoked within that tradition. Much of this is, in fact, regarded as orthodoxy in the post-Freudian era and so seems unexceptionable even though there are a number of assumptions and constructions hidden within it that should be explored *en route* to a more adequate account of the psyche. A more or less realist interpretation of Freud's (1986) theory is problematic, but is a good basis for that inquiry.

> To sum up: *exemption from mutual contradiction*, *primary process* (mobility of cathexes), *timelessness*, and *replacement of external by psychical reality*—these are the characteristics which we may expect to find in processes belonging to the system Ucs. (p. 160)

Philosophical problems with the unconscious

The discursive theory of subconscious content drawing on Dennett and Lacan is best developed by pursuing the philosophical problems of psychoanalytic theories.

MacIntyre (1958) notes that Freud thinks of the unconscious not merely as unformed libidinous material but as 'the realm of repressed memories and emotions' so that it has determinate meaningful content in the form of a range of ideas each of which is 'a discrete unit of mental life, associated in various ways with other such units'. Freud posits that certain experiences in infancy produce such ideas: 'Freud conceives of the memory of the trauma as . . . an 'idea' . . . laden with feeling to greater or lesser degree' (p. 11).

A child's experiences normally enter consciousness clothed with meaning by the language-based mechanisms operating between Pcs and Cs, and ideas are only relegated to Ucs when they are 'traumatic ideas' such that to introduce them into Cs in their fully explicit form would cause disruption, conflict, or suffering so that such a psychic move is resisted.

> Thus, certain types of reaction to the world around him prove so painful to the child that the memory of them together with the emotion which expressed the instinctual desire behind the reaction are suppressed from consciousness.

> (MacIntyre, 1958, p. 26)

But recall the status of the entities, mechanisms, and processes here so confidently discussed:

> In explaining the meaning of 'traumatic', reference has already had to be made to resistance, and like 'traumatic', 'resistance' is not a description but an explanatory, theory-laden expression. The patient does not remember certain experiences of childhood; when in his own free associations he approaches them, he is thrown into a state of some agitation or betrays emotion in some other way. When the analyst suggests that he is avoiding reference to them [and] he repudiates this interpretation of his behaviour with some force, from all this, the analyst will infer that the patient is resisting the recall to mind of some memory. But the patient is *ex hypothesi* unconscious of the fact of resistance.
>
> (MacIntyre, 1958, p. 14)

The Freudian doctrine of the unconscious therefore embodies certain key claims:

> 'The Unconscious' is the name of a system of mental acts. The justification for belief in the existence of this system is twofold: first, we are able to account for behaviour which cannot be accounted for in terms of conscious intentions; secondly, if we assume in psychoanalytic practice the existence of the Unconscious, we are able to bring into consciousness contents of which the patient was unaware, and in so doing, we help to bring about the healing of his mental disorder.
>
> (MacIntyre, 1958, p. 33)

MacIntyre critiques this position in a traditional and fairly realist way but Cavell, drawing on Wittgenstein's later philosophy, offers a more radical (anti-realist) critique.

Traditional criticisms

The first criticism, echoing Karl Jaspers, concerns Freud's mechanistic or causal hypothesis.

> One may ask 'Why?' and expect an answer in terms of reasons, intentions, purposes, and the like; or, one may ask 'Why?' and expect an answer in terms of physiological or psychological determining antecedent conditions.
>
> (MacIntyre, 1958, p. 52)

Freud (1940) portrays events that are meaningful for the subject and uses their meaningful content to characterize psychic entities standing in causal relations with each other so that the psychic reality described—comprising id, ego, cathexes, and anticathexes—are seen in physiological terms with almost 'Newtonian' interactions between the posited states and events:

> Nervous or psychical energy occurs in two forms, one freely mobile and another, by comparison, bound; we speak of cathexes and hypercathexes of psychical material, and even venture to suppose that a hypercathexis brings about a kind of synthesis of different processes—a synthesis in the course of which free energy is transformed into bound energy. (p. 43)
>
> The *ego* has been developed out of the id's cortical layer, which through being adapted to the reception and exclusion of stimuli is in direct contact with the external world (reality). (p. 77)

MacIntyre (1958) notes the presumed psychophysical correlations as a point of criticism in that they reify both the mental states and events posited and presumed states and events correlated with them in the unbroken stream of neural activity in the human brain (p. 66). Nevertheless, despite the Victorian ontology, certain psychoanalytic theses are worth noting. First, there is the 'correlation between certain types of childhood experience and later adult behaviour' (p. 67). This is fairly unexceptional and need not be linked to the associated neurodynamic theory. 'The legacy of childhood' (Cavell, 1993, p. 176) does not imply that there are distinct memories existing in an unconscious domain of thoughts and feelings and other mental states, a realist thesis that is particularly dangerous when interpreted as the claim that repressed memories of actual experiences are powerful in influencing behaviour and can be recovered as evidence to be used in proceedings related to the posited childhood events[3]. Third, McIntyre questions the idea that bringing to remembrance a childhood state of affairs and consciously talking about it can change the adult psyche. But Freud (1986) also suspects the naive and simplistic hope that 'making conscious' will neutralize the harmful psychic effects of conflictful material, arguing that there has to be a connection of the conscious idea 'with the unconscious memory-trace' (p. 151) allowing the ego to entertain and explore the elements previously excluded from it through the therapeutic relationship and its associated emotional (transference) 'work' on the effects maintaining dysfunctional ego defences.

MacIntyre notes the 'evidence' for repressed material: present discomfort when certain areas of psychological life become the topic of discussion such that the person concerned will not say why these areas cause discomfort and is presumed not to know. Freudian theorists conclude that the material concerned is present, contentful, and active but resides at a different psychic location from that accessed in the present conversation, but that conclusion embeds a strong doctrine of the nature of the unconscious mind that is deeply problematic. MacIntyre (1958) remarks:

> This difficulty over 'repression' extends for the reasons I have suggested to 'the unconscious'. The issue about 'the unconscious' can now be restated. Either the unconscious is an inaccessible realm of inaccessible entities existing in its own right or it is a theoretical and unobservable entity introduced to explain and relate a number of otherwise inexplicable phenomena. If it is the first, then being a real existent it requires evidence for its existence to be credible. But *ex hypothesi*, it cannot be observed and so we cannot possibly have evidence of its existence. If we dismiss this alternative as too naive, although Freud's talk of the unconscious as the *ding-an-sich* behind the sense data is naive in just this way . . . then the other alternative demands that we inquire what precise explanatory role the concept of the unconscious plays. And here I find myself at a loss. (p. 71)

Macintyre notes the dilemma: either we are discussing real structures in the mind or brain or we are discussing explanatory entities or hypotheses to account for certain data. The difficulty is well illustrated by Cavell's (1993) discussion of cases such as *Little Hans* and *the table cloth lady* (p. 188) in which the trains of ideas explaining the behaviour do not really make sense as intentional explanations, even though they have

---

[3] Of this, more in Chapter 10.

the flavour of doing so when read in the context of a discussion of the primary process as an interpretive device. But the explanation is illuminating quite apart from its posited mechanism with (articulated) functional parts:

> To say that something is repressed is not to draw attention now to the pushing of a memory from one realm into another but to some stratagem whereby the personality defends itself in psychologically painful or dangerous situations . . . Freud's indispensable terms are 'unconscious' and 'repression', used descriptively; except insofar as illuminating description may count as a kind of explanation, their place as explanatory terms is highly dubious.
>
> (McIntyre, 1958, pp. 78–79)

MacIntyre's phrase 'illuminating description' evokes a set of images and metaphors woven into a narrative exploring the accommodations of the self to the strains of psychological adaptation in a vexed world of interpersonal relationships and multiply intersecting significations. That narrative is coherent in a queer kind of way captured by Freud's term 'primary process'.

> Associations like these point to different mental processes from the ones we variously call reason, but not to ones that are temporally prior.
>
> Primary process is primary in that it is the earliest mental processes and the most primitive in form, remaining as a substrate of even the most adult and normal mind.
>
> (Cavell, 1993, pp. 171, 175)

The characteristics of primary process are to be expected when we adopt a post-structuralist (and associationist) account of signification and the psyche. The difficulties for psychodynamic philosophy and psychology arise when we forget the Multiple Drafts model and think of ourselves as describing events, states, and processes really existing in a mentalist (quasi-physical or causal) realm of psychic being connected in roughly the ways found in stylized discourse. The problem for causal realism about the unconscious is nowhere more clear than in the evident contradiction between freedom and therapeutic change that it entails.

> The sharpest distinction in Freud's clinical practice is presumably that between the suffering neurotic and the successfully analysed patient. The former goes through compulsive rituals, is harassed by delusive beliefs, cannot understand his own behaviour, and cannot control it; the latter is characterized by what Freud calls 'self-knowledge and greater self-control'. Thus, 'cure' for Freud means more than 'the mitigation of neurotic symptoms', which is what it tends to mean for those who apply physical methods in psychiatry. To be cured is to have become reasonable, aware of the true nature of one's situation, able to cope with it instead of being overcome by it. But curiously, this whole distinction, lacking which the whole project of psychoanalysis would be meaningless, is obliterated by the determinism of Freud's general theory.
>
> Thus, the psychoanalyst as therapist contrasts compulsive and unfree neurotic behaviour with normal free choice, but as theorist, his conception of unconscious causation leads him to deny this contrast by seeing both as unfree.
>
> (McIntyre, 1958, pp. 90–91)

Even without the strong view that mental disorder can be cured by analysis, this is a damaging paradox often neglected in discussing psychodynamic arguments against free will. As the present account of the psyche unfolds, partly under the stimulus of this paradox, it becomes clear that psychological determinism involves grave conceptual errors.

Church, in discussing irrationality, reformulates an understanding of the unconscious while preserving some traditional Freudian insights in a more tightly worked philosophical guise that makes useful distinctions between 'subconscious content' and conscious mental life. She criticizes Davidson's account of irrationality (1980) that distinguishes the causal efficacy of intentional states from their rational (or meaningful) credentials.

> The alternative I am proposing maintains that irrational beliefs, desires, and actions are just those that are ill-coordinated with reflective states and reflective forms of reasoning.

> (Church, 1987, p. 360)

For Church, reflective aims or intentional states are 'those which are themselves objects of awareness at a given time' (p. 357), and her view of coordination reflects Freud's (Kantian) 'synthesis' as a characteristic activity of the ego. Reflective awareness potentiates a judgement by the subject based on epistemic, conative, or other evaluative criteria such that if the mental state concerned is a belief, then the evaluation in question is epistemic—is the state a legitimate way to signify a given set of conditions in the world according to the norms of some discourse or another. In the case of a conative (appetitive) judgement—<I want ___> or <I like ___>—the evaluation concerns the affirmability of the intentional state given the commitments and current interests of the subject (for instance, if I am to be a sensitive new-age guy, I should not think of women according to some blonde bombshell stereotype.) Church, I think rightly, suggests that the fact that a state is or is not a candidate for reflective (or second-order) judgement is an important feature of conscious mental content in that reflection on one's own states is an important feature of phenomenology and the norms according to which a subject configures him or herself according to his or her discursive position (as a self mirrored by others).

Cavell (1993) takes us further towards a discursive (post-structural) account of the unconscious by (as Kierkegaard does) jettisoning the claim that there are determinate meanings in any sublinguistic domain of the psyche: "outside language", there are neither contradictory nor different 'terms'; there are simply things, waiting to be conceived, named, sorted out' (pp. 167–168). These things and events may affect us in various ways, but meaningful trains of thought cannot get underway without the participation of discourse and its norms of signification coming into play and these do not hold sway where primary process rules.

Cavell is also sceptical about the idea of subjective content with effects in the subconscious mind becoming conceptualized by being linked to a distinct relatum—a signifier—contra certain Cartesian realist readings of the Saussurian doctrine of signifier and signified (p. 169).

Cavell (1993) summarizes the defensible claims available to a theory of the unconscious as follows:

(1) There is a primary process not subject to rational constraints that works by loose associations and assignments of significance.

(2) There is a dynamic unconscious in which the inaccessibility of contents is motivated by the organism's need to protect itself from psychic distress.

(3) Childhood has a legacy in the adult psyche that escapes the norms an adult would impose on mental contents. (pp. 175–176)

I have urged that a reflective attitude towards one's own responses, judgements, and thoughts is a discursive technique formed in a domain of imperatives where one reacts to and responds in terms of the reactions of others (Lacan, 1977, p. 106). Discursive techniques focus on both unsignified and signified experience as a being-in-the-world-with-others. Signification is an immediate or prereflective (to use a phenomenological term) response to lived experience and reflection is a secondary response to signification. On the discursive view, signification and reflection, similar to all other discursive techniques, are produced in a public sphere of personal interaction where one latches onto the responses of others in terms shaped by their responses to things around them, to my responses, and to me as a thinker. I learn to frame myself as subject of the same kind of judgement that others make about me (thus, I attain self-knowledge). There is, to echo Strawson or Wittgenstein, an internal (conceptual or essential) relation between <I am angry>, <I am thoughtful>, <I am considerate>, or in general, <I am M>, where M is a mental predicate, and judgements directed towards myself (by others) of the form <You are M>. These judgements have both descriptive content and an evaluative tone conveying things about me besides the descriptions I instantiate (angry, thoughtful, considerate . . . M). Through learning to make such judgements about myself, I construct a 'second-order mental life' in which my (first-order) perceptions, feelings, attitudes, and responses are potentially subject to self-evaluative reflections and commentary (drawn from the mirror world constituted by others).

The Freudian superego makes a similar point, but notice that the judgements concerned are modelled on interpersonal transactions that explicate lived experience making it articulate, communicable, and conscious. If the reflective judgements associated with certain events and situations are disturbing because their evaluative loading intimates something disruptive, dangerous, or disturbing, then some encounters are never properly explicated and cannot be reflected upon. Compare this process, reflecting degrees of articulation (or explication), to exploring a dangerous maze in which a direct encounter with what is there at a certain point could have dire consequences. In such a case, full exploration is understandably tempered by a fairly sensitive response to hints of danger. By analogy, the moments of the psyche exist on a continuum from unsignified or indeterminate forms, through forms in which their content is clear but second-order judgements are not articulated, to forms in which the encounter basks in the full light of reflection and integration with other autobiographical mental content.

This view is made even more plausible by an anti-realist critique of Freudianism, Dennett's account of consciousness and brain processes, and Lacan's account of subjectivity.

An anti-realist critique

Freud (1986) himself hinted at an anti-realist critique of psychoanalytic theory, comparing it to the state of physics before the quantum era (p. 185). He refuses to describe the essence or nature of psychic entities (in themselves), and rather asserts their existence and causal relevance in terms of psychological explanation. An anti-realist critique points out that a causal realist account of the unconscious mind and the states and events within it reifies entities that are abstractions from discourse and discursive understandings of human activity. Conscious thought is determinate because it is, *ex hypothesi*, part of a narrative and therefore configured according to the discursive techniques articulating that narrative. The subconscious contents of present or past experience do not have that clarity. The problem goes beyond Church's claim that certain experiential or intentional states are unreflective and instead proposes that we are affected in ways that are discursively influenced, but perhaps inchoate. The fact that reflectively uncoordinated material has (quasi-psychic) content and determinate effects on behaviour even though it is not reflectively endorsed, refined, or explored still allows that it can figure in explaining behaviour, but Searle's (1992) scepticism about the unconscious seems closer to the mark: 'the ontology of the unconscious is strictly the ontology of a neurophysiology capable of generating the conscious' (p. 172). The last phrase should perhaps read 'a neurophysiology from which conscious experience is generated by the discursive subject' given Dennett's deconstruction of the bottom-up view of the determination of the mental by the physical and the current (discursive) orientation, but the form of the account is sound.

The anti-realist view of the interface between brain activity and mental processes is that the intentional content of brain activity is fixed by human discursive skills that shape it according to the meanings and stories available around here. The painting isn't finished until it is finished (just like a baseball game) and what looks like a swan at one point may transform itself into a skull at another depending on the picture unfolding as the painter works. In an analogous way, the discursive autobiographer goes to work on the flux of interaction between himself or herself and the world, and the content of that interaction evolves as he or she works so that, in a sense, it is never finished. This is a particularly strong theme in Lacan's study of the unconscious.

4.4 Lacan: the signifier and the unconscious

Lacan (1979) has modified, or some would say transformed, the dynamic theories of the Freudian school of psychoanalysis in the light of the structuralism of de Saussure (in linguistics) and Levi-Strauss (in anthropology) on the basis of Heidegger's existential phenomenology. Freud discusses the 'object presentation' distinguishing the word presentation and the thing presentation (as Kant does), the former available to Pcs and Cs, and the latter only to Ucs caught up in the primary process mode of psychic activity. Lacan both develops and extends these concepts to illuminate the relation between language, the human milieu, and the psyche. From de Saussure, he derives the insight that language is a structured system in which meanings arise from the contrasts and connections between signs, and from Levi-Strauss, he takes over the idea that language has a totemic or mythical function and form. Vygotsky (1929/1962), Husserl (1950/1999), or Luria (1973) could be invoked to support certain of his claims about language, interpersonal transactions, and the unconscious in that each stresses the social nature of language and the importance of interlocutors in the formation of mind.

Lacan's claim 'the unconscious is structured like a language' (1979, p. 20) directs our attention to the network of signifiers collectively transcending an individual psychological history and inscribing the individual mind through the subject's immersion in a speech community.

> The psychoanalytic experience has rediscovered in man the imperative of the Word as the law that has formed him in its image. It manipulates the poetic function of language to give to his desire its symbolic mediation. May that experience enable you to understand that it is in the gift of speech that all the reality of its effects resides, for it is by way of this gift that all reality has come to man and it is by his continued act that he maintains it.

> (Lacan, 1977, p. 106)

Lacan notes that we do things to each other by speech and that interpersonal discourse constitutes reality for the subject who then uses discursive techniques to grasp the reality in which she or he is engaged. She or he then remains a user and product of the symbolic and poetic function of language that articulates his or her life events so that they form a good-enough narrative to live in (or by means of). Notice how far this has moved away from the simplistic view that language is a set of signs carrying information about an objective world.

Only some aspects of the subject's immersion in discourse are transacted at a conscious level so that in order to understand them 'one should see in the unconscious the effects of speech on the subject' (Lacan, 1979, p. 126). To explore the psyche is, in part, to map the network of signifiers shaping it (Lacan, 1979, p. 45) so that when we consider the way that an individual personality is formed, it is the precipitated (or congealed) residue of a lifetime of encounters with others (as Frame has it) and we should beware of the objectifying tendency in this formulation. The subject is not fixed but is active, so that it is 'in the relation between the subject's ego (*moi*) and the 'I' (*je*) of his discourse that you must understand the meaning of his discourse' (Lacan, 1977, p. 90).

Lacan critiques the error of believing that there is a 'truth' about the psyche comparable to the real essence (Locke) of a natural species. The real essence of a natural object gives us a way of understanding its modes of interacting with the world in terms of its intrinsic properties and their engagement with laws of nature. But, in psychology, there is no essence of the soul or personality determined independently of the subject's way of being in the world as a creative and fluid project (discerned perhaps in the process of analysis). The Lacanian view is both anti-realist and emancipatory in that 'the unconscious is the sum of the effects of speech on a subject, at the level at which the subject constitutes himself out of the effects of the signifier' (1979, p. 126). Lacan speaks of the 'illusion that impels us to seek the reality of the subject beyond the language barrier' and the mistaken idea that the truth of the personality of the subject 'is already given in us and that we know it in advance' (1977, p. 94). True speech when it emerges in analysis involves 'the realization by the subject of his history in his relation to a future' (1977, p. 88). It is therefore self-constitutive and not deterministic.

Note the self-constituting role of the subject and also the implicit constraints imposed by

(a) The intrinsic connections between the signifiers; and

(b) The particular resonances that the signifiers have gained in speech transactions involving the individual concerned.

We should also note that there is always more to a conversation than words. The 'more' is, *ex hypothesi*, inexpressible and unsignified but plays its part, alongside the signifier, in forming the subject and thereby influencing behaviour. This view can be derived from almost any post-Husserlian conception of the differentiation of figure and ground in experience because that which is omitted from the signification of the figure or theme in any particular experience still has psychic effects even though they may be difficult to determine. The whole (signified and unsignified) impact of any experience on the subject comprises the individual encounter or *tuche* (touch of the real; Lacan) that constantly affects and is affected by one's participation in the human life-world as a being who contributes to it.

A myriad of such encounters culminate in a word or phrase taking a place in the psychic structure of the individual that is replete with associations and that psychic structure is marked by names or signifiers and the subject's assumption or refusal of those names (Lacan, 1977, p. 86). The immediacy and indeterminacy (cf. Kierkegaard) of the subject's contact with the world is rendered by signification so that it takes on a (determinate) structure. Beyond signification, psychic content (as argued by Cavell and Church) is unregulated by the norms of discourse that constitute intentional states as reasonable, contradictory, coherent, or legitimate.

Lacan (1977) refers to the *tuche* transcending the generalizations and assimilations involved in explicit signification or interpretation so that it can only be captured (in its lack of determinate content) as the '*petit a*'. The *petit a* (an abbreviation of '*l'autre*' or the 'unsaid')—the inaccessible—takes place within a framework of comprehensible discourse and struggles to be understood through the 'technique of speech' (p. 93). It is found in the elusive original encounter that can never fully be signified and constitutes the 'opacity' of the trauma to the subject and the analyst (Lacan, 1979, p. 129). Opacity or persistent incomprehensibility (as evidenced, for instance, by repetition) is a clue to psychic formations active in the discourse of the subject but resistant to signification and beyond 'the limits of remembering' (p. 129). A similar point is made by Freud's (1986) conception of the 'thing presentation' that, along with the 'word presentation', comprises the totality of the 'object presentation', a partially signified 'lumpy' whole giving rise to a memory (p. 178).

Repetition fills out this picture: 'what cannot be remembered is repeated in behaviour.' Repetition, in a sense, is the core of the unconscious. Lacan (1977) illustrates the phenomenon (as does Freud) by invoking childhood 'games of occultation' or repetitive games of hiding and showing an object, 'games in which subjectivity brings together mastery of its dereliction and the birth of the symbol' (p. 103). The child, in these games, causes the object to appear and disappear in a way that contrasts with his lack of control over 'the encounter with the real' or *tuche* at the heart of a trauma and also at the heart of his own exposure to the world. The intransigence of the real keeps dragging the subject, through the medium of his own need for mastery, back to itself. Lacan (1979) remarks, 'the signifier will never be able to be careful enough in its memorization to succeed in designating the primacy of the significance as such' (p. 61) precisely because it is a signifier (or mode of representation) and not the thing in itself. The subject is drawn back to that which has touched him or her because of the unsatisfactoriness of signification (and even repetition) in reproducing the actual original encounter.

Consciousness (con-scio—with-I know), according to Lacan, constitutes a signified and therefore transformed field of phenomena (as in the theory of PAs prevalent in post-empiricist philosophies of mind [e.g. see Bolton & Hill, 1996, pp. 34–36]). The encounter with the real as a core of unconscious experience is given form (in part) by the subject's use of signifiers with their multiple associative traces (this distances him from a representational theory of the psyche.) Signified experience derives from the language-like network that forms the unconscious in its image, a network reflecting the evaluative and discursive formations forming the subject. For Lacan, as for Foucault, signifiers channel the subject's access to the encounter with the real so that repetition reflects the complex interaction between a particular subjectivity, a discourse, and a situated life of encounters with the real world.

The Lacanian account meshes well with the 'Multiple Drafts' model of consciousness with a twist added by the discussion of reflective and unreflective content. It also supplies a psychodynamic and socially situated elaboration of the somewhat individualistic and organismic no-self (or self-as-illusion) neurophilosophy of Thomas Metzinger. The developing account of the psyche is supplemented by insights available from short diversions into the study of dreams and Jaspers' critique of psychoanalysis.

4.5 **Dreams: Freud and beyond**

What are dreams? I will assume that we have such things and set aside for the minute the silly view that there is no more to dreams than stories people are disposed to tell when they awake (Malcolm, 1959). In case you think my way with this view is a bit short, I would argue that the phenomenon observed—narratives on waking—should inspire the question, 'Why is this person disposed to tell this story at this time?' An answer to that question, on the basis of the account of the unconscious I have favoured, is not too different from an answer to the question, 'What has happened to this person while they were sleeping to cause them to report just these experiences?' In order to answer to these questions, we can begin with Aristotle's view and then move on to Freud's theory of dreams, not as historical curiosities but because they encapsulate widespread beliefs about what happens in a dream.

Aristotle (1984) does not clearly pronounce on questions that seem important, such as 'Do dreams express the wishes and passions of the heart?' and 'Do psychic mechanisms cause dreams?' He remarks, 'dreaming is an activity of the faculty of sense-perception but belongs to this faculty qua imaginative' (459a 22, p. 730), and goes on to explain that images may reside in the deeper parts of the sensory organs long after the stimuli causing them have ceased to impinge upon us (a view that is prescient in terms of contemporary cognitive neuroscience).

> From this it is manifest that the movements based upon sensory impressions, whether the latter are derived from external objects or from causes within the body, not only [occur] when persons are awake but also occur when this affection which is called sleep has come upon them, and at that time, they appear more. (p. 733)

These movements in the sensory organs (or perceptual systems) sink inwards during sleep and 'appear more' because they are all the psyche has impinging upon it; thus, 'what has little similarity to something appears to be the thing itself'. This is only a psychic presentation; but 'if, however, he is not aware of being asleep, there is nothing which will contradict the testimony of the bare presentation' (p. 734). Aristotle espouses the view that dream content is related to waking perception, as is Freud. He also regards the content as not subject to the critical faculties of waking life and therefore as having certain characteristics Freud attributes to the primary process. Aristotle is not clear, however, on whether there are psychological 'causes within the body' operating to influence the residues of waking perception that are dream images (as the frontal lobes seem to). It is not too much of a leap to say that the psyche, as the organ of rational adaptation, does not control dream images and their content in the light of the reality principle (or its ongoing contact with the real world of organismic adaptation). It remains for Freud to explore the question of the significance for the psyche of dreams and their content.

Before we discuss the actual concepts Freud applied to dream content, we should recall the context of dream analysis. The dream analysis is only one aspect of a prolonged encounter in which a person has presented to Freud with a disorder and the dream to be analysed has emerged as one source of material seeking expression in Pcs and Cs. The meaning of the dream is, therefore, just one way of arriving at the complex causing the problems afflicting the patient. It may provide an entrée into the problem, but the interpretation of the dream is not an end in itself and will not by itself indicate what the problem is. The dream, particularly if it is a recurring dream, may manifest repetition that is occurring in Ucs, but only does so in a form that is able to evade the censor that is actively excluding the disturbing psychic complex from the ego. We should also notice that the dream reflects a source of unease that is currently present in the daytime life of the subject but is not apprehended clearly for whatever reason.

Freud (1986) believes that dreams are an area of mental life, par excellence, where the censor, constituted by the selective functions of Cs, does not control the ideas and connections that operate according to the primary process in Ucs. There is always a stimulus to the dream in the waking life at the time when it occurs so that 'dreams are never concerned with things which we should not think it worthwhile to be concerned with during the day' (p. 101). He remarks of an interpretation of one of his own dreams as follows:

> By following the associations which arose from the separate elements of the dream divorced from their context, I arrived at a number of thoughts and recollections, which I could not fail to recognize as important products of my mental life. (p. 87)

Freud makes free use of the idea that the actual contents of a dream may not reflect the psychic contents that can be discerned in it and accounts for this by the fact that traumatic psychic content is often obscured by the primary process. From Lacan's treatment of repetition, we can discern that the need to obscure and bypass the censor indicates a point where a trauma or encounter with the real causing psychic conflict is being revisited and keeps drawing the subject back to it much as a wounded animal may repeatedly lick a wound. Freud (1986) remarks, 'The situation in the dream is often nothing other than a modified repetition, complicated by interpolations, of an impressive experience' (p. 103).

After Lacan, we could say that the dream continually reworks the principal emotive and cathectic content of an encounter that has not been satisfactorily signified and integrated into the lived narrative of the subject. The modification of psychic material in the dream involves moves reminiscent of those found in the primary process such as 'condensation, displacement, and pictorial arrangement of the psychical material' (p. 108) but also the formation of a narrative or 'dream composition'. Freud (1986) claims that the obscurity of the dream narrative reflects the state of repression accompanying the relevant psychic material and accounting for the transformation of the real subject of waking concern that occasions the dream (p. 114).

We can illustrate these features of the dream interpretation by examining a recurring dream recounted by one of my students that stood out for her as an unusual occurrence:

> She dreamt she was nauseated and went to the bathroom to vomit; but when she got there, she found that her family had vomited all over the bathroom and the smell was quite horrendous. She had to clean the entire bathroom before she could relieve her own nausea. She awoke at that point and was not nauseated at all.

It emerged that she had been feeling abject and very much taken for granted by her adolescent family at the time she had the dream. The multiple minor irritations of having to pick up after them, having to look after their needs, the feeling that she was taken for granted and not appreciated, the feeling of being used and having always to put her own feelings second are condensed and displaced or transformed in the dream into her own nausea, something to which she was not prone in waking life. The cathexis of this detritus of repeated mundane abuse of her care is transformed into the family's vomit, which she found all over the bathroom. This was one of the most vivid images of the dream and it was primarily 'olfactory' not visual. The bathroom was also pictured very clearly. In that way, the dream narrative presents, tells the story of, and cloaks her psychic distress and its causation.

Thus, the dream reveals unassimilated but psychically connected and active trains of thoughts, feelings, and wishes that inhabit the Ucs. Freud posits a censor that normally excludes material in the Ucs from appearance in Pcs or Cs and that relaxes in sleep so that sensitive material is presented to the ego in a form that is often displaced from the nucleus of the psychic conflict. There is, Freud (1986) argues, 'a causal connection between the obscurity of the dream content and the state of repression' (p. 114). Thus, dreams are one further instance of a process that is noted again and again in psychoanalytic accounts of mental disorder.

Repression—relaxation of the censorship—the formation of a compromise, this is the fundamental pattern for the generation not only of dreams but also of many other psychopathological structures. (p. 117)

For Freud, the content of the Ucs is meaningful and formed, and he aims to disclose its nature so as to lay bare the way that it explains events in Cs. Dreams allow the complexes in Ucs to erupt into Pcs and Cs in symbolic form so that with the aid of free association, allowing the subject to elaborate on aspects of his or her story, attending to little anomalies such as slips of the tongue, and applying the key concepts of dream analysis, an analyst can discover the conflict provoking repetition and causing the particular dream to be presented during the analysis.

4.6 Freud's reification of unconscious content

Lacan's view, as we have repeatedly noted, is deeply rooted in Freudian theory even though Lacan rejects Freud's objectification and realism about unconscious content and the psychic subject. Jaspers' (1913/1974) critique is that Freud is not talking about causal connections and extraconscious mechanisms as they figure in Jaspers' own analysis. 'In Freud's work, we are dealing in fact with *psychology of meaning* not *causal explanation* as Freud himself thinks' (p. 91). Jaspers (1913/1974) summarizes Freud's contribution by linking it to Nietzsche:

> Freud teaches us many new individual meaningful connections and does it in a convincing way. We understand how complexes repressed into unawareness re-emerge in symbolic form. We understand the reaction-formation to repressed instinctual drives, the differentiation between the primary real psychic events from the secondary ones, which are merely symbols or sublimations. Freud takes up Nietzsche's teachings and develops them in detail. He penetrates deeply into the unnoticed parts of psychic life, which through him is brought into clear consciousness. (p. 91)

Jaspers' Freud is really unravelling connections in the life experiences of his patients and providing meanings in which to articulate them. Jaspers accepts that real events configure the psyche, but is careful not to identify them with the representational (and realist) interpretation given to them in Freudian theory, recalling Lacan's observation that the signified content is not the truth about any event. Jaspers (1913/1974) is also suspicious of Freud's attempts to construct a substantial (internal or Carteisan realist) psychological theory.

> An error in the Freudian teaching consists in the increasing simplification of his understanding, which is connected with the transformation of meaningful connections into general theories. Theories tend to simplification. Understanding finds infinite variety and complexity. (p. 92)

The view that Freudian theory cannot distil from itself a general or relatively parsimonious scientific theory of the unconscious (as a causal domain) is widely trumpeted but less often pursued metaphysically. In fact, this objection suggests that meaningful connections are not the right kind of thing for a systematic theory in traditional or positivistic terms and are more conducive to particular or qualitative approaches to psychology. This criticism, avoided by Lacan (who attempts only to identify the network of signifiers and interconnections that reveal the structure likely to determine an individual's psychic formations), should warn us against fixed or objectifiable structures within an individual psyche, because the network and the signifiers themselves are being constructed in and through the analytic experience and the attempts of the patient to deal with phenomena such as the repetition.

For Lacan, the imperfect match between the child's experience and the categorized and standardized language in which he is immersed leads to an interesting schism in the unconscious in which real lived experience, the *tuche*, replete with interpersonal meanings and relational content, is never fully captured by signification or symbolization and thus moves the subject in ways that cannot be neatly captured in any narrative. The subject is always negotiating the shifting space between, on the one hand, the inchoate or primitive impact of events and their ongoing influence on his or her being and, on the other, the signified events that, in their transformed guise, exert their influence. Both are subject to misconstrual (meconnaissance) especially reifying (or realist) misconstrual. Thus, there is a sense in which a person is constantly composing the moments of his or her mental life from material that does not fully determine it, a thesis that is important for topics such as Multiple Personality Disorder (MPD) and coheres well with the 'Multiple Drafts' model of consciousness.

4.7 Consciousness, Multiple Drafts, and the extraconscious

Freud (1986) makes a very revealing remark in discussing external stimuli occurring during a dream: 'Every dream which occurs immediately before the sleeper is woken by a loud noise has made an attempt at explaining away the arousing stimulus by providing another explanation of it.' (p. 121)

He (or she) is thinking about the loud noise that occurs externally at the point where the dream narrative has a shot occurring as part of the unfolding events. He (or she) also mentions applause for a play he (or she) had written in his (or her) dream that coincided with somebody beating a carpet or a mattress. The dreamer gives the external event significance as part of the psychic events of the dream by inserting it into the narrative as if it belonged there (when, in reality, it was external and had nothing to do with the dream narrative). This suggests that a subject telling the story of conscious or quasi-conscious events such as dreams smoothly integrates into the story the events impinging on him or her whatever their source and links to the person's lived (and enacted) story.

The discursive view holds that consciousness is a 'field' of personal activity in which a stream of events is given explicit content so that it can be reflected on by the subject. The narrative is, without doubt, influenced by factors beyond consciousness, but is an autobiographical production in which the person makes sense of and takes ownership for his or her life, a view deeply congenial to Dennett's account, in which conscious experience is a selective and interpretive activity based on

(i) The flux of impingements of the world on the subject; and

(ii) The responses, reactions, and spontaneous activity in the information-processing systems of the subject accompanying that flux of events.

To call this flux 'a stream of events' is to go beyond the bare fact that the environments, outer and inner, in and through which a subjectivity moves are reflected in a stream of embodied informational transactions with the world signified by the subject as instancing certain points of significance. The significance is negotiated in the light of its context (both synchronic and diachronic) so that an intelligible form is imputed to the person's subjective trajectory in the world. For any subject, the stream of conscious experience is smoothed over and moulded for maximum coherence according to scripts of the kind considered legitimate 'around here'. When uncontentious things such as commonly perceived conditions involving mundane objects and events are in focus, the legitimated story is similarly uncontentious and what appears in experience is material that any human individual or group would tend to signify in similar (inter-translatable) ways. When the material concerned is more ambiguous, emotionally loaded, or politically sensitive, the judgements of significance show exactly the same characteristics. Typically, interpersonal events have the more loaded nature and are subject to factors arising from the subject in a local discourse that give rise to varying readings of 'the same events'. This becomes particularly important when the material lurks in the Unconscious.

Lacan's account of conscious thought and its relation to experience, combined with the 'Multiple Drafts' model, yields the conclusion that the impingement of life on the subject is only partially signified and transformed into material for reflection despite the whole flux of incoming information affecting activity in the neural network. The implications of events and their symbolic effects on a subject are therefore likely to be quite sensitive to the explicit signified content of those events, but the full impact of any situation outstrips its signification. The most marked of these effects (from the unsignified), *ex hypothesi*, arise from those conditions that the discursive mind avoids in scripting one's lived 'good enough' consciousness.

Here, we can recall the categories Freud applied to operations on the subconscious contents of the mind when he divided them into the preconscious and the unconscious, the latter comprising contents not admissible to the consciousness in any explicit form. The preconscious contents are subject to 'the work of the function of speech, which brings material in the ego into a firm connection with mnemic residues of visual but more particularly of auditory perceptions' (Freud, 1940, p. 43). For Freud, the preconscious has access to both consciousness and the speech mechanisms and contains material derived from the id and the superego.

By contrast with Freud's divisions, Jaspers (1923) refers to the 'extraconscious mechanisms which are the understructure of our psychic life' (p. 364). Some are clearly neurophysiological, 'such as habituation, memory, aftereffect, fatigue, etc.' (p. 365), but others more psychic, such as 'symbolic gratification' and 'sublimation'. Jaspers (1923) denies that the effects concerned are mediated by the explicit meaning of events as consciously interpreted by the individuals concerned and invokes aspects of individual experience that are best explained in terms of their human meaning (such as the death of another person and the fear of death):

> Everything we experience and do leaves its trace and slowly changes our disposition. People with the same disposition at birth may eventually find themselves in entirely

> different grooves, simply through their life-history and experiences and the effects of their upbringing as well as of their own efforts at self-education. Once such development has taken place, there is no point of return. In this lies the personal responsibility involved in every single experience. (pp. 369–370)

Jaspers' existential leanings are evident and imply that the construction of the subconscious mind is not totally outside of the control of the subject. He uses the term 'complex' to refer to residues of an experience or type of experience that 'influences the later psychic life in a way that is meaningful in terms of the original experience' (p. 371).

Metzinger (2003, 2004) has offered a sceptical account of the self according to which the self is not an inner entity but a construction based on *mineness* (the sense of ownership), *selfhood* (the conscious experience of being someone), and *perspectivalness* (a phenomenological reflection of egocentric and located space). His view coheres with (and traces the cognitive neuroscience of) Lacan's claim about the *imago* (image-ego). Metzinger demurs from explanations in terms of the self for 'the hard sciences', but the imago plays a role in shaping one's being-in-the-world and providing a structure on which *meconnaissance* can be predicated so that all the mis-construals of the self that bind us to ways of being with others that are maladaptive and unsustainable can be understood and their discursive structure exposed for the purposes of 'argument' (therapy for the soul). One does not talk to brains but one engages with people and the imago; however, the imago is realized in terms of cognitive neuroscience, affecting the terms of engagement so that, for clinical psychiatry and psychology in general, it had better affect our thinking (if we intend to display the truth about being human).

We might therefore offer the following synthesis: a person enters situations partly constituted (in their significance) by his or her ways of seeing things and, as a result, certain elements of experience come into engagement with the symbolic content of the speech mechanisms and the multitude of intersituational connections mediated by that content. Any such signification is a selection in which a subjective figure (or theme or topic) emerges from the ground that is the immersion of the subject in the situation. What is selected for signification has an effect on the unfolding narrative of the subject as does what is not selected (despite it being inexpressible and inarticulate, or immediate and indeterminate). Thus, as Janet Frame notes, 'The future accumulates like a weight upon the past,' turning an unfolding narrative into an enacted individual history and increasingly defined personal character. The self-constituting narrative rests on the 'bedrock' (Wittgenstein) of extraconscious mechanisms underpinning the human psyche, and the effects of signified and unsignified content are inscribed on the subjective body. As a result, a set of reactions and habits is formed shaping the unfolding personality and its modes of experience (as is evident from cognitive experiments showing priming effects, interference effects, fixation on initial suggestions, incubation effects, and gaps in reasoning, all neurocognitive processes influencing the direction of the conscious stream but without determinate propositional content).

When one locates an individual in a discourse (however widely or narrowly defined), certain acts and inner determinations become explicable on the basis of features of that discourse and the interactions it potentiates (as seen in certain aspects of Oscar's story [see Chapter 2] and recurring features of the treatment of psychiatric patients). The complex picture of situated subjectivity allows us to extend and develop our treatment of psychiatry and its patients, one increasingly distant from the (Victorian, quasi-industrial) neural hydraulics of the Freudian view.

4.8 **An even more discursive view**

Sartre (1958) denies that there is psychic material sequestered from consciousness in an unconscious system and argues that blaming things on unconscious motives and mechanisms is just bad faith, a view radically opposed to the 'inner causes' approach to the psyche:

> A young woman is sitting in a cafe talking intently to a young man who slips his hand over hers. She ignores the implication of this gesture and is later surprised when his sexual intentions become clear. (p. 55)

Freud's synthesis is that her knowledge that his gesture has a sexual meaning is channelled into Ucs by the censor operating between Cs and Ucs so that it is not available to her consciousness and the sexual move genuinely surprises here. Sartre (a Frenchman), on the contrary, claims that the sexualization of the relationship is evident, but she chooses not to admit to herself what his gesture means. She is therefore in bad faith or denial when she is surprised because the whole idea of the unconscious is just a way of excusing ourselves from actions for which we do not want to take responsibility.

Sartre's view involves a radical (some would say unrealistic) attitude to human psychology. Sartre's subject sees clearly the choices before her and always *puts herself* in a position instead of merely *finding herself there*. But life is not like that. In a chess game, you might choose every move but find yourself in an unenviable position that you would never have chosen to be in had you clearly seen what you were doing. Life is more like chess or a box of chocolates; one makes choices based on an understanding framed by the discourses one inhabits and the resulting shape of the psyche (shaped within me and without me). I might still find that a situation surprizes me because some aspect of it has not struck me until I am positioned in a certain way. I make choices and my choices are self-formative, but I may find myself trapped, uncomprehending, and silenced by what has happened to me. A retelling of Freud's story of post-hypnotic suggestion illustrates the discursive view.

Think of the situation from the patient's point of view. The doctor, a powerful figure, comes into the ward and says some things including the command 'When I come in again, you will come to meet me with my umbrella open and hold it over my head.' He goes out and then comes back again. The patient does what he says. The doctor then says to him, 'What's this you're doing? What's the meaning of all this?' What is the poor patient supposed to say? This, to use Laing's phrase, is mystification. The patient cannot think (the God-forbidden thought) that *the doctor is stupid*; but if not, why would he ask a question the answer to which was so obvious? No wonder that the patient's words in this nonsensical situation are likely to be 'embarrassed . . . some lame remark . . . made up on the spur of the moment' (Freud, 1986, p. 188).

The patient as subject and the power relations surrounding him in the asylum transform the story from one about post-hypnotic suggestion (indeed, that is an unnecessary hypothesis) to one about alienation and mystification by discourse. The subjectivity and silence of the umbrella story should alert us to the fact that the evidence for the unconscious can be reinterpreted to suggest something quite different from the Freudian layers of the psyche.

In fact, Freud (1986) himself signals the way in which moral and other discursive considerations can and do obscure the mental acts we call unconscious in interpreting one of his own dreams:

> I might draw closer together the threads in the material revealed by the analysis, and I might then show that they converge upon a single nodal point, but considerations of a personal and not of a scientific nature prevent my doing so in public. I should be obliged to betray many things which had better remain my secret, for on my way to discovering the solution of the dream, all kinds of things were revealed to me which I was unwilling to admit even to myself. (p. 87)

The discursive account suggests that the unconscious is that whereof we cannot speak, for whatever reason. For Freud, things about his dream must be kept silent for personal reasons. In the umbrella story, the complex relation between power, position, subjectivity, and discourse silences the asylum inmate. Such complexities abound in the human life-world.

Take, for instance, the material of childhood experience. A novice narrator is mastering discursive and narrative techniques in the midst of the experiences to be integrated into his autobiography. He is unclear how things should be named (under the name of the father), how to use the many possible connections between signifiers to locate them in his evolving story, how to cope with any disturbing events befalling him, and how to make discursive judgements about those teaching him the skills of discourse and upon whom he is dependent for his psychic growth (the adults in close relationships to him). There are no signposts apart from the smoke and mirrors of his interaction with others (with its occultations, multiple identities, and reappearances), an ongoing interaction with the world mediated by language and etched in the brain. In the process of turning this material into psychic content, the subject exercises discursive skills (with their built in norms and evaluations). A loving, nurturing environment imparts the skills and provides experiences that produce a satisfying and well-integrated story. Otherwise, the story may become disturbed and fragmented, containing indigestible (nauseating) lumps of experience unfit for assimilation into the narrative. When this happens, the psyche, or the subject—its narrator, tries to digest the lumps—the alien material, *l'autre*—resulting in repetition, defence formation, and so on, all vain attempts at closure and the restoration of meaning or integrity in an autobiographical narrative.

'Subconscious psychic material' and its progeny signal 'I do not know what to say about myself at this point.' There may be many reasons for that and the person concerned may choose any one of a number of discursive techniques if they find themselves able to explore that silence in the context of conversation and argument (the therapy of the soul). Chemical bullying is unlikely to be a good way of going about the unfolding of fragile silences even though a different kind of silence may yield to chemical abreaction. It is vital to the suffering person that a narrative sensitivity engages with the 'unconscious' conflicts and plays a part in working them out.

Narrative sensitivity is something we can all develop. Each of us takes shape among narratives and constructs them (cooperatively) from birth to death. Narratives have content and context, construed inclusively to embrace emotion, power, moral commitments, symbols, the structure of language revealed in and through our speech, and the whole multifaceted discursive reality forming a being-in-the-world-with-others. Subjectivity, position, and power are constants or givens of the human life-world and give rise, in their myriad machinations, to the unnamed and the unavowed, two basic categories of the non-conscious psyche.

4.9 **The primal wound**

A case study for any theory of the unconscious is the 'primal wound' (Verrier, 1992): 'all adopted children begin their lives having already felt the pain and, perhaps, terror of separation from the first mother' (Verrier, 1992, p. 9).

> While adopted parents may refer to the child as 'chosen' and to themselves as the 'real' parents, the child has had an experience of another mother to whom he was once attached and from whom he is now separated, which he can never completely ignore. (p. 9)

Conceptualized in traditional terms, the experience mentioned here and the abiding awareness of separation is deeply problematic (lost in 'infantile amnesia'). Many adoptions occur within the first few days of birth so that they do not enter into the episodic or narrative memories of an infant, yet Verrier (1992) claims that the 'primal wound' is basic to the psyche of an adopted child.

> Adoption for these children isn't a concept to be learned, a theory to be understood, or an idea to be developed. It is a real experience about which they have had and are having recurring and conflicting feelings, all of which are legitimate. These feelings are their response to the most devastating experience they are ever likely to have: the loss of their mother. The fact that the experience was preverbal does not diminish the impact; it only makes it more difficult to treat. It is almost impossible to talk about, and for some, even difficult to think about. (pp. 16–17)

Whether Verrier is correct and has identified a real psychiatric phenomenon is a matter for empirical study, but we should ask, 'Could this possibly be true?' The philosophical question is prior: 'Is the primal wound conceptually incoherent or a viable thesis about adopted children?'

If the primal wound could not be a claim about conscious experience or explicit narrative memory, it must concern 'unconscious' aspects of the psyche, inexplicit or narratively inaccessible, material with a marked effect on the mental life of the person concerned. Verrier (1992) acknowledges all the problems implicit in such a thesis.

> How many of us remember very much about the first three years of our lives? Does our lack of memory mean that those three years had no impact on us . . . our personalities, perceptions, and attitudes?

The present account begins by conceptualizing conscious material (the not-Ucs) as

(1) Signified or rendered in an interpreted form;

(2) Accessible to reflective endorsement or evaluation; and

(3) Integrated to some extent in an autobiographical narrative.

I have used the metaphor of inscription to suggest that such experiences inscribe the body with their effects and argued that there are several forms in which psychic material may be cast. One form is as consciously active material both signified and available to second-order attitudes such as reflection. Another range of material is discursive and signified but not subject to explicit second-order scrutiny or evaluation. Yet another range of material is inchoate, unsignified, the other (*l'autre*), and even though it may (implicitly) fit a certain intentional form (e.g. rejection, abandonment, and so on) and its effects may be understood according to those significations, it is not discursively accessible (or explicit, determinate) in that form.

The primal wound, on this reading, is an experience of loss, rejection, and abandonment (with psychic immediacy) causing loss of trust and a sense of being alone and cast adrift. However, the subject cannot think it through in those terms because it happened in a preverbal stage of development and has never been named (the words of the adoptive parents may explicitly deny any such thing). One cannot autobiographically understand this rift at the centre of self because there is no situation to be conscious of with the necessary discursive characteristics even though a situation of that type 'lies beneath' and (inchoately) informs one's experience of everything else. The wound happens before drafts are available to be retained for later narrative work, so it is lost to signification or is silent; the traces are there but cannot be understood. Similar to a lost archaeological or textual source, the effects are inexplicable until a conjecture or discovery keys the narrative and the gap in one's self becomes signified and rendered accessible to discourse. At that point, a puzzle (or knot) in the psyche starts to unravel.

> Adult adoptees, whom I have seen in treatment, most of whom did not act out in childhood, speak of having a sense that the baby they were 'died', and that the one they became was going to be different, to be better, so that he would not be abandoned again. Many became 'people pleasers', constantly seeking approval . . . Locked inside them was pain and the fear that the unacceptable baby who died would come back to life if they were not vigilant. They could never truly bond with anyone.

> (Verrier, 1992, p. 32)

This account is structured by discursive metaphors associated with a belief in the posited wound, but nevertheless has an authenticity suggesting that it might not be wholly misguided. It makes sense of the behaviour (and subjectivity) of an adoptee and rings true with a kind of imaginative or empathic leap into the experience of one who might have been wounded in that way. That the wound could be subconsciously active in conditioning all post-natal experience is plausible and that it could exist within and without the autobiographical narrative makes sense on the present account. Therefore, it is a hypothesis worth exploring and a good example of the way that an adequate theory of the unconscious might open the way for genuine and therapeutically relevant discoveries about the human psyche and its range of discontents.

4.10 **The role of psychiatry**

The brain is a physiological information processor. As such, it is sensitive to biochemical disruptions and therefore to disorders affecting mental function by altering the biology of information transmission in the brain. These dysfunctions are evident in the severely disordered phases of psychotic conditions such as Manic-Depressive Psychosis or acute schizophrenia when the patient's cognitive dynamics seem to resemble an electronic system buzzing with interference effects so that the content that is manifest is fragmented, uncoordinated with ongoing activity, and at odds with normal responses to situations. We refer to thought that is disordered in form and/or content[4], and the most obvious therapeutic response is to minimize or reduce the biological disruption that is confounding cognitive processes by two means:

(i) Corrective pharmacological control to offset as far as possible the biochemical turmoil that is wreaking havoc in thought and personality function; and

(ii) Help in the reorganization of thoughts and attitudes so that mental economy can be restored and personality reconstructed.

Psychiatry therefore needs an inclusive stance to understanding the three-way interaction between biology, cognition, and interpersonal activity. Such a stance allows us to act at any and all of the points where a person—as a rational, social, and biological being—is vulnerable. The maladies of the soul may arise from inborn processing biases (perhaps evident in many affective, personality, and neurotic disorders), chemical aberrations (probably giving rise to the major psychoses), and social and personal factors that shape one's subjectivity affecting every psychopathology and possibly causing some varieties of soul-sickness.

Social and personal factors through their effect on the perceived contingencies of the environment inscribe the body (particularly the brain) under the influence of reactive attitudes and may produce a mental disorder as resistant to change as any other type of dysfunction. Brain processing networks realize the cumulative effects of experience so that personal interactions (the mirror world of self-formation) literally produce one's subjective being-in-the-world-with-others. Thus, disorders arising from such processes have effects just as real as and perhaps even more enduring than any biological aberration that brings a person to the attention of psychiatric services.

I have taken a view in which the mind is a narrative told by a person on the basis of the engagement between their brain and the world. The person, as the teller of this tale, is primarily and inescapably a discursive being and the discontents of the mind are disorders of relational, narrative beings who depend on their brains as the information-processing organ realizing and mediating their interactions with the physical, interpersonal, and cultural world around them.

---

[4] It is the main topic of Chapter 5.

The telling of a narrative can be disrupted or 'broken' (Brody; Freud; Zaner, 1998). This can happen because something extraconscious has thrown the storyteller 'out of whack', perhaps a chemical storm or perhaps a genetic predisposition to be unable to cope or to dissociate. The resulting reactions may be appropriate or inappropriate to the person's evolving narrative, but 'positive-feedback loops' influencing mood or disposition make it hard for the storyteller to mobilize sufficient discursive skills to rescue it so that the narrative of an 'alien' may spiral downwards into a greater and greater discontent, disintegration, and abjection. Correcting the chemical imbalance may be the first step in restoring a person's ability to resume the disrupted narrative task of reintegration. A desperately depressed mother and homemaker might need a course of Prozac so that she begins to get her life together enough to deal with the psychic wounds inscribed upon her and disrupting her story, but that is likely to be no more than a beginning in reconstructing a narrative to live by. The therapeutic task, in most cases, needs the kind of sharing and nurturing of discursive skills that create the ability to care for the self.

These skills are many and varied. They may consist in letting a person see that a position he has put himself in is the position he now is surprised and discomfited at finding himself in (as in the chess game). We are not gods (not even the doctors among us) and the way it looks from here might not be the way it looks from else-where, but narrative skills enable one to see 'differently' or even to 'look awry'. When we learn to see ourselves as others see us, the mismatches between positions into which one puts oneself and those in which one finds oneself begin to disappear. Any lived experience transcends the individual, and once the reality of being-with-others is a source of inspir(it)ation, the discontents of the mind subside and the inscribed body presents an unwounded or healthy aspect (a harmony of the lively demons). Experiences written within that kind of narrative resonate with and make more clear the lines of autobiographical self-definition and free the soul from the cathectic wounds that, like a dog, one keeps licking at, so that the person can say 'I am whom I am, and I am OK'.

4.11 Conclusion

A discursive theory of the dynamic unconscious differs from other theories of the unconscious in that it is sceptical about the psychic content of states not part of the discursively constructed autobiographical experience of the individual. Dennett's Multiple Drafts model and Lacan's theory of signification and the encounter combine to yield an account in which the brain–world exchange potentiates meaningful experience, but determinate mental states do not exist without consciousness. The body is causally affected in a number of ways by encounters in the human life-world, certain features of which make up an individual history and become available for reflection to the discursive subject. The subject (particularly the scientific or philo-sophical subject) is, however, prone to misconstrual (and reifying the structures of self) and so constantly substitutes a mechanism-like thing within to do the work of living and relating to others. Thus, features of the self are never made available to clear reflection and their contents are never cast into a determinate intentional shape; they remain immediate and inchoate in reality and distorted in the world of representation.

The unconscious is not a set of informational states lying in a room beneath consciousness and moving the subject through psychic levers (as in Wittgenstein's thought experiment); rather, conscious lived experience is a selection from what happens to one as a situated subjective being. Some things that happen to me and move me may be inchoate, inadequately signified, or even just immediate in their effects on me. As such, they are integrated into one's life narrative post-hoc (and sometimes very poorly) and thus may trouble me until I am able to rework them and bring discursive skills to bear on them. The drafts defining self are candidates for adoption, but understanding their selection and non-selection, as Freud astutely observes, is the beginning of the project of dealing with the mind and its discontents.

Chapter 5

Thought in disarray

I will tell you what to do, to think, to feel, to change, to reason, and awaken. Happiness is better than pleasure, peace better than war, strength is better than weakness, and sanity is better than insanity. Now I will tell you the truth about me who catches the world and twists it around till I am too confused to perceive the truth. I am the bullshit substitute. I remember the past, I give double meaning, I am for the young and ignorant, I slander the truth and there is no reason to experiment in your mind with my mistakes. I'm the hypocritical bastard.
(Gates & Hammond, 1993)

5.1 Introduction: philosophy and psychosis

The psychoses are dramatic malfunctions of the psyche. Therefore, 'the inside story' making full use of discursive formations that render it, to some extent, comprehensible offers a unique view of psychic phenomena such as perception, belief, consciousness, motivation, reason, thought, understanding, and self-consciousness (each of which has a considerable philosophical literature).

The common philosophical view of perception is that we encounter various things in the world around Dus and form representations allowing us to think about those things. The phenomenological analysis teaches us not to make the mistake of thinking of the mind as being directed, in experience, on inner objects (reified ideas or images), but as in touch with the world so as to 'track' aspects of it (cf. perceptual tracking), a cumulative and interactive data-gathering exercise that informs the subject's actions and reactions.

The standard empiricist epistemology is quite unhelpful here—as distinct, for instance, from phenomenology or Wittgenstein's (1953) account of perception (Section II part xi)—both of which notice that in perception a subject engages cognitively with a domain of action. Locke (1689/1975), for instance, holds that objects in the world cause (simple) impressions in the mind that are the basis of the person's ideas, both 'simple' (such as the idea of *red* or *extension*) and 'complex' (such as *parrot* or *Paris*). Complex ideas are the most common type because objects both interest us and instance a number of qualities. By and large, the empiricists hold that thought and belief are based on 'input', in some sense passively received from (or caused by) the world affecting the subject through the sensory systems, a 'passive picture theory' of inner representation (Millikan, 1993) that neglects the problems of form and intentionality (we see the frog as a frog and 'fill in' or deploy schemata accordingly.) Empiricists take imagination and perception to have the same content but different causal histories: perceptual ideas are caused by input to the sensory systems whereas imagination deals with 'phantasms' produced by the brain. A mind producing phantasms but unaware that it is (as in psychosis) is therefore analysed causally (to do with faulty brain mechanisms) rather than providing an entrée into the lived experience of a 'disembodied spirit or deanimated body' (Stanghellini, 2004) or someone with 'a profound disorder of the self' (Sass & Parnas, 2003).

The empiricist view gives rise to the sceptical argument about hallucination:

(1) Hallucinations are sensory experiences that have no basis in the external world.

(2) One can imagine a hallucination so vivid that a person would mistake it for reality.

(3) A person having an hallucination can sometimes not tell that it is not real.

(4) It is possible that at any moment what I take to be reality might be an hallucination emanating from my own brain.

(5) I can never know if I am seeing something real or having an hallucination.

However, other analyses are more revealing and allow psychosis to shed light on our lived experience as beings-in-the-world by drawing our attention to the cognitive skills and structures of the self that are part of being an experiencing subject (Zahavi, 2004).

5.2 **Consciousness, perception, and imagination**

Post-empiricist views (Bolton & Hill, 1996) begin by noting that perception and consciousness are complex skills enabling a creature to preserve itself in a domain replete with 'affordances' (Gibson 1966) and abounding in objects with which it has 'dealings' (Heidegger, 1953/1996). Note the two important features:

(i) Perception and consciousness are active and exploratory, and hence the term 'skills' (as in Kant, Wittgenstein, and Merleau Ponty).

(ii) We are alert to *affordances* or aspects of things relevant to needs and self-integrity as a central focus of our knowledge-acquiring skills (as in Gibson and Heidegger).

Phenomenological analyses prompt questions as to why and how a human being is motivated to gather certain information and how she or he makes sense of it. That inquiry potentiates an understanding of the structure of the information emerging from the behaviours it informs, recalling Wittgenstein's sympathy for pragmatism about truth and knowledge (Gillett, 1990a). Situations structured to be 'no-win' or systematically ambivalent frustrate the development of perceptual skills because the pay-offs are unsystematic (Bolton & Hill, 1996, p. 314ff), an insight convergent with the thesis that action or doing and thinking rightly (being able to make sense of a shared world) are closely entangled and crucial in understanding mental illness.

This orientation to intentional content resonates well with the case of 'Lucie Blair':

> Her affect is flattened. She has auditory hallucinations, ideas of reference and influence, varying delusions of persecution. She says she is tormented and torn to pieces: she feels people put unpleasant sexual ideas into her head . . . suffers from vague and woolly thoughts. She speculates on religious themes: she is perplexed, puzzled about the meaning of life.
>
> (Laing & Esterson, 1970, p. 51)

Lucie, up to her psychiatric admission, has lived with her mother and father. Her father persecuted her and rules the family in accordance with his own rather paranoid ideas:

> [He] told her that if she went out alone she would be kidnapped, raped, or murdered . . . He would ridicule any feelings she had: he would discourage her from getting any ideas of being able to follow a career, and he would say that she was making a fool of herself, that she was 'simple', etc., if she thought anyone liked her or took her seriously. (p. 55)

Mrs. Blair does not agree that anything is wrong with her husband, particularly when Lucie says so, and never, in her husband's presence, disagrees with him. Her lack of validation of Lucie's perceptions and thoughts has an understandable effect:

> I can't trust what I see. It doesn't get backed up. It doesn't get confirmed in any way—just left to drift, you know. I think that's probably what my trouble is. Anything I might say, it has no backing up. It's all due to imagination, you know.
>
> (Laing & Esterson, 1970, p. 58)

The result of this no-win situation is predictable:

> I sort of lost faith in myself, naturally—get no support, no support in anything I want to do. I feel that it's sort of collapsible, sort of in a collapsible state. Can't get any firm backbone at all. (p. 65)

This loss of belief in self and one's agency occurs against a background of insecurity whereby the home is represented as essential to Lucie's health and integrity.

Laing and Esterson's (1970) accounts were written before the era of publicity about childhood sexual abuse, but even so (and especially if Lucy had been abused) it is unsurprising that she was terrified of being torn to pieces by her father and of losing 'the link' between herself and her mother. Lucie felt that she could not survive without her father and mother (p. 68), a mixture of dependence and hostility characteristic of abuse and analysed by Laing through an existential understanding of her schizoid world. Lucie's paranoid disorder is characterized by passivity and 'deanimation':' . . . there doesn't seem to be any solution to it—it doesn't leave you any kind of er . . . hopeful move at all' (p. 74). The existential–phenomenological orientation profoundly illuminates her psychosis.

5.2.1 Perception as active and intentional

Kant, the first post-empiricist, challenged the empiricist view of perception as a passive receipt of impressions, arguing that the mind applies concepts in making sense of the flux of sensory matter from the world. Contemporary cognitive science (as in Neisser, Lakoff, and Bruner) is built on this thought:

> Human beings behave very differently and are by no means neutral or passive towards the incoming information . . . They select some parts for attention at the expense of others,

reconding and reformulating them in complex ways ... For this reason, a really satisfactory theory of the higher mental processes can only come into being when we also have theories of motivation, personality, and social interaction.

(Neisser 1976, pp. 7, 305)

Husserl, Sartre, and Heidegger realized that an active search for themes and figures relevant to the perceiver delineates the life-world of the human subject so that the mind is active in both perception and imagination, but in perception the subject engages the subject in an interaction that is transformed into a series of structured representations or significations. In imagination, although the same processes and principles are at work, their content arises from the mind itself and is not dynamically constrained by the interaction between the subject and world.

Kant pictured the mind as a respository of rules deployed by a faculty of judgement that applied the rule to the instance so as to provide the subject with meaningful experience. As a conscious subject masters the skills of judgement, she or he achieves a sense of what is sensible, objective, and liable to be validated by any rational observer suitably placed. In *The Critique of Pure Reason*, Kant (1789/1928) argues that a thinker's subjective and practical test of the adequacy of his or her determinations about what is really going on in the world is convergence in judgements with other rational subjects (B848).

> It is also a subjectively necessary touchstone of the correctness of our judgement and consequently of the soundness of our understanding that we relate our understanding to the understanding of others, and not merely isolate ourselves within our own experiences.

(Kant, 1798/1978, p. 117)

Discursive psychology stresses the normative role of discourse in determining rules of judgement and reasoning, thereby locating the rules governing experience in a public sphere of interpersonal activity. Husserl (1950/1999) remarks:

> I experience the world (including others) . . . not as (so to speak) my private synthetic formation but as other than mine alone [mir fremde], as an intersubjective world actually there for everyone, accessible in respect of its objects to everyone. (p. 91)

Kant identified a breakdown in the intersubjective process as fundamental in psychopathology, which we can gloss as a dysfunction in the operation of discursively mediated skills enabling a subject to make sense of experience. 'Reality, the objectivity of things, is not just given: objectivity rather is the achievement of a subject' (Spitzer, 1990c). Spitzer notices the role of an integrated and well-functioning subject in right thinking such that, considering the importance of the validating judgements of others in the shaping of a cognitive system, self-integrity can be seen as a product of intersubjectively moderated existential engagement as a being-in-the-world-with-others.

The theme is pursued by the phenomenological school beginning with Brentano's (1924/1973) claim that intentionality—directedness to an object forming the focus of consciousness or thought—is the critical feature of mental phenomena. Thus, for instance, the focus of my thought <that chair is red> is the chair—the object on which the thought is directed. But the intentional object is not equivalent to the actual physical object being thought about, as is seen when a person, say Jon, meets his new boss at his office party and, not realizing to whom he is speaking, remarks 'I have heard the boss is a real tyrant.' Now, although (in one sense) Jon has insulted his boss, this characterization misses out a crucial fact—that the object of Jon's thought is *this man at the party* and not *my new boss* even though, in fact, both are the same person. There is therefore a distinction between the objects of a thought and its contents, where the latter records the way that the object is presented (or signified). Frege (1892/1952) refers to this as the difference between *sense* and *reference*, where the *sense* is the *mode of presentation* or *cognitive significance* of the object to the thinker answerable to the real world in that it tracks or follows this object and is open to correction by the way in which others think about the object and the *reference* is the object itself (as it is in itself).

Husserl (1962), in discussing the objects of experience, speaks of the focus or topic of thought and the incidental or background features as 'thematic' and 'automatic' aspects, respectively, of the way the subject directs experience or attention to an object (p. 109) such that it has a meaning or significance for the thinker (terms that should recall Gestalt psychology and the idea of figure and ground in any given act of perception). *Noesis* (the activity that enables us to know about things) is bound by *noemata*, supraindividual or ideal forms governing our thoughts about a shared world so that what counts as an oak is the same for everybody but whether you do or do not recognize and think of an oak as an oak is a matter of the operations of your own *noetic* abilities and capacities. Thus, a particular object is differentiated from its general context in some particular way depending on the cognitive skills of the thinker. There are approved or legitimated ways to think of objects and there is room for creativity such that one can depart from these norms (for instance, in poetry and metaphor).

According to Gestalt psychology, the subject transforms experience by picking out figures that are significant to him or her. There are many ways of cognizing any given experience (and some arrays are especially designed to accommodate more than one, such as the Ishihara colour vision stimuli). The Rorschach inkblot test (used in dynamic psychology to try and identify the motivational and unconscious factors influencing the constitution of mental objects) is one way of focusing on a person's subjectivity and what influences it, but we should not forget the norms governing *noemata* (the forms instanced by objects such as a chair) and their objective, or intersubjective, features.

Husserl discusses the noematic rules governing experience, thereby emphasizing the social or validated aspects of perception and, helped by Wittgenstein, can forge a link between the 'Platonic' world of ideal forms (or norms or rules) governing experience and the 'down-to-earth' world of everyday cognitive business.

The rules determine not only the type of object that is meaningful to folk around here but also the complex ways in which meanings interconnect so that if I remark on a dog bounding across the street I am committed to the stance that I am seeing an actual animal, furry, with teeth and four legs, a bark, and so on. The concept *Dog* and the rules governing it (as taught to me and current in my conversations with others) determine the contents of my mind in this situation and I realize that the truth of the situation transcends my own view of it (in its *'thereness for everyone'* [Husserl]) such that the correctness of my view of it is governed by criteria not intrinsic to my own experience. My adherence to these criteria (through the exercise of certain neurocognitive skills) reflects my normality or integrity as a thinker.

Wittgenstein's (1969) 'bridge' between the ideal, normative, or prescriptive world and the actual world rests on the thought that conceptualization is a rule-governed skill relating signs or repeatable markers to a world of objects so that meaning and truth are internally related: 'The truth of my statements is the test of my understanding of these statements' (¶ 80). Judgements such as 'That is a cat,' 'The atmosphere here is very tense,' 'She does not like me,' 'He is trying to control us,' and so on are shaped and corrected by others and a person's grasp of the significance of an experience depends on having mastered the skills of applying (intersubjectively determined) meanings to it. Conceptualizing objects correctly is, therefore, not a matter for private (or even subjective) determination but requires the discursive subject to fit into the praxis that is language, something formed long before I got here and into which I am born (Lacan, 1977, p. 103).

Speculative questions about whether schizophrenic experiences might be valid or truthful reports of aberrant experiences (Spitzer, 1990c, p. 50) should be linked to questions about the discursive skills of giving true reports and making true judgements, both of which may also be impaired in the psychotic patient. Therefore, a delusional report could be (i) a true report of the lived experience of an unusual existential situation, or (ii) a graphic and potentially misleading report of an inept and mystified intentional construction of a situation, or (iii) an absurd or disordered event in consciousness the meaning of which has no relation to the situation of the patient.

These three possibilities are not mutually exclusive in that some combination of them might characterize psychotic subjectivity as an alienated mode of being in a life-world, a possibility that motivates a discursive analysis of the phenomenology of psychotic thought and pursues Laing's seminal work into the writings of Husserl and Foucault.

Foucault uses phenomenology to differentiate between the experienced world of a psychotic patient and pathological meaning-giving techniques, but given the relational conception of consciousness, the mismatch between subject and world is more important. If one's indwelling world is bewildering, frightening, and obscure, then psychotic incomprehensibility (notionally) transcends the subject but psychotic alienation occurs in a shared world, implying that processes intrinsic to the subjectivity of the individual are in play. Foucault (1954/1987) notes certain features of the psychotic perception of space: 'clear space' blurs into 'obscure space', the space of fear and night, or rather, they come together in the morbid world instead of being separated, as in the normal world (p. 52).

We all, on occasion, experience the space around us as obscure and threatening—perhaps as a result of fear, unfamiliarity, or the darkness of night—so we can appreciate the effect when such blurring is interwoven into everyday, normal reality. Unlike most of us, a psychotic may experience alienation, disruption, and threat in the familiar and predictable ways of life that articulate the social world.

Others may cease to be partners in a dialogue or discourse and present themselves against a background of bewildering social implications and (hidden) relations of power according to which they lose their reality as *socii* and become, in this depopulated world, Strangers. Recall the Lone Ranger's remark to Tonto, 'Relax, we are among friends,' to which Tonto replies, 'Only trouble is, they ain't ours.' The insecurity of seeing others in a social context from which we feel alienated and adrift so that the shared social context cannot construct the background of one's life world is alienating and unsettling; it demands attention as a problematic aspect of one's subjectivity, disrupting our 'dealings with' things around us so that nothing is clear, everything holds hints of obscurity and complexity. Such is the disturbing world of psychosis.

We are confronted by the loss of the individual in a threatening and bewildering world in which one's existence as a coherent subjectivity negotiating a meaningful life trajectory of affordances and opportunities is derailed, thrown out of kilter, or falls apart. Laing plays the theme in *forte* mode but, in *piano* mode, it is pervasive in human experience (often vastly outweighed by our assurance of the subjective normality of the real world and our being-in-the-world-with-others). The strange world surfaces in, for instance, the works of Kafka, who manages to 'articulate fears which lurk in the recesses of the mind in all of us' (Storr, 1989, p. 61). The psychotic world and the world experienced psychotically are therefore two sides of the same coin in which a fundamental 'self-disorder or ipseity disturbance' characterized by 'distortions of the act of awareness: hyperreflexivity and diminished self-affection' (Sass & Parnas, 2003, p. 427) unseat the relational or intentional being of the person who lives within the psychotic experience. What Spitzer (1990c) has conceptualized as a 'valid account of what is different in their experience' (p. 50) implicates one's being-in-the-world and the normal interchange between that and what is inscribed on/in one's subjective embodied life.

The alienation, unreason, fragmentation, and irrationality characteristic of psychotic thought disengages the intersubjective rules operating in the human life-world, breaking up and disorganizing or disarticulating thought so that it becomes incoherent and impenetrable to the non-psychotic witness. But, armed with an appreciation of the disruption of self that is psychotic, the possible extraconscious mechanisms, for instance, attention and information-processing deficits, at the cognitive heart of psychotic disorganization and disconnectedness cry out for investigation.

5.3 Thinking and reason

Sequential and interwoven trains of thought conducted according to normal rules of cognitive coherence reflect the complexity of simple moments of conscious experience. Having rejected an uncritical acceptance of some version of the passive picture theory whereby sound belief and well-grounded reasoning rest on a series of transparent, causal, and/or rational transitions in thought based on observational evidence, we need to go beyond the Empiricist Representational Theory (ERT) of mind (Gillett, 1992) and examine more closely the active meaning-making skills of the (intersubjectively engaged) human subject.

Note that the poet or novelist may show idiosyncratic and singular transitions quite unlike those of normal patterns of inference but not have a thought disorder as, for instance, in *The Trial* where Kafka (1953) depicts the man who waits at a door to be given access to the Law (perhaps, after Lacan, the imperative of the word under the name of the father). He repeatedly asks if he will be allowed to enter; he is told by the doorkeeper, 'It is possible, but not at this moment.' 'In the first years, he curses his fate aloud; later, as he grows old, he only mutters to himself. He grows childish' (p. 236). As he is about to die, he summons the doorkeeper:

> 'Everyone strives to attain the law . . . How does it come about, then, that in all these years no-one has come seeking admittance but me?' The doorkeeper perceives that the man is at the end of his strength and his hearing is failing, so he bellows in his ear, 'No one but you could gain admittance through this door, since this door was intended only for you. I am now going to shut it.'

(Kafka, 1953, p. 237)

This passage, and its paranoid but deeply meaningful conversation, at a stroke, both recalls the 'thought disorder' or chronic paranoid schizophrenia and is deeply revealing about our shared human experience. Psychotic accounts hold no such insights.

> The love/peace/hate battled around the source of power that biology had intricately constructed in his veins. His heroes in his brain knew of peace and war. He had come from Valhalla and nobody knew the Sphere child flew at night to the darkness of fright. He flew around the electric wires of anxiety.

(Gates & Hammond, 1993, p. 68)

This (disordered) thought is shifting, disconnected, and elusive, sketchy, indeterminate, perhaps amenable to a Rorschach-type response that manufactures a meaning from a formless stimulus but no better than that. The book it is from is difficult to read because the connections constraining and linking moments in thought, though evincing rules that are difficult to pinpoint and specify and making sense in a way that engages with skills learnt in ordinary human discourse, slip away as one tries to grasp them.

Thought is driven and formed by praxis: 'Concepts lead us to make investigations [that] are the expression of our interest and direct our interest' (Wittgenstein, 1953, ¶ 570). What one does and how one's life hangs together keeps thought on the (relatively permissive and multidirectional) rails that direct its normal course. A derailment occurs when the link between *noesis* and our dealings with actual world objects is severed. Our cognitive skills are attuned to objects equally accessible to self and others (Kant, Husserl, Wittgenstein) so that the rules governing them articulate a shared actual world experience of doing things together (as Foucault's *socii*) within intersecting experiential trajectories.

The realization that a thinker must use a given concept rightly (make true judgements in a range of different conditions) to count as understanding it grounds theories that reveal the link between meaning (or understanding) and truth—a link providing the warrant for sane thoughts that things are thus and so. 'Reality testing' depends on that link and proceeds as an aspect of a dynamic intelligent action and the informal (rather than statable or codifiable) rules that connect it to the world.

Kant denies that we can teach and learn rules for the use of the rules relating concepts to the objects instancing them (representations to what is represented or signifiers to what is signified). Consider the use of the term 'leaf': imagine that someone could not learn to apply it and try to formulate a rule to delineate a correct response.

> !Apply the term 'leaf' to parts of a plant which are flat and approximate an oval with pointed ends, or sometimes a blade, or sometimes a heart shape!

But we have a problem of multiple ambiguity (so that the rules cannot get started anywhere): 'What is a plant?' 'How approximate?' 'What sort of a blade?' 'How can something be both like a blade and a heart?' and so on. There looms an infinite regress of rules governing other rules so that Kant (1789/1929) concludes that we need judgement—a skill refined in practice and governed by norms (*noemata* [Husserl]) informing the psyche—'the faculty of mother wit the lack of which no skill can make good' (B172).

The present account reworks the appeal to mother wit and intrinsic abilities by noting that human beings have innate tendencies to catch on to the praxes of other human beings and build on them through training in judgement (creating in them a 'second nature'). This picture does not fit the Cartesian view that is so entrenched in traditional empiricist thought and the present account of psychosis contrasts it with more familiar varieties of 'common sense . . . as a network of beliefs (i.e. social knowledge) and as a basic individual attunement with the social world' (Stanghellini. 2004, p. 14).

In the era of artificial intelligence, the idea of rules is often mistakenly analyzed in terms of dispositional regularities or mechanisms within the thinker (Bolton & Hill, 1996). The philosophical flaws in such an account emerge when we realize that the rules obeyed in thinking and reasoning are not causal (Kripke, 1982) or formal (Kant, Wittgenstein) but normative and prescriptive—standards for a person to follow as an embodied subjective, intelligent, and creative individual. Human rule following is marked by

(i) The correct way to go on—something decided independently of my responses and tied to (intersubjectively accessible) objects in the world; and

(ii) The way I actually go on—an individual performance reflecting whether I am following the rule.

These are, respectively, normative and descriptive elements of human rule following. Whereas the latter element may be explained in terms of cognitive mechanisms, the former (noematic [Husserl] or normative) feature cannot be: it yields a standard for meaning that my performance—produced by inner mechanisms—is judged against. Kripke offers a communitarian or sociocultural solution to this normative problem, but any simplistic version of that solution neglects the possibility of an embodied thinker forming an articulated system of dealings with things guided by public usage and the good tricks shared by a human group (Gillett, 1995; Heidegger, 1953/1996).

Rationalists claim that axioms and self-evident logical transitions underpin valid trains of thought, claiming that these impose an order on the unstructured flux of experience, arguing that sensory input engages with cognitive structures but does not generate the rational processes and ordered categories characteristic of human thought. Many rationalists (such as Piaget) consider these operations to be innate even if they require experience to mobilize them and the idea that a priori (in the innatist sense) causal structures do much of the work has received fresh impetus from the work of Chomsky (1972) and others (e.g. Pinker, 1994) in this tradition.

Such thinkers recognize the need for the mind to engage with the world but tend to overlook the nature and source of the rules governing thought and the use of concepts. Even Kant, who merged the strongest claims of rationalism with the obvious strengths of empiricism, neglected any systematic development of his insights into the intersubjective validation of mental contents (Strawson, 1966, p. 151) and therefore failed to provide a *via media* between the dubious credentials offered by innate or biological mechanisms on the one hand and sociocultural constructionism on the other.

A phobia about cultural relativism predisposes a rationalist towards innatism and an 'inner set of goings-on' theory of mind but then obscures sight of the fact that the norms or rules operating in thought are discursively located and that thinking is a product of skills and techniques honed by living in the world as an embodied subject among others (Merleau Ponty, 1964; Wittgenstein, 1953). Thus, aberrations in thought are often regarded as arising from a computational or biological change underpinning the life of the thinking subject, thereby effectively relegating irrationality to extraconscious causal mechanisms unrelated to the meaningful aspects of mental content. An adequate understanding of insight and delusion might, however, lead us beyond such an individualistic view and show us how 'epistemic virtue' (Blackburn, 1984, p. 245)— the ability to distinguish between right and wrong beliefs—is fundamental in human mental life and tied up with self as a product of intersubjectivity (Staghellini, 2004, p. 61). Such an understanding reveals the skilled nature of right thinking and the structures of embodied subjectivity that underpin the relevant skills.

If we think of the cognitive apparatus as a way of processing data from the environment according to a range of causally configured operations, the thinker as an active person making meaning of the world tends to take a backseat. Thus, psychotic phenomena can only arise from the thinker receiving false data or processing it badly due to faulty internal connections. But the view that we are all attuned to a shared world so that each embodied self is the 'incarnated profile of common sense' broadens the scope of explanation beyond three simplistic alternatives, viz.,

(i) Either the disordered mind is causally in disarray because of some irrational and inexplicable biological influence, or

(ii) The rational mind is subject to that kind of distortion in which wishes, needs, and vulnerabilities overbalance the psyche, or

(iii) The individual rational mind can adopt a marginal and discredited position because of sociocultural factors in signification.

Neither rationalism (according to which self-evident axioms held by all reasoning beings are applied in a quasi-mathematical way to 'experiential data') nor the ERT can explain everyday or psychotic irrationality and the alienation that pervades psychotic experience. A discursive and phenomenological approach illuminates the misfit between thought and the actual world because it identifies a set of discursive skills articulating the interaction between the brain and the (intersubjective) world around it. Discursive or interpersonal reality locates the human subject in a life-world that is (*ab initio* and a priori) a shared fleshly world grounded in intersubjectivity as the basis of 'getting it right'. This orientation yields an understanding of right thinking and the distortions of self, which are discussed in terms of insight and delusion in psychosis.

The problem of insight, 'inner awareness' (Lewis, 1934), or self-reflective thought is often regarded, in clinical practice, as more difficult for a patient than thinking about others or the outside world. David (1990) goes so far as to say that 'insight into another's illness may be preserved despite the loss of personal insight' (p. 800). But, to a philosopher trained in traditional epistemology, that is very odd.

The Cartesian view holds that knowledge of one's own mind is immediate and incorrigible so that 'most persons can enter readily into their supposed or possible motives' (Lewis, 1934, p. 19). But self-knowledge is often profoundly disturbed in psychosis, so we need an understanding of self-reflective thought that accounts for the disturbed *ipseity* (or self-hood) seen in the clinic (Sass & Parnas, 2003).

5.4 Thinking, judgement, and reasoning: a set of skills

Kant and Wittgenstein provide insights that can be melded together with an anlysis of thought informed by phenomenology to understand cognitive skills as techniques of embodied subjectivity that are developed and maintained intersubjectively. Thinkers grasp the rules governing the use of concepts (both in their applications and their role in cognition) by modelling the activity of fellow human beings and articulating their activity in ways that reflect a shared common sense. As a result, one learns, in 'those situations where language is taught and learnt' (Quinton, 1955), a range of skills or techniques that inform subjective experience and reflect the cumulative results of adaptive skills shaped in human forms of life (not merely the functioning of computational operations).

The psyche is fluid, dynamic, and open to interpersonal effects, its operations informed by norms imparted through discourse (through correction and training), so that the relationships between persons (*qua socii* [Foucault]) who obey principles such as the principle of Charity (Davidson), allowing mutual comprehension, make a thinker who she or he is. Discourse produces cohesion, a 'fusion of horizons' intrinsic to a 'form of life', and 'Sociality unfolds itself in the realm of action' (Stanghellini, 2004, p. 85) providing a consistent context for cognition and interpersonal behaviour, a frame that is suspended in the Kafkaesque world of some institutional settings (or even some families).

The norms governing speech and communication are pervasive, governing judgements about the contents of an experience, techniques of belief formation, and the conduct of mental life in general. Thus, an individual story—the product of a good-enough autobiographical consciousness—is built on intersubjective techniques that are both informal and difficult to define or specify but which human beings latch on to by being-with-others in situations and relationships where linguistic terms or signs mark certain ways of responding to the world and act as a mirror for one's lived subjectivity (Gillett, 1992, 2008). In that way, any given individual obeys shared prescriptive norms and appreciates that there are right and wrong ways of articulating experience so that the *noematic* (normative or ideal) pervades the actual world of human discourse and an individual (functioning sufficiently well to develop an adequate set of cognitive skills) embodies the (intersubjectively shaped) norms that articulate his or her life-world.

Self-reflective thought arises as a thinker learns to use concepts influenced by the way that others react to his or her judgements: for instance, when he or she says 'That is a car' and is told 'No, it is a van,' he or she adjusts his or her performance. As he or she learns to imitate their responses to objects of mutual attention, so does he or she learn to mimic their responses towards him or her so that, in the process of mastering concepts, a thinker develops the ability to judge for himself or herself whether or not he or she is getting it right; 'with every mental activity—or act—there is an observing or registering of its apprehended quality apart from the material upon which the function in question is being exercised' (Lewis, 1934, p. 19). Any judgement about the world (by a subject who is an incarnation of common sense) therefore also potentiates a reflective (second-order) judgement on oneself as a thinker. That one is a possible object of one's own judgements is implicit in the fact that others treat one as such an object. Freud emphasized the moral or conative role of self-reflective judgement when he discussed the formation of the superego and the defence mechanisms protecting the ego from the unacceptable, and Lacan (1977) speaks of the mirror stage as 'an identification . . . the transformation that takes place in the subject when he assumes an image' (p. 2). Reflection and self-knowledge require the subject to focus on his or her own responses and assess them according to parental, social, and cultural ('mnemic') residues. The stance is pervasive and produces, as it were, a normative (and evaluative) commentary grounded in the (imagined and/or imitated) judgements of others both on what one says and does and, implicitly, on oneself.

One might therefore expect the techniques of self-judgement to be more difficult to master than those involved in straightforward judgements about things out there and to be loaded with emotive, conative, or evaluative nuances and implications. Many features of the Freudian superego therefore mark self-reflection: it is evaluative, subjective, and lived in a way that austere structuralist readings of Lacan's play of signifiers do not quite capture. The imperative of speech captures the formative influences of parents and others who speak into existence the 'imago' (image and ego), the quasi-stable psychic basis of individual identity and self-development. Small wonder, given its elusive and dynamic target, that self-knowledge is prone to disruption in disorders of thought and judgement, especially in the context of disordered or pathological interpersonal discourse.

The present account sees human thought and action as essentially relational skills used by a human being to negotiate a shared life-world illuminated by the activity of others. A human individual does not slavishly conform to others' ways of seeing things or to majority judgements but, by analogy with chess, certain basic techniques must be mastered before one can devise anything original or intelligent such as a stratagem. The shared rules of a human discourse delineate a range of techniques based on symbolically mediated interaction that equip a person to deal with novel situations and articulate them (Gillett, 1993c). In fact, Kelly (1955) analysed personality and individuality in terms of one's articulation by personal constructs best viewed as products of the interpersonal and relational discursive techniques that form us.

Kelly bases his 'personal constructs' on relations between people significant in the mind of the subject such that each construct emerges from a conceptualization of similarity and difference between significant others. A personal construct is a dimension in terms of which two individuals are similar and contrast with another. For instance, a teacher who is admired might be contrasted to the subject's mother and father and suggest that a dimension of intellectual acuity and a skeptical view of social mores might be part of that subject's hierarchy of constructs. Being connected to and intersecting with other constructs would help to explain the person's cognitive and experiential world. One's complex and intersecting set of personal constructs frames conscious experience and invest it with a personal orientation to the world and those who inhabit it. Notice that the framework is implicitly evaluative, self-locating, and affecting, drawing on the ways in which one has lived and moved among others and through one's embodiment and realtionality, shares one's social world and its meanings with them.

My own personal approach to the world is deeply influenced by an implicit contrast between two mentors (an English teacher and a philosopher whose ability to analyse and articulate everyday thoughts was deeper and more revealing than I had previously encountered) and my family (solid representatives of a suburban and pedestrian life-world). My mother, father, and other relations probably saw many things of which I was unaware, but the dimension of analytic perspicuity, a continuum defined by my English teacher and my first philosophy lecturer, has remained dominant in my hierarchy of constructs and values ever since.

The discursive and phenomenological view of consciousness and perception fleshes out the themes dominating this work. A human thinker commands a wide range of skills in making sense out of the world; they articulate experience, informing (and reflecting) it according to (discursively embedded) constructs that

(1) Validate the existence of the thinker as a subject who experiences being-with-others as an essential mode of consciousness;

(2) Reveal the key person–signification dyads articulating consciousness;

(3) Structure experience in the light of values conveyed and acquired through existential (subjective embodied) being-with-others.

A serious fracture or dislocation between one's own subjective life and that of others therefore creates existential doubt about who one is and one's place in the world. The lived being-with-others underpinning conscious experience is disrupted, rendered confusing, distracting, and potentially frightening, a domain of alienation[1] in which one's existence is constantly in question because the intrinsic inhabitability of intentional relations between the self, others, and world breaks down.

> The most basic features of the world and of the self become deeply strange and opaque. Because the syntheses which constitute a continuous and unitary self have become seriously weakened, the self disintegrates and begins to be experienced as conjoined with aspects of the non-self.
>
> (Wiggins *et al.*, 1990, p. 33)

---

[1] Discussed in Appendix D.

It is against these broad-brush outlines that we should try and understand psychotic phenomenology including hallucinations, delusions, irrationality, and thought disorder.

They are equally relevant to the experience of human beings whose world of meaning is other than that inhabited by their fellows through dreams and visions or a spiritual life or through any other source of 'mirror images' of the world not shared by their fellows.

5.5 **Hallucination: false perception**

A common theme in phenomenological analyses of conscious experience is the phenomenological difference between imagination, perception, and memory. The differences radically affect the *gestalt* of a conscious event such that a normal thinker does not mix them up: such things as the lack of surprise or ongoing discovery in imagining things means that imagination, memory and perception are phenomenologically distinct from each other (Sartre, 1972). Such distinctions underpin the absolutely basic skill of convergence in judgements with other observers about 'objective' or 'intersubjective' reality, a skill so basic that 'we are self-aware through our practical absorption in the world of objects' (Sass & Parnas, 2003, p. 430).

Added to this basic distinction between perception and imagination, other features of the imaginary conscious experience distinguish it from the perceptual experience.

> Imagine a policeman walking towards you.
> Now, ask yourself what colour his hair was. If you cannot answer such a question, then either you have to do a bit more creative mental work or the question is unanswerable. In either event, if you are restricted to commenting on your original imagined policeman, you are caught in the following trap.

Q. You imagined a policeman?	A. Yes
Q. He was not a bald policeman?	A. No
Q. Therefore, he had hair?	A. Yes
Q. He was your creation?	A. Yes
Q. Therefore, you created his hair?	A. Yes
Q. All hair is coloured?	A. Yes
Q. Therefore, you must know what colour it was?	

The fundamental phenomenological distinction is (in part) constituted by the fact that an imagined object is a mental creation so that there is nothing more to discover about the imagined image or experience, and it cannot surprise us: what is there is psychically created (so that the claim that imagination and perception have identical content but different causal origins is wrong). We can be mistaken about the objects of consciousness in altered states of consciousness (such as dreaming), but normal perception and thought about the world is so basic to 'the relationships between subjectivity and the material and natural order' that confusing the two (subjectivity and actuality) results in a special kind of 'perplexity or bewilderment' (Sass & Parnas, 2007).

This realization confronts us with the reality of hallucinatory disorders of thought. They indicate that a twofold feature of our nature as subjective beings-in-the-world-with-others (*the sensus communis*—as synthetic awareness of whole objects at hand and shared social knowledge—and *self-affection*—normal absorption in and awareness of a shared world) is deeply disturbed in psychosis. So basic are these to our nature as thinkers that hallucinations are symptoms of a profound disorder of the psyche.

Most hallucinations, at least in psychosis, are verbal and are represented as voices.

> They say all different kinds of things to me. Sometimes nice things, sometimes bad things, sometimes just repeating whatever I say. They tell me about other people, before I even meet them. The voices didn't tell me about you. But now they're talking about you and listening.

(Jaynes, 1990)

The phenomenological quality of hallucinatory experiences is that they are private and personally directed to the subject, inaccessible to those around him or her. This is not the case with real voices in a conversation; therefore, hallucinations are only mistakenly thought to support the argument for the indiscernibility of proximal content (images arising on the mind side of the mind–world divide) from distal content (images caused by the external world) as something separate from its origins appealed to in many empiricist accounts.

The claim that there are contents of experience qualitatively the same in hallucination, imagination, and normal perception and that the mind infers from various clues what has given rise to that content is a long way from the truth. The psychotic may, in fact, be quite specific about the voices: 'The voices come from in my head. Actually from in my right ear.' But there is often unclarity—'about three weeks ago, the voices started and I would look around to see if anyone was there but there never was' (Jaynes, 1990, p. 160)—even if they are quite distinguishable (and recognized to be so once the psychotic has learnt the distinction) from normal conversation in the way they affect the person; 'he could not control these voices and they did not let him control his own mind' (Jaynes, 1990, p. 161).

Many explanations have been given for the form and content of the voices, but they are often imperative and accusatory, expressing morbid thoughts consistent with the distress and schizoid self-reflective attitudes of the patient inviting an existential phenomenological interpretation in terms of interpersonal dynamics and a threat to the self. Laing suggests that the schizoid splits in the self reflect two aspects of the self in the world, 'an awareness of oneself by oneself and an awareness of oneself as an object of someone else's observation' (cf Sartre, 1962, p. 106). In the schizoid state, the apparent transparency of self to the other is accompanied by a paranoid attitude whereby others are seen as threatening and disapproving so that the most common type of hallucination—persecutory voices—is a commentary upon self, from the (phantasized) perspective of the other. But the realization that it is (in some sense) self taking this role is self-knowledge not available to the patient (a disturbance of the self characteristic of psychotic experience and its disturbed ipseity).

The disruption of conscious mental life producing psychotic hallucinations strikes at the essence of oneself as an integrated person reciprocally attuned to others in a shared world of things with ready-to-hand meanings (Stanghellini, 2004, pp. 91, 22). This offers no support for the neat and tidy philosopher's 'hallucination stereotype': an odd perceptual event appearing in a normal consciousness as an ordinary object-experience distinguished only by its lack of correspondence with an actual thing.

A similar pervasive disorder of the lived incarnation of common sense characterizes delusions.

5.6 **Delusion: false belief**

In the *Diagnostic and Statistical Manual of Mental Disorders IV* (DSM IV; APA, 1994a), a delusion is defined as

> A false belief based on incorrect inference about external reality that is firmly sustained despite what almost everyone else believes and despite . . . incontrovertible and obvious proof or evidence to the contrary.

When the delusion involves a value judgement, the judgement must be 'so extreme as to defy credibility'. But the definition is widely recognized to be flawed. Delusions are not just false beliefs resistant to evidence because a delusion can be true: the famous Othello syndrome is a case in point whereby a man believes his wife to be unfaithful, she is unfaithful, and yet his belief is a delusion. An evaluative delusion may, in fact, converge with the judgements of others and yet have the characteristic flavour or tone of a delusion, and other delusions are impossible to assess as true or false. If a patient believes that God is sitting in judgement on him for his past deeds, then it is crass to categorize this as simply false because 'religious beliefs are neither true nor false, at least in the scientific meaning of the words' (Spitzer, 1990b). Along with this oversimplistic definition, we have lost sight of the 'personal' and self-directed nature of nearly all delusional thoughts when they are explored by the therapist (as noted in the DSM III-R).

Some delusions are problematic in that they present us with a psychiatric version of the antinomy of the liar, as in the case where a patient believes he is insane (Fulford, 1989, pp. 204–205). Here, the patient says and believes that he is suffering a mental illness so that if he is correct, then his belief is not false, and if we rely on its falsity to classify it as a delusion, he is not deluded (indeed, he has insight and, given the key place of insight in conceptualizating psychosis, we might argue that he is not insane at all). Thus, if he is correct, he correctly judges that he is insane and therefore he must be insane, but if he is wrong, then he is deluded about being insane and therefore is insane. The paradox depends on delusion being a false belief and in and of itself sufficient to indicate insanity (so genuinely innovative scientists, watch out!), but other major criteria, such as negative symptoms, usually mean that the paradox does not, in practice, arise.

The paradoxical example trades on the view that a false belief of the right kind is a delusion, but if the criteria for being deluded go beyond the truth or falsity of the belief concerned, then something else is recognized by an experienced psychiatrist when faced by a psychotically deluded patient. This further fact seems to distinguish genuine delusions from false or overvalued beliefs (Mullen, 2003). Problems also arise in the definition of irrational thinking in that delusory beliefs may not be recalcitrant to reasoning or impervious to correction by others but may accommodate contrary content in a bizarre way rather than exhibiting normal corrigibility and sensitivity to information. In fact, psychotic patrients may be more rather than less rational in their thinking according to formal or syllogistic reasoning (Czynewski, 2007) and some delusions are not completely insulated from real life (Brett-Jones *et al.*, 1987); rather, the relevant evidence is offset by defects such as overreadiness to accept inadequate confirmation for a delusional system or pseudorational explanations for conflicts between delusions and presented evidence. Thus, even though delusory thinking is not totally insulated from normal evidential–inferential confirmation, it is often not susceptible to the reality testing that a 'normal' subject would impose as an embodiment of common sense in our everyday interpretive order (but what of the prophet, genius, artist, visionary?).

The freeing of oneself from normative constraints on inference and belief formation seems to be related to a further feature—'cognitive recklessness': 'deluded subjects predicted future events more readily and on the basis of inferior standards of proof in contrast to normal and psychiatric controls' (David, 1990, p. 803). Again, the thinker has abandoned normative commitments and is no longer concerned about 'getting it right' in terms that reflect a commonsensical view (or shared social knowledge).

An extreme manifestation of this problem is the ability of deluded patients to believe impossible things such as 'existing in the past as well as the present . . . having inside one's body something larger than oneself (e.g. a nuclear power station), being in two places at one time' (David, 1990, p. 804), and so on. In attempting to give reasons for their beliefs, persons show how far they have strayed from the canons comprising the *sensus communis* underpinning both *sophia* and *phronesis*.

As in hallucination, delusional thought should alert us to a deep disorder in the mind disrupting skills of thought rooted in the communication and convergence in judgements that organize our experience of and action in the world. Therefore, delusion is neither just false belief nor an immoderate evaluation of a situation: it reveals a deep disquiet in the mind manifest in subtle and manifold ways often affecting the form and content of thought. The 'Cartesian attitude' of immediacy and incorrigibility towards judgements that normal people subject to established epistemic or evaluative procedures linked to a balanced view of one's trajectory through a social and practical world (Spitzer, 1990, p. 389) seems to go wrong in delusions of control, thought insertion, or broadcast thought in which the individual is alienated from the structures of his or her own narrative. Such ideas resemble suspicions that common sense usually dismisses as absurd. In psychosis, they reflect disrupted ipseity engendering a failure of a person's integrity as a subjective being, a subject of thought but also of action and intention (Bolton & Hill, 1996; Sass & Parnas, 2007; Stanghellini, 2004; Zahavi, 2005).

If belief formation depends on an active set of techniques based on rule-governed use of concepts, the mentally disordered patient has, in greater or lesser measure, a defect of the validating, balancing, and self-reflective skills normally active in perception, concept use, the evaluation of experience, inferences, and modification of behaviour. Each area of cognitive activity is vulnerable to both meaningful and biological influences because of the complementary roles, in the psyche, played by one's being among others and one's neurocognitive function. A human being as a being-among-others is deeply threatened by the loss of these skills so that psychotic thinking has not only experiential but also existential significance for a thinker.

5.7 **Irrationality**

The following argument was abstracted from the statement of a woman who had killed her infant daughter.

(1) All human beings die and are judged.

(2) They are judged according to their sins.

(3) If they are found innocent, they live with God in heaven.

(4) Living with God in heaven is better than life on earth.

(5) My baby has committed no sins.

(6) If he dies, he will be innocent and go to heaven.

(7) Therefore, I killed my baby.

There is irrationality of a very profound kind here, but it is not clear just how to categorize it. Premises 1, 2, and 3 are believed by a great many people and therefore each belief is 'one ordinarily accepted by other members of the person's culture or subculture' (DSM IV; APA, 1994a, p. 765). Premise 4 is found in some of our great religious works (e.g. Paul, Philippians 1:21). Premise 5 is plausible to many people who think in those terms, and 6 is merely a logical entailment of 2, 3, and 5. The practical conclusion comes as a surprise but, given the argument, is not surprising on purely rational grounds. One nods in agreement (or is it relief?) on learning that the argument is produced in justification of child murder by a woman diagnosed as suffering from psychosis (rather than a moral philosopher).

Reciprocity between persons and an assumption of charity—that people largely believe what is true and want what is desirable—underpin the attribution of thoughts to others and, along with shared views about coherence and rationality within a belief system, form 'the interpretive view of mind' (Doring, 1990), an idea attributed to Quine (1960) but recently championed by Davidson (1984).

> Suppose you came as an explorer into an unknown country with a language quite strange to you. In what circumstances would you say that the people there gave orders, understood them, obeyed them, rebelled against them, and so on?
>
> The common behaviour of mankind is the system of reference by means of which we interpret an unknown language.
>
> (Wittgenstein, 1953, ¶ 206)

The interpretive view in its analytical (post-empiricist) form is based on the possibility of interpreting the utterances of speakers by a careful (and gracious) observation of the relations between their statements and their activity in the world (also found in the idea of life-worlds [Husserl], forms of life [Wittgenstein], dealings with things [Heidegger], and post-structuralism). Davidson's views on meaning, truth, and rationality are based on the interpretation of linguistic utterances in terms of their conditions of utterance and their place in an overall theory of the behaviour of a language-using group. On this account, language users are seen as holding true statements that enable an interpreter to make valid links between utterance types and conditions of utterance. Davidson's version of the account makes explicit use of the *principle of charity* whereby we reckon most language users to be correct in most of their beliefs (thereby justifying the a priori link between statements, conditions of utterance, and states of affairs or truthmakers).

Wittgenstein's remarks, as we have noted, link a person's understanding and the truth of a sufficiency of her or his basic statements (1969, ¶ 80) and he also notes the fundamental role of agreement in judgements in the determination of meaning (1953, ¶ 242).

These theorists offer us an account that can lose itself in rational closure according to logical rules and principles even though it aims at a realistic view of the best explanatory fit between the behaviours of individuals and their environment as the basis of mental attributions. That it must be loosened from a rigid adherence to logical constraints is evident when we look at the insufficiency of logic to capture the problem in the case of the woman who committed infanticide (and the general syllogistic competence of schizophrenic patients). In the real world, there are numerous conflicting constraints on belief formation and the weighting of information so that rationality is holistic, reflecting the fusion of horizons and reciprocal attunement that marks adaptive immersion in a social world and a shared interpretive order. Hidden factors and unforeseen events may derail what seems like a watertight and logically coherent plan of action. We therefore understand the Russian peasant who, approached by a Moscow-based researcher posing the following type of problem, strikes a blow for down-to-earth common sense.

> In the Far North, where there is snow, all bears are white.
> Novaya Zemla is in the Far North.
> What colour are the bears there?
> The peasant thinks carefully and then remarks, 'You ought to ask my cousin Uri; he lives near Novaya Zemla.'
>
> (Luria, 1976, p. 107)

Most poorly educated respondants gave this kind of response, firmly grounded in well-attested relevant experience. The world of tricky words, abstractions, and propositions is not their world and they express 'a complete denial of the possibility of drawing conclusions from propositions about things they had no personal experience of' (p. 108); they live by honesty, integrity, and truth to experience (embodied being-in-the-world) so that they are engaged with actual 'ready-to-hand meanings' far removed from the alienated rationality of syllogistic models of human cognition (Doring, 1990). In fact:

> Differences in reasoning between deluded patients and controls are surprisingly small. Patients are somewhat more prone to endorse invalid or fallacious responses, especially when emotive themes are involved.
>
> (Kemp *et al.*, 1997)

The study explored the effect of emotion on the psychotic group (Kemp *et al.*, 1997, p. 401), highly relevant when one considers the subjective distress and existential insecurity of psychosis, and confirmed the general finding that emotional disturbance disrupts cognition (especially already impaired cognition). A human being has a place in discursive reality and, on the basis of 'the essential structures of human experience and existence', 'operative intentionality' or our 'practical absorption in the world of objects', a human being develops a liveable identity and a good-enough autobiographical integration (Sass & Parnas, 2003). Therefore, we cannot merely document the 'objective' situations that the world presents to an individual because the subtlety of the coherent conscious narrative must be borne in mind as we strive to understand psychotic thought. What also should be borne in mind is the neurobiological disruption of thought by factors that tend to loosen association and induce incoherence.

Incoherence and the loosening of associations are almost certainly an absurd, extraconscious, or physiological factor in the formation of psychotic thought patterns (similar to the motor effects commonly seen in psychosis). Such cognitive effects are manifold, including flight of ideas, disorganization, and loosening of associations or *Zerfahrenheit* seen in the 'paralogies, neologisms, bizarreness, mannerisms, stereotypies, perseverations, iterations, verbigerations, viscosity' (Sass, 1992) of psychotic thought.

> One of Gruhle's patients, in a specific affective state, noticed three marble tables in a cafe and was suddenly convinced that the end of the world was imminent.
> His explanation is as follows:
> The character of direct evidence, which originally is only justified for the perception (three tables) is now expanded and adapted to the totality of the idea. (Sass 1992, pp. 153–154)

Recent work confirms that purely incidental or meaningless connections occur more frequently in schizophrenic patients (Spitzer, 1992); but, in fact, 'Jung investigated word associations in healthy people under normal and distracted conditions and noticed that conceptually driven associations decreased while clang associations increased' (Spitzer, 1992, p. 170). Jung's explanation of this phenomenon centres on the role of attention in 'maintaining a particular idea within consciousness and stabilizing its direction or goal' (Spitzer, 1992, p. 171). More recent work on lexical decision making confirms this view and shows that semantic priming in psychosis reveals 'a larger semantic priming effect in thought-disordered schizophrenic patients' that becomes less as the acute disorders of thought are brought under control (Spitzer, 1992). Spitzer concludes:

> Inhibitory processes by which irrelevant associations are normally excluded from consciousness are defective in schizophrenic patients. As the maintenance of an organized sequence of thought and of organized language utterance requires the operation of a goal-directed organization of thoughts . . . it can only be accomplished by active inhibition (exclusion) of associations that are irrelevant to the intended utterance. (p. 187)

A human thinker develops a set of focused and directed intentional skills (learnt from others and underpinning a repertoire of rule-governed techniques) to respond to the conditions that ground the use of concepts and structure behaviour (Gillett, 1992). But in psychosis, the crucial ability to screen stimuli or develop selective attentional skills is impaired by neurophysiological or neurochemical abnormalities (Solomon *et al.*, 1981): 'schizophrenia is characterized by a weakening of the influence of regularities of previous input on current perception' (Hemsley, 1992, p. 236). The defect means that 'patients with schizophrenia do not habituate readily or use contextually appropriate, memory-based schemata to orient perception and disattend to familiar stimuli or irrelevant information' (Sass & Parnas, 2003, p. 432) and explains the hyperacuity of schizophrenic patients who sometimes notice all sorts of things about their therapist that 'see through' the many little strategies the therapist and normal people have for hiding their imperfections or disaffections in a conversation. It seems that prevalent social conventions (adapted to through 'reciprocal attunement') do not operate in someone who is hyperattentive to incidental and 'irrelevant' stimulus cues. This 'tuning out' from the normal conventional patterns of attention and preoccupation is also seen in mystic practices where people allow the mind, often after meditation, to go where it will and show patterns of behaviour such as glossolalia and trance-like automatisms.

The fundamental neurochemical disorder responsible for loosening of associations may also be discerned in schizophrenic motor disorders, affecting practiced rhythmic activities where the inherent redundancy of the task allows it to be performed in a more or less subattentive mode (Manschrek, 1992). It may be that the disorders of attention of schizophrenia allow incidental psychic material to intrude into and disrupt this quasi-automatic activity involved in normal subjective 'indwelling' of perception, social activity, and action.

Schizophrenia also affects voluntary movement, and abnormal involuntary movements are correlated with more severe and prognostically gloomy varieties of schizophrenia where the pervasive attentional defects may have broken up and severely attenuated well-established 'Hebbian' patterns of neural activity. In fact, work on attention in the 1960s prefigured the recent experiments and their interpretation.

5.8 Pathology of attention

In the 1960s, McGhie (1969) and others investigated the complex connections between attentional mechanisms and the disorders of thought and perception in schizophrenia, following hints in earlier observations by Kraepelin and Bleuler:

> Even though uninterested and autistically encapsulated patients appear to pay little attention to the outside world, they register a remarkable number of events of no concern to them. The selection which attention exercises over normal sensory impressions may be reduced to zero, so that almost everything that meets the senses is registered.
>
> (McGhie, 1969, pp. 44–45)

A number of phenomenological reports support this general orientation.

> It's as if I'm too wide awake—very, very alert. I can't relax at all. Everything seems to go through me. I just can't shut things out. (p. 45)
> I take more time to do things because I am always conscious of what I am doing. If I could just stop noticing what I am doing, I would get things done a lot faster.

> My trouble is that I've got too many thoughts. You might think about something, let's say that ashtray and just think, oh yes, that's for putting my cigarette in, but I would think of it and then I would think of a dozen different things connected with it at the same time. (p. 48)

McGhie posits a crucial role of attention in thought and experience as follows:

> By the process of attention, we thus break down and effectively categorize both the information reaching us from the environment and that which is internally available in the form of stored past experience. By such processes, we reduce, organize, and interpret the otherwise chaotic flow of information reaching consciousness to a limited number of differentiated, stable, and meaningful percepts from which reality is constructed. (1969, p. 49)

This passage assumes special significance when we consider the analysis of experience and meaningfulness underpinning the links between common sense, ipseity, intersubjectivity, and social attunement. The importance of signification and selective construction in shaping a person's lived conscious narrative suggests that attention and its pathologies are particularly important in understanding mental disorder.

McGhie (1969) differentiates between the classical hebephrenic type of schizophrenic, with the disintegration and fragmentation of experience and narrative involved, and the contrasting intense paranoid type whose inappropriate focusing of attention seems driven and narrowed by a delusional system or systems. In either case, there is a loss of 'mother wit' and its dynamic balance between flexibility and intentionally focused cognition so that a 'schizoid gap' develops between the adaptation of a normal subject to the world and that of a psychotic patient. Attentional mechanisms organize the normal engagement between mind and world so that neither exploration and novelty nor focused attention interfere with the exercise of lived subjectivity. In the schizophrenic experience, 'the gap' alienates the subject from the world, unsettling every aspect of experience so that even conversation becomes difficult:

> When people talk to me now, it's like a different kind of language. It's too much to hold at once. My head is overloaded and I can't understand what they say. It makes you forget what you've just heard because you can't get hearing it long enough. It's all in different bits which you have to put together again in your head—just words in the air unless you can figure it out from their faces.

> (McGhie, 1969, p. 62)

Again, it seems that schizophrenic patients cannot use the normal contextual, structural, and rhythmic clues based on redundancies and stimulus parsing that normally disambiguate linguistically structured information (McGhie, 1969, p. 63).

5.8.1 More recent evidence

McGhie's (1969) work has stimulated and is convergent with a great deal of ongoing experimentation into attentional mechanisms in schizophrenia based on the idea that 'flooding by excessive and poorly inhibited enteroceptive and exteroceptive stimuli leads to cognitive fragmentation' (Venables,1960, p. 78). Many workers researching cognition and schizophrenia now accept that deficits of attention found in schizophrenia and seen in non-schizophrenic relatives of those with schizophrenia are a manifestation of the primary neuropathology of schizophrenia and the basis of functional impairment (Birkett *et al.*, 2005; Ikebuchi *et al.*, 1999). The ego-impairment index, for instance, is claimed to be 'an effective, direct assessment of how a subject uses internal constructs to interpret exteroceptive stimuli' (Perry & Braff, 1994, p. 366) and is correlated with impaired inhibition of auditory startle responses. The hypothesis that defects in inhibition and attentional screening of information interfere with performance on current tasks is supported by the finding that the severity of impaired selective attention performance in schizophrenic patients is correlated with the degree of disorganization in behaviour evident clinically (Carter *et al.*, 1992). The same general posit is also found in neural network models used to explain the difficulty experienced by schizophrenic patients 'in maintaining contextual information over time and using that information to inhibit inappropriate responses' (Servan Schreiber *et al.*, p. 1105). McGhie's conjectures therefore seem confirmed by recent experiment and theory in cognitive neuroscience.

The understanding of Schizophrenic Disorders of experience in terms of discursively honed skills of attention and selective information use, and the neural and cognitive processes underlying them, also converges with recent phenomenological analyses. Taken together, they suggest that human subjectivity depends on cognitive skills (undergirding the conscious use and integration of information) that we all take for granted and explain why a profound disturbance of lived experience is caused by a biological disorder affecting those skills and their component functions. Laing plays the phenomenological and existential themes in *forte* mode, as do Stanghellini, Sass, and Parnas, but those who are more biologically oriented put the emphasis elsewhere and relegate analyses of the psyche to a more *piano* role. Both approaches are needed to characterize the discontents of psychosis.

5.9 Insight and self-consciousness

The ability to achieve a correct set of beliefs about oneself and others has a pivotal role in clinical psychiatry, as is evident in the widespread acceptance that a lack of insight is a distinguishing feature of major psychiatric disorders. The non-psychotic patient has insight into the fact that she or he is ill and that the illness has affected her or his mind, and is aware that certain experiences and thoughts are pathological in a way that resonates with the phenomenological-existential analyses of reflection and self-consciousness (note the link between mirrors or the mirror world and reflection).

Insight is defined in many ways. However defined, it concerns beliefs about one's own mental life and is of deep interest to philosophers because a tenet of post-Cartesian philosophy of mind (particularly of the Empiricist Representational stripe) is that a thinking subject has immediate, privileged, access to the contents of his or her own mind. It is linked, in the clinical sphere, to defects in what some psychiatrists call 'reality testing', and seriously disordered patients have problems in both areas—knowledge about one's own thoughts and knowledge about the external world. The idea of disturbances of ipseity relates the two through the disorders of thought giving rise to them by focusing on the fact that a human being is primarily a being-in-the-world-with-others who is mirrored in a shared framework of meanings.

Having insight is adopting 'a correct attitude to morbid change in oneself' (Lewis, 1934) based on an ability to monitor, review, and evaluate one's own thoughts (vis-à-vis the reality they allegedly concern and the constructions of self and reality current around here). The subject tests whether thoughts are true or false and clarifies their contents in terms of a shared social horizon (Stanghellini, 2004, p. 85) that forges a conceptual link between the grasp of mental content, an appreciation of its truth (in certain conditions), and one's own worthiness or rectitude as a thinker. The link, between understanding a thought, the ability to judge its truth in the actual world (Davidson, 1984; Quine, 1953; Wittgenstein, 1969), and to locate oneself in the symbolic matrix realized in the words of others (Lacan, 1977), produces the human subject but also seems closely related to the problems of schizophrenia.

The importance of insight and reality testing is evident when we realize that a patient who cannot tell the difference between the 'phantasms' of his or her own mind and reality is more severely afflicted than one whose attitude, mood, disposition, or adjustment is impaired but who still knows what is actually going on in relation to his or her being-in-the-world. Psychotic patients lacking insight do not seem reliably to recognize whether events are real or unreal, have deficient knowledge of self, and may not appreciate that they are mentally deranged. However, patients who are not psychotic but, say, depressed as a result of some physical illness may not realize that they are depressed so that if we define insight as a 'correct attitude to a morbid change in oneself' (Lewis, 1934, p. 17), such a patient looks not to have it.

Perhaps the difficulties of defining and articulating 'insight' and 'delusion' arise from the ERT and, given that they seem useful in the diagnosis, management, and monitoring of psychoses (David, 1990; Fulford, 1989), we should look to an epistemology (focused on the tacit and interpersonal skills that go into the construction of knowledge about the world and oneself) based on a phenomenological understanding of self-knowledge and self-consciousness that locates human subject in a radically intersubjective world of being-among-others.

If we characterize insight as the recognition that one is suffering an illness affecting the mind so certain events one experiences have to be relabelled as pathological (David, 1990, p. 798), we can see what post-structural phenomenology has to say about the key notions—recognition, realization, and relabelling. The analysis goes beyond 'looking inwards rather than looking outwards' (Lewis, 1934, p. 17) and converges with the claim that skills such as evaluative judgement and coherent action are central to mental illness (Fulford, 1989) by seeing lived experience of oneself as being intertwined with agency and the images reflected back from a social world that produces meaning.

Sartre (1958) defines the ontological dimensions of human existence as *being what one is, being what one is not, being-in-the-world,* and *being-for-others.*

> Human reality is being in so far as within its being and for its being it is the unique foundation of nothingness at the heart of being. (p. 79)

This puzzling passage should be read in the light of Sartre's existential ontology of consciousness (following Heidegger, his teacher) such that the human being is a being for whom the question 'Who am I?' is always already pressing to be answered against a fused (or shared) horizon of historical existence. Pointing at myself at a given moment in time achieves nothing more than 'I am me' and can be negated by 'that is not me as I am doing the pointing' or 'that is not really me because I am going to be different.' What is more, such a gesture contains no sense (meaning, articulate content) even of self-affirmation. The existential subject is always becoming something rather than resting content with a fossilized self-designation based on who it has been up to now and at this moment, but the being for whom its being is always already in question is not static nor empty and does not exist in (Cartesian) isolation.

Thus, I am continually refining and redefining myself through my interactions with the world and others and seeking to find reflections of the self (in the mirror world of others and shared social meaning). But because I am not alone and, apart from the things I encounter, there are also other people who encounter me with *the look*, I am shaped by the word as law so that the looks of others fix or determine me. In the look of another, something else profound happens and my world, up to that (logical) moment experienced as centering around me, is decentred from a single centre of consciousness to an intersubjective play of mutual consciousnesses. My world is our world; I am not just what I think of myself as being, but I am also a being for others, and particularly for you, who thinks of me as being thus and so and relates to me in certain ways. That interchange holds me in being; I cannot escape any of these onto-logical dimensions of my being, but each of them generates constructs none of which completely capture my being-in-the-world.

Therefore, I have a certain history and identity and am continually outliving the historical object that is me, the me that is defining myself by interacting with the world, and the me that is defined by the way that others see me. Those are the elusive truths of my complex existence as a being-in-the-world-with-others and it is profoundly difficult to achieve right knowledge of the being who is oneself. Insight, as a summation of what Jaspers (1923/1997) calls 'the modes in which the self becomes aware of itself' (p. 121), is therefore genuinely complex (*pace* the Cartesian picture).

At this stage, it is worth mentioning a few more clinical features of insight and delusion:

First, insight is a matter of degree (David, 1990, p. 800); it concerns 'the amount of realization the patient has of his own condition' (Lewis, 1934, p. 16). Early on in the development of an illness, some patients realize that they are mentally abnormal, and often experience profound anxiety as a result. Over the course of treatment, many come to an increasing realization of the extent to which they have been mentally deranged so that many of their supposed experiences were fanciful and their constructions of the world flawed or deficient in terms of the fused horizon they share with others.

Second, the relation between insight and prognosis, such that 'patients with more insight were significantly less likely to be readmitted over the course of follow-up' (McEvoy *et al.*, 1989), is explained if insight is a cognitive achievement that demands a great deal of anyone (rather than being immediate, incorrigible, and self-sustaining).

Third, insight can occasion greater psychological distress in a patient because it reveals the patient's condition to himself and so 'may involve a painful struggle against psychotic disturbance' (David, 1990, p. 801). One young patient remarks, 'I cannot picture anything more frightful than for a well-endowed cultivated human being to live through his own gradual deterioration fully aware of it all the time. But that is what is happening to me' (Lewis, 1934, p. 28).

Fourth, the phenomenon of pseudo-insight, where the patient produces utterances that seem to capture what is wrong with him or her but that are not integrated into his or her general thought and self-reflexive abilities, is a mere sham of the real thing: 'the patient merely regurgitates overheard explanations arising out of different theoretical perspectives' (David, 1990, p. 801). This phenomenon lays bare the difference between a properly indwelt and articulate lived experience and a compliant, superficial, or unthinking level of (mimetic) conversational interaction. To discern whether the patient recognizes or understands that there is a disorder in the various existential modes of being and relation of the self, we must enter the patient's sphere of reflexivity and self-affection.

The rich phenomenology and existential complexity of the self results in a conceptualization of insight, delusion, and belief that explains why schizophrenic self-focused thought disorders (of *ichstorung* [Jaspers] or *ipseity*) indicate a seriously disordered psyche, and exhibit disruption of both meaningful and causal connections constitutive of being-in-the-world-with-others.

We already have touched on Laing's discussion of the self and the false self and the ontological insecurity that arises in the distressing alienation of an individual in a schizoid state. But becoming *somebody* is not negotiable for a human being.

> Kafka, the man with no identity, forever ironic, gentle, self-effacing, was, in his inner world, courageous, uncompromising, ruthlessly honest. If his fate was to live under the harrow [a lethal torture device], that was where he had to be, and he was not going to wriggle out from it. As a writer, he not only did not flinch but also discovered his real identity.
>
> (Storr, 1989, p. 75)

Self-knowledge, insight, consciousness of self, and reflection as somebody identifiable by others are all complex and skilled epistemological attainments and can be disrupted at many points, so it is no wonder that such disruption is characteristic of psychosis. But right thinking about oneself is a much wider and more prevalent affliction than psychosis, although in other settings, it takes distinct and different forms; indeed, one could be tempted to think that disturbed thinking about oneself is the most pervasive psychic discontent, and when the spotlight is turned on any of us, we find that the fabric of life is criss-crossed throughout with small deceptions (foci of *meconnaissance*) about the true nature of self and its relationship to others.

The complexities implicit in veridical experience, rationality, and genuine knowledge should alert us to the difficulties of providing a conception of right thinking in general and of defining insight, because what constitutes getting it right about myself depends on a holistic and informal set of discursive norms and techniques. I define myself irrevocably by my actions, and yet remain someone who is yet to act, who must navigate a path through a world conceptualizable in many different ways, and who must form sustainable relationships with others allowing me to function in all of these modes of being. In developing a conception of who I am, I am always already acquiring the relevant skills and learning the techniques of negotiating interpersonal relationships through my immersion in discourse with others, especially those closest to me. In fact, clinicians probably use the interpersonal sense derived from this kind of activity to discern when somebody is disordered in their thinking and make diagnoses 'without being able to tell how they do it' (Spitzer, 1990b).

It is, in fact, no wonder that the same holistic interpersonal or participatory skills that underpin a judgement that someone lacks insight are manifest in all our judgements about others, the logical conditions for which are more or less impossible to specify (Gillett, 1989; Morris, 1992). Lewis (1934), reflecting on clinical judgement, remarks, 'we will observe his demeanour and see how far it corroborates or gives the lie to his statements. It is to his total attitude, possibly over a long period, and not to his verbal statements or his so-called intellectual acceptance of a point of view that we pay attention' (p. 25). That the recognitional skills operating in everyday human 'forms of life' were evident to Kant surfaces when he invokes 'mother wit' in the use of concepts.

What is more, it is clear that the skills enabling insight and rational belief formation are susceptible to both biological and interpersonal forces in that selective attention is a cybernetic psychomotor activity susceptible to biological 'spanners in the works' that unhinge, loosen, or dedifferentiate associations, disestablish patterns of expectation and detection, and derail orderly trains of inference and judgement thereby disrupting thought as it attempts to align the ideal (*noematic*) and the actual so as to form ground *noesis* in experience. Focused attention and the inhibition of distraction by competing elements in the stimulus conditions are important in the exercise and maintenance of these skills of self-attunement to a human life-world (Gillett, 1992; cf. Wiggins *et al.*, 1990).

Alienation from the interpersonal milieu to which human beings are attuned plausibly impairs not only the skills of mental ascription and self-ascription crucial in forming right beliefs but also reflective self-knowledge. The most vulnerable skills, those that are most difficult to master, are, I have argued, implicated in 'introspection' or reflection about my own self-location and the multiple ambiguities and uncertainties that are inherent in the existence of any subjective self-questioning being.

The elements of right thinking are, however, so closely tied to adaptive activity and so shaped by dispositions to make sense of things in terms of what normally happens around here that the system is constantly nudged back on track unless there are serious biological derangements of cognition. As long as such derangement does not fragment thought, as in significant dementia, it is understandable that the subject produces well-formed delusions and aberrant perceptual phenomena focused on the vulnerable (and existentially vital) knowledge of one's place and value in the world.

It is not true that 'most mental disorder can be considered to be a social role' (Wing, 1978, p. 150) and a phenomenological analysis reveals a primordial or organismic component in most major mental illness. However, it is inescapable that 'there is always some degree of interaction between social and biological factors, not only in the causation of deviance or disease but also in treatment, in prevention, and in long-term management' (Wing, 1978, p. 165).

Thinking about things (placing them correctly in the mirror world articulated by logic and signification) rests on rule-governed ways of responding to things around one mastered within a panoply of formative discursive interactions with other thinkers. They require one to use techniques of selective attention, assessing salience, weighting information, and assembling 'montages' of 'biology and representation' that are 'carriers of meaning and relation to others' (Kristeva, 1995, p. 30). The approvals and disapprovals of others convey the structure of right thinking (through the imperative of the word as law) so that there is a holism about human mental, moral, and spiritual life. Relational or connected aspects of our being, so heavily imbued with conative and moral overtones, help form the epistemic and existential aspects of our being through exchanges focused on one's being as an embodied person and are rendered (made comprehensible and/or torn apart) in terms of the mirror world (the distinctive medium of the human psyche).

A mental life is a narrative construct or product of the integrating activity of a concept-using subject as a person in relation to others. It relies on a cognitive and hodological (action-related or purposive and interested) map of the world and a repertoire of cognitive techniques using that map to negotiate situations in which one finds oneself. Thus, acting and relating are the foundations of the psyche rather than merely receiving, assembling, and connecting representations (*In amfang war die Tat*), and in the intersubjective milieu that is the human life-world, the insane person stands out as alien (and alienated from self and others) by his or her whole way of being-in-the-world.

5.10 Insight, irrationality, and delusion revisited

We can now lay out some conclusions about insight, insanity, delusion, and alienation.

Insight is best seen in terms of 'a rough notion of the patient's sanity of judgement, or commonsensical attitude towards his illness', and insanity is marked by 'a disturbance which makes it impossible for the patient to look at his data and judge them as we, the dispassionate, presumably healthy outsiders do' (Lewis, 1934, p. 25). A sane human being does not just have a set of beliefs which happen to be true: she or he uses a range of cognitive and discursive skills to become attuned to the world. Some of these skills are elusive and they all depend on the attunements and sensitivities of those who nurture one and shape one's cognitive structures (so that one way of being alienated is to be attuned to a different reality from that of the rat-race or the dog-eat-dog world of competitive survival). Attunement to the human life-world is disrupted by insanity, creating a schism between the self (as lived subjectivity) and others.

Psychotic thinking is disrupted by faulty cognitive mechanisms and aggravated because one is 'thinking only along one's own lines without caring for dialogue and intersubjective feedback' (Spitzer, 1990, p. 392), a defect more far-reaching than not 'agreeing with the interpretations, however extraordinary, offered by your analyst' (Editorial, 1990, p. 408). Insight is not only right thinking about oneself, the competent and coherent use of self-reflective techniques of judgement and concept use, but also being rightly related to a world of fused horizons. Mental 'illness' disturbs one's adaptation to the world (Fulford, 1989, p. 216), reflecting the fact that one lacks the normal warrants for cognitive acts because one is alienated from the intersubjective activity holding those warrants. Evaluation, prescription, and interpersonal norms, intrinsic to such activity, engage one as a psychosomatic unity whose soul is entangled with one's being-with-others and impairments in that unity can have many causes (or even origins).

5.11 **Intersubjectivity, truth, and social constructionism**

Thinking and the concepts or significations framing our particuipation in a shared life-world are governed by rules imparted in interpersonal contexts through normative judgements of others about one's own judgements. The good 'trick' of taking a normative attitude to one's own judgements, given that one's thought is not perpetually dependent for feedback from others, allows one to turn the same reflective light on the judgements of others as one turns on himself or herself and so to become (potentially at least) as much a social critic as a self-evaluator. A social constructionist view of knowledge neglects this fact and fails to notice that the 'situations where language is taught and learnt' (Quinton, 1955) are sufficiently diverse and idiosyncratic that the mastery of a basic repertoire of meanings is compatible with a wide range of creative uses of those concepts. Recall the rules of chess enabling one to make creative moves although, in making those moves (and perhaps outwitting one's teacher), one follows the rules one has been taught. Szasz (1996), sceptical about disorders of thought in schizophrenia, assimilates disorders of thought to 'faulty speech'.

> What counts as faulty speech depends on the criteria of correct speech. I do not deny that many so-called schizophrenic patients have identifiable speech patterns that may be called 'deviant' . . . The point is that speech defects . . . are the manifestations of the speaker's incorrect use of the muscles of his mouth and tongue, not of his disordered thinking or diseased brain. (p. 534)

A discursive theorist notices that language and thought are elaborated in social contexts and obey certain social norms but also notes that we are engaged in an actual world imposing real contingencies to which we must be attuned and engage our speech (and therefore, our thoughts and ourselves). We relate to things themselves and not just representations or conventional depictions of them. Reductive (antipsychiatry, or social constructionist) orientations discount the existential and dystonic reality and 'illness' of psychosis, features that give rise to fierce rebuttals of Szasz's synthesis.

> Szasz claims that a hallucination is a variant of the normal thought process. The patient and his family take a different view. Otherwise, family and friends would not hasten to seek an appointment with a psychiatrist as a matter of urgency. And if the patient interpreted the symprom as some minor and transient anomoly in his thinking, he could correct by trying to avoid self-scrutiny or some other strategem he would not respond as he generally does with a blend of perplexity, agitation, and anger.
>
> (Roth *et al.*, 1996)

Perplexity, agitation, and anger, discontents of the psyche in its fundamental structures of existence, lie at the heart of Foucault's analysis of the distress produced by insanity and the alienation that marks its frantic scramble to recover meaning in a surd world.

The social constructionist view of mental disorder is countered when we recall, with Wittgenstein, Husserl, Heidegger, and many others, that concepts are instruments or tools used for certain purposes in a world in which we are born 'incomplete and premature' and needing techniques to make sense of it (Wittgenstein, Lacan). Even if concepts are produced by social and cultural activity, they are the means of competence and individual adaptation through *praxis* or operations articulating one's engagement with real contexts of lived human activity. The phenomena of the mental world may be conceptually articulated (and therefore with an origin in the mirror world), but they are also embedded and functioning in our natural history (including our social being). The psyche cannot therefore be understood apart from *da-sein* and the intuitive, interactive, and interpersonal skills used in everyday being there and our dealings with what we find there.

Rational, insightful, thinking is distinct from insanity on the one hand and social, cultural, or political deviance on the other. A grasp of the rules linking thoughts to conditions potentiates normative procedures of self-correction and adaptation learnt from others but tested in reality. Aberrations in one's thought may be explicable in terms of a conceptual structure imparted by one's primary cognitive group or a certain societal role, and then we need not invoke individual aberrations to explain deviance in thought. For instance, a young man admitted with a set of troubling symptoms spoke of having seen ghosts in his room. He said they were the ghosts of relatives who had come to reassure him in his illness. A 'right-thinking' psychiatric team might, depending on the exact form of the phenomena, conclude that he is hallucinating or deluded but, in his cultural context, ghost visitations are common at times of stress, so his experience was 'normal' for his human group (the phenomenology was also not that of psychotic hallucinations).

Despite the importance of cultural context, an individual can transcend the received or validated opinions and power relations of a group or subculture because each of us participates in a number of discourses in the normal course of living—family discourse, peer discourse, work discourse, gender discourse—and the voices legitimated in these various discursive contexts do not necessarily agree with one another. Power relations in one may not be mirrored in another. As a centre of subjectivity, one has the difficult task of integrating these diverse voices in the face of various aspirations, commitments, and contexts of belonging. The integration that emerges, in the midst of a set of relationships, at a certain point in time and in a given cultural context is understandably (more or less) unique. A normal human being is good enough at the integrative trick most of the time and, in the process, learns successfully to negotiate the highly complex life-world carved out by human activity on the face of the already complex natural world. The resulting psychosomatic unity is inscribed by many different discursive formations in dynamic equilibrium the point of balance of which can shift gradually or change schismatically at any point in a lived autobiographical narrative.

5.12 Conceptions of psychosis

The complex biopsychosocial phenomenon that is mental disorder can be understood in a way that attends to brain dysfunction and interpersonal or relational violence as effective causes of twists and turns in the personal narrative of any individual. We can therefore best explore psychiatric phenomenology by making full use of causal, meaningful, and existential analyses of the human condition (Gillett, 1990b). Causal analyses focus on brain mechanisms, physiological disorders of neural function, psychological determinants of temperament and behaviour, and social influences. Meaningful or discursive analyses reflect the world of signification in which the patient is immersed, and a person's trajectory in that world is existential, urgent, and a subject of concern or care (*sorge*) suggesting alternative approaches to clinical phenomenology and the patient's predicament.

The present view accommodates historical and cultural explanations for phenomena such as witch-hunts, Windigo psychosis, and koro and a somewhat different type of explanation for more-or-less universal psychiatric syndromes (Wing, 1978, p. 165). Various mixtures of these quite different explanations illuminate different aspects of psychosis, hysteria, and anorexic syndromes, all of which may involve false thinking about oneself, one's relationships with others, and the states of one's body. Understandings of insight, rationality, and delusion, indeed of mental life and content, incorporating discursive analyses are both dynamic (in a broad sense) and person-centred, focusing attention on persons and their engagement (both articulate and tacit or primordial) in a shared life-world. That framework becomes even more apparent as we move on from psychosis to autism, and the development of personality.

5.13 **Philosophical questions**

A raft of perennial philosophical questions concern perception, consciousness, belief, motivation, reason, thought, understanding, and self-consciousness, all of which have figured quite prominently in the present discussion.

Perception as reception

The 'passive picture theory' of perception characteristic of traditional empiricism (Bolton & Hill, 1996) still holds sway in some philosophical accounts (Millikan, 1991). The human subject is seen as a receiver of impressions caused by conditions in the world from which inference constructs a picture of what has caused them. Post-empiricists note the role of judgement, organization, packaging, attentional selection, and the sorting of information in conscious and unconscious thought and our modes of attunement to a shared world (cf. Bolton & Hill, 1996; Hundert, 1989).

> During the last while back, I have noticed that noises all seem to be louder to me than they were before. It's as if someone had turned up the volume ... I notice it most in background noises—you know what I mean, noises that are always around you but you don't notice them. Now they seem to be just as loud and sometimes louder than the main noises that are going on ... It's a bit alarming at times because it makes it difficult to keep your mind on something when there's so much going on that you can't help listening to.
>
> (McGhie, 1969, p. 46)

This is perhaps as close as we can come to an account of what it would be like to be a passive perceiver even though the picture is confounded because of the *noetic* activity structuring the networks of information processing that receives and channels the incoming information. Normal perception relies on active cognitive skills, otherwise.

> Consciousness would be flooded with an undifferentiated mass of incoming sensory data, transmitted from the environment via the sense organs. To this involuntary tide of impressions, there would be added the diverse internal images, and their associations, which would no longer be coordinated with incoming information . . . If the incoming flood were to carry on unchecked, it would gradually sweep away the stable constructs of a former reality.

> (McGhie, 1969, p. 49)

A somewhat more sophisticated picture of sensation and perception (as in phenomenological analyses) informs contemporary cognitive science whereby distinctions between 'thematic' and 'automatic' consciousness and the differentiation of figure and ground inherent in the noetic phase of experience as a being-in-the-world allow us to appreciate the techniques involved in any significant experience (Gallagher, 2005; Wittgenstein, 1953 [esp IIxi]).

The argument from hallucination

Recall the sceptical argument from hallucination.

(1) Hallucinations are sensory experiences which have no basis in the external world.

(2) A hallucination could be so vivid that a person would mistake it for reality. Or,

(2a) A person might have a hallucination of such clarity and distinctness that he or she cannot tell that it is not real.

(3) It is possible that at any moment what I take to be reality might be a hallucination emanating from my own brain.

The present analysis of psychotic experience blocks the move from 2 or 2a to 3 by inserting defeating premises.

(2ax) A person having hallucinations has great difficulty in correctly discerning the content of experiences so as to derive from experience what Descartes calls 'clear and distinct ideas'.

(2bx) This is because people having psychotic experiences have impaired skills of ordering experience and discerning its significance.

(2cx) Normal people, including myself, use these skills to form clear and distinct ideas that distinguish perceptions from imaginary and/or psychotic experiences everyday.

Therefore,

(3a) It is not possible that at any moment what I take as reality might be a hallucination.

The argument accepts a reductive (rather than holistic) reading of psychosis and the disruptions of experience and this mistakenly allows the assimilation of hallucinations to normal perceptual experiences in a way which is untrue to the phenomenology of both normal and psychotic consciousness.

Insight and belief

The fact that patients with schizophrenia may lack insight into their own condition and be plagued by bizarre beliefs about themselves and the world they inhabit is sometimes treated as a question to be dealt with in terms of simple truth and falsity. The problem with psychotic thinking is not that it is false or ill-grounded but that the whole process of belief formation and indwelling one's experience of the world is derailed by a dysfunction of those skills engaging self with the world in the balanced, flexible, and responsive way that is natural for human beings. Traditional epistemic categories of true versus false and rationally sound versus inferentially unsound therefore do not capture the ways in which a human being can be alienated from the world. Negotiating a correct assessment of one's experience and sensitively using that in understanding according to the informal rules governing meaning and inference in everyday discourse is unhinged in psychotic thought even though fragments of clarity and intact performance may survive. The intersubjective elements of being-in-the-world also come into prominence in relation to the very different dysfunctions found in autism and Asperger's syndrome.

Thus, schizophrenia, in its various forms, is an actualization of the perils of the human condition in which social mystification and biological disturbances can operate singly or in combination to confound the well-travelled paths of cognition articulating lived human subjectivity. A profound biological disturbance seems to be necessary to produce schizophrenia, but whether its primary aetiology is always and only biological is not so clear. Perhaps, there are cases in which the cumulative effects of biology and a highly abnormal discursive environment engenders both the biochemical and psychic manifestations of psychotic disorder by unsettling a person's attunement to the human life-world (perhaps only temporarily).

Chapter 6

The black dog and the muse

I raced about like a crazed weasel, bubbling with plans and enthusiasms, immersed in sports, and staying up all night, night after night, out with friends, reading everything that wasn't nailed down, filling manuscript books with poems and fragments of plays, and making expansive, completely unrealistic, plans for my future.

I lost all interest in my schoolwork, friends, reading, wandering, or daydreaming. I had no idea what was happening to me, and I would wake up in the morning with a profound sense of dread that I was going to have to somehow make it through another entire day. I would sit for hour after hour in the undergraduate library, unable to muster up enough energy to go to class . . . When I did go to class it was pointless. Pointless and painful. I understood very little of what was going on, and I felt as if only dying would release me from the overwhelming sense of inadequacy and blackness.

I kept on with my life at a frightening pace. I worked ridiculously long hours and slept next to not at all. When I went home at night, it was to a place of increasing chaos; books, many of them newly purchased, were strewn everywhere. Clothes were piled up in mounds in every room, and there were unemptied shopping bags as far as the eye could see . . . The chaos in my mind began to mirror the chaos of my rooms. I could no longer process what I was hearing; I became confused, scared, and disoriented . . . I could not follow the path of my own thoughts. Sentences flew around in my head and fragmented first into phrases and then words; finally, only sounds remained. . . One evening, I stood in the middle

of my living room and looked out at a blood red sunset spreading out over the horizon of the Pacific. Suddenly, I felt a strange sense of light at the back of my eyes and almost immediately saw a huge black centrifuge inside my head. I saw a tall figure in a floor length evening gown approach the centrifuge with a vase-sized glass tube of blood in her hand . . . Then, horrifyingly, the image that had previously been inside my head now was completely outside of it . . . The spinning of the centrifuge and the clanking of the glass tube against the metal became louder and louder, and then the machine splintered into a thousand pieces. Blood was everywhere. It splattered against the windowpanes, against the walls and paintings, and soaked down into the carpets.
(Jamison, 1996, pp. 36, 44, 78–80)

This is a first-person account of a sufferer of bipolar disorder who is also a clinical authority on Manic-Depressive Disorder/Bipolar Disorder (MDD/BD). Among other things, she discusses the curious link between BD and creativity, and her writings reveal the sense of well-being that often accompanies mania, phenomena with profound ethical implications. A third theme is the nature of moods, mental states without objects, highly relevant to an account of the mind and its disorders based on intentionality (the object-directedness of thought).

6.1 **Bipolar disorder**

Winston Churchill, like his ancestor the first Duke of Marlborough, suffered prolonged and recurrent fits of depression. His own name for his depression was 'black dog': a nickname suggesting that it was an all-too-familiar companion (Storr, 1989, p. 5). Churchill's family had a history of mood disorders (or disorders of affect), the most notorious being Manic-Depressive Psychosis or bipolar II disorder (DSM IV [APA, 1994a]), a disorder of mood or affect exhibiting both manic or mixed (manic and depressive features) and depressive episodes. The major fluctuations in mood are often associated with significant disturbances of thought and mental content of the type illustrated by Kay Redfield Jamison's autobiographical reflections.

The disorder is dramatic; manic episodes are marked by 'a persistently elevated, expansive, or irritable mood' accompanied by one or more of 'inflated self-esteem or grandiosity, decreased need for sleep, pressure of speech, flight of ideas, distractibility, increased involvement in goal-directed activities, or psychomotor agitation' (DSM IV [APA, 1994a, p. 328]):

> During hypomania and mania, mood is generally elevated and expansive (or, not infrequently, paranoid and irritable); activity and energy levels are greatly increased; the

need for sleep is decreased; speech is often rapid, excitable, and intrusive; and thinking is fast, moving quickly from topic to topic.

(Jamison, 1996, p. 13)

Depressive episodes plumb the depths of human misery as is evident in Jamison's description and the list of features in DSM IV: 'depressed mood', 'loss of interest or pleasure in nearly all activities', 'feelings of worthlessness or guilt', 'recurrent thoughts of death or suicidal ideation, plans, or attempts' (p. 320), and '[p]atients sometimes speak of a black cloud pervading all mental activities' (Gelder *et al.*, 1983, p. 187). There are also 'vegetative' or biological features such as psychomotor retardation, loss of weight, loss of appetite, sleep disturbance, loss of libido and lethargy (Gelder *et al.*, 1983, p. 187) and, in some cases, anxiety, irritability, agitation, and restlessness, and marked impairment in social functioning or frank psychotic features (DSM IV [APA, 1994a, p. 333]), symptoms that signal for some a spiritual crisis in their lives.

These events may be precipitated by stress, but there is a tenfold increase of risk in first-degree relatives and a concordance rate for monozygotic twins (whether reared together or apart) of 67% (Gelder *et al.*, 1983, p. 203) even though it seems likely that stressful life events, illness, or substance abuse might act as the 'last straw' in precipitating an episode. Jamison (1993) assembles a number of convincing genealogies of prominent artists and writers with mood disorder or related conditions even though the phenomenological link with spiritual crises suggests that we should look beyond the purely biological synthesis of the disorder.

The co-morbid conditions associated with mood disorders are significant: intrafamilial abuse and violence, academic or occupational failure, marital breakdown, substance abuse, antisocial behaviour, and suicide all appear in the list (DSM IV [APA, 1994a, p. 354]).

> In addition to drinking and using drugs to excess, individuals with depressive and manic-depressive illnesses are also far more likely to commit suicide than individuals in any other psychiatric or medical risk group.

(Jamison, 1996, p. 41)

The clinical profile of BD can be devastating, but also can be obscured by the fact that the individual with bipolar disorder, when hypomanic, may be highly amusing and exciting to be with and between episodes is often both interesting and engaging (particularly in bipolar I disorder). Many artists and highly intelligent and achieving people suffer from the disorder and yet maintain an active and productive life, somehow sustaining their personal relationships and commitments despite the considerable obstacles to doing so.

> The clinical reality of manic-depressive illness is far more lethal and infinitely more complex than the current psychiatric nomenclature *bipolar disorder* would suggest. Cycles of fluctuating moods and energy levels serve as a background to constantly changing thoughts, behaviours, and feelings. The illness encompasses the range of human experience: thinking can range from florid psychosis or 'madness', to patterns of unusually clear, fast, and creative associations, to retardation so profound that no meaningful mental activity can occur.

(Jamison, 1996, p. 47)

Again, we see a glimpse of a state of being that plumbs the depths of human disaffection and scales the heights of inspir(it)ation. Michel Foucault (1973) devotes considerable attention to a form of madness that sounds very much like bipolar disorder, contending that '[t]he possibility of madness is . . . implicit in the very phenomenon of passion' (p. 88). He describes a state poised between mania and catatonia.

> There comes a moment in the course of passion when laws are suspended as though of their own accord, when movement either abruptly stops, without collision or absorption of any kind of active force, or is propagated, the action ceasing only at the climax of the paroxysm. (p. 89)

Foucault remarks on the psychosomatic unity of such states: 'the affection of the brain is of the same quality, of the same origin, of the same nature, finally, as the affection of the soul' (p. 88). He speaks, paradoxically, of the liberty from everyday constraints as a force that binds the madman in the grip of madness (p. 93), drawing attention to a freedom that, by its lack of disciplines or rules, is a kind of bondage. His insight, grounded in the idea that the disciplines through inscribing us constitute the soul (1984, p. 177), reinforces the link between defects of rule following and disorders of thought suggesting the connection between madness and imagination that surfaces in the vivid and disturbing images of Jamison's melancholic delusion. Foucault's comments on the connection between artistic achievements and madness precede and go beyond most contemporary discussions of that problem (Jamison, 1993).

BD has a familial incidence, particularly evident in relation to the creativity that often seems to be associated with it in certain families who are prominent in the creative arts, such as those of Tennyson, Schumann, Henry James, and Virginia Woolf: 'The families . . . share in common certain themes of madness, suicide, destructive patterns of drug and alcohol use, and financial chaos; however, uncommon ability and originality are often present as well' (Jamison, 1993, p. 235). This fact alone provokes difficult clinical questions about treatment and the positive and negative evaluations placed on suppression of symptoms or manifestations of BD. There is little doubt that BD is a serious and life-threatening disease; there is, for instance, probably a more than 100-fold increase in suicide rates (10–17% compared with 4–40/100,000 in the normal population). Therefore, treatment may be indicated on these grounds; 'mortality studies . . . carried out on lithium-treated patients . . . have shown that the mortality of manic-depressive patients given long-term lithium treatment is markedly lower than that of patients not receiving such treatment' (Schou, 1997, p. 11). However, there are downsides to this harm prevention and lithium treatment has its detractors (Moncrieff, 1997).

The ethical question about treatment turns not only on issues of morbidity and mortality but also on issues related to the possible suppression of positive and creative features of a life otherwise marred by BD. To explore these, we turn to the nature of creativity and the association between the creative or artistic life and BD, attending closely to first-person accounts of the phenomenology of BD and first-person evaluations of the relative merits of life with and without treatment. There is also the more radical question about what is revealed to the person who violates the codes of conduct and taboos of society to the point that their adaptation to the shared human life world is disrupted.

6.2 **What is creativity?**

The link between creativity and unreason has a long intellectual history.

> For the poets tell us, don't they, that the melodies they bring us are gathered from rills that run with honey, out of glens and gardens of the Muses, and they bring them as the bees do honey, flying like the bees? And what they say is true, for a poet is a light and winged thing, and holy, and never able to compose until he has become inspired, and is beside himself, and reason is no longer in him.

> (Plato, 1961, p. 219)

Kant (1790/1951) argues that aesthetic genius 'is the exemplary originality of the natural gifts of a subject in the free employment of his cognitive faculties' (p. 161). 'Freedom' here goes beyond the spontaneity that distances reason from the causal effects of being-in-the-world (so that thought is governed by 'oughts' and logical requirements) and embraces the play of thought in the domain of representation (the mirror world).

> The mental powers, therefore, whose union (in a certain relation) constitutes genius are imagination and understanding. In the employment of the imagination for cognition, it submits to the constraint of the understanding and is subject to the limitation of being conformable to the concept of the latter. On the contrary, in an aesthetical point of view, it is free to furnish unsought, over and above that agreement with a concept, abundance of undeveloped material for the understanding, to which it applies, though not objectively for cognition yet subjectively to quicken the cognitive powers and therefore also indirectly to cognitions.

> (Kant, 1790/1951, p. 160)

Kant scholars probably find this passage pellucidly clear, but certain clarifications may be needed for ordinary mortals. Kant uses the term 'cognitive' both in a technical sense (as the empirical understanding of experience by which we come to knowledge of the actual objective world and the events and laws of nature that operate within it) and in a more commonsensical way (as the thinking involved in all mental activity). Kant holds that, in ordinary empirical knowledge, the imagination marshals images and possible images conforming to the discursive constraints of a concept that tell us whether the concept is instanced in current experience. He acknowledges that artistic creativity, as a species of general thought or cognition, ranges freely over the resources of the imagination to furnish images that may have no actual world correlate but which inspire thinking unconstrained by the demands of everyday (law-governed) empirical knowledge. The freedom in artistic cognitive activity is liberty or license and not *spontaneity* in the rather special sense he uses that (to defeat a crass causal naturalism about human reason). Kant is prepared, in a way resonant with Plato, to see a certain liberty or even unconstrained profligacy of cognitive activity as having a role in art (and perhaps in metaphor and revelation, whether scientific or theological) that it should not play in ordinary reasoning and knowledge of facts according to the paths of reason.

The present work, contrasts the constraints of reason with the impulses and unreflective associations of the primary process on the one hand and the loose associations of psychosis on the other. Some find the escape from reason common to both of these aspects of mind suggestive in terms of a theory of psychosis and it is indeed tempting to link the primary process and the hunches, insights, and moments of inspiration connecting contiguities and condensations of images in artistic creation.

> It is not easy for dry academicians to accept that syncretistic primary-process techniques rather than analytic clarity of detail are needed by the creative thinker to control the vast complexities of his work.
>
> (Ehrenzweig, 1976)

Ehrenzweig suggests that the kinds of links made in the unconscious (leaps from point to point in the network of signifiers and associated significations) are used by the artist in the creative process. This implies that the relevant techniques are not organized according to the rule-governed transitions prevalent in ordinary thought (based on the narrow needs for survival and adaptation, or the survival of a particular theoretically driven view of the world). However, even if they do not obey the normal rules of discourse, there are real connections here that are neither obvious nor easily identified. These connections are mediated according to the primary process, and therefore meaningful to all of us, but with a structural connection to the free play of imagination, and an idiosyncratic character making each artistic work unique and original. Thus, there is a relation between creativity and the unconscious: 'creative activity is not a direct relation of deliberate intention; much of its impetus and significance remain hidden from the individual creator and, quite possibly, from those in his or her community as well' (Gardner, 1993, p. 24).

A further insight arises from studies of the personality, relationships, and the unconscious aspects of mental life discerned in the psychology of creative women. 'Ambivalence towards the mother, the need for autonomy, and the development of strong symbolic interests, a father who seems to have modelled the use of intellectual activity for self-expression and for purpose in life—this constellation recurs' (Helson, 1976, p. 248).

The influence of Chodorow's (1978) thesis that girls naturally gravitate towards identification with the mother is evident, suggesting that creative women are unconventional in that they both identify and are attracted to the father and his intellectual status, and yet are also alienated from him. The unconventionality of such attitudes of the psyche might be expected to lead a creative woman not to accept common stereotypes and thought patterns and to turn that difference to good effect in her creative achievements.

Creatively intelligent children are similarly unconventional in that 'high creativity children, whether high or low regarding intelligence, are more willing to postulate relationships between somewhat dissimilar events' (Wallach & Kogan, 1976, p. 215). Gardner (1993) refers to 'divergent thinking' (p. 20) in keeping with Ehrenzweig's observations about syncretism and the non-orderly associations arising in the unconscious, yet somehow resonating with human structures of meaning (and their complex layers of connection).

Creativity goes along with a qualitative and quantitative increase in ideas prompted by cognitive tasks (such as the challenge to create figures out of geometrical elements, the possibility of closing incomplete figures in novel or non-obvious ways, and the imagining of a purpose for objects constructed from simple components): 'children scoring high on tests of creative thinking initiated a larger number of ideas, produced more original ideas, and gave more explanations of the workings of unfamiliar science toys than did their less creative peers' (Torrance, 1976, p. 223). Creative individuals also evince far less stereotypy and commonality in their responses than that shown by subjects rated relatively low on creativity (Mednick, 1976, p. 231). Taken together, these studies suggest that creativity is more common where fertile and unconventional cognitive fields inform the individual (through a conscious and unconscious 'network of signifiers').

The idea that a creative individual has an unconventional mental world is reinforced and extended when we consider the relationship between the creative individual and his or her context. Gardner (1993) argues that there needs to be a fruitful asynchrony between the creative *individual's personal talents*, the *accepted ways of proceeding* in the domain in which the individual works, and the *individuals and institutions* comprising the relevant field (pp. 40–41). The asynchronies may involve any of the three nodes of 'the creativity triangle' (Gardner) or a novel mismatch between them such that there is 'an unusual profile of intelligences within an individual', or 'a domain which is experiencing a large amount of tension', or 'a field that is just beginning to shift in a new direction' (p. 41).

Other factors relate to motivation, affect, and interest in creative individuals:

> Such individuals engage in a wide and broadly interconnected network of enterprises; exhibit a sense of purpose or will that permeates their entire network, giving direction to their daily and their yearly activities; favour the creation and the exploitation of images of a wide scope . . . and display a close and continuing affective tie to the elements, problems, or phenomena that are being studied.
>
> (Gardner, 1993, p. 23)

This energy and breadth of thought are highly reminiscent of Jamison's reflections on mania. These philosophical and psychological reflections reveal aspects of creativity and the psyche but do they help answer the vexed question of BD and creativity?

6.3 **Creativity and bipolar disorder**

Jamison (1993) argues that there is a relation between creativity and bipolar disorder: 'the manic-depressive and artistic temperaments are, in many ways, overlapping ones . . . causally related to one another' (p. 237). Despite problems with causal accounts of the psyche, this relation is deeply instructive.

> Many of the changes in mood, thinking, and perception that characterize the mildly manic states—restlessness, ebullience, expansiveness, irritability, grandiosity, quickened and more finely tuned senses, intensity of emotional experiences, diversity of thought, and rapidity of associational processes—are highly characteristic of creative thought as well.
>
> (Jamison, 1993, p. 105)

Jamison (1993) mentions two aspects of hypomanic cognition also encountered in creative thought: 'fluency, rapidity, and flexibility of thought on the one hand and the ability to form new and original connections on the other' (p. 105). The loosening of associations and release of the attention mechanisms from stereotyped social grooves in psychosis suggest that creativity might be enhanced by BD (which does not imply that acute psychotic states such as mania or severe agitated melancholia are conducive to creative work, because in such states the creative energies are so unfocused and the mind so disordered that it would be difficult for anything significant to be produced).

That aside, the syncretistic, adventitious, and opportunistic trains of association in psychotic thinking and the global drivenness of mild mania seem likely to potentiate periods of sustained and prodigious creative output. The crucial fact that distinguishes unstructured ravings from creative output has nothing to do with measures applied to the behaviour but with its vital and grounded connection both *to the truth* (perhaps literary or artistic truth) and *with others* to whom it speaks.

The other and darker side of BD also has implications for creativity. 'Profound melancholy or the suffering of psychosis can fundamentally change an individual's expectations and beliefs about the nature duration and meaning of life, the nature of man, and the fragility and resilience of the human spirit' (Jamison, 1993, p. 117).

Many of the creative works that we most admire put us in touch with the darker side of human nature and are melancholic reflections on human life and meaning. Fyodor Dostoevsky, William Blake, Victor Hugo, Sylvia Plath, Percy Bysshe Shelley, Robert Schumann, Herman Melville, and Vincent van Gogh (all mentioned by Jamison) are authors who, in sometimes 'dark' works, offer sensitive and insightful commentary on the human condition. For some, the pain that is a bipolar crisis of either kind may only be resolved by a voyage of discovery rather than a quick fix, ignoring its depth and the healing available in the true meaning of human life.

If the resonance of human experience creates a narrative sufficiently rich to indwell, then at least some reflection of the depths of human misery might be essential to it. In fact, the metaphor of depth conveys something of what we mean by insight in human thought.

> Depression forces a view on reality, usually neither sought nor welcome, that looks out onto the fleeting nature of life, its decaying core, the finality of death, and the finite role played by man in the history of the universe.
>
> (Jamison, 1993, p. 119)

Mood gives tone and colour to our ways of seeing and signifying situations, as Jamison (1993) notes:

> Manic patients . . . tend not only to speak more, and more rapidly, but also to use more colorful and powerful speech, including more action verbs and adjectives . . . Manic patients tend to use vivid and highly contrasting colors; depressed patients, on the other hand, use primarily black and cold darker colors. (p. 127)

It is hard to resist concluding that the fact that an artist suffers from BD is significant in his or her art and entire way of being in the world.

Foucault (1973) also finds in the visions of artists a striking connection between, on the one hand, the irrational nature of madness and, on the other, insight, creativity, and inspiration:

> And this madness that links and divides time, that twists the world into the ring of a single night, this madness so foreign to the experience of its contemporaries, does it not

transmit—to those able to receive it, to Nietzsche and Artaud—those barely audible voices of classical unreason, in which it was always a question of nothingness and night, but amplifying them now to shrieks and frenzy. (p. 281)

Amplifying to shrieks and frenzy can mean that madness and art stand in opposition to one another because art comes into being at a point of delicate balance where the individual glimpses things that are profound and unsettling, about him or herself and human beings in general, but does not succumb to the disruption of the psyche that these insights threaten to provoke and that would render him or her incoherent. A kind of 'divine madness' may be at the heart of artistic and creative inspiration, but it does not destroy the adventure or symbolic significance of the act of creation, 'an act placed in the bipolar field of the sacred and the profane, the licit and the illicit, the religious and the blasphemous' (Foucault, 1984, p. 108). The act of creation, for Foucault, is at a limit where significance and meaning are almost but not quite caught up in disorienting and dizzying possibilities, a fragile point of creativity central to understanding the link between BD and the artistic process.

Foucault (1984) not only discusses the creative arts but also innovations in scientific thought. He argues that Freud, for instance, 'made possible not only a certain number of analogies but also (and equally important) a certain number of differences' (p. 114), recalling Gardner's suggestion that a mismatch or asynchrony in 'the creativity triangle' (whereby analogies and differences begin to intend multiple novel possibilities) is part of the creative process. Foucault (1984) poses an interesting question about this liminal space, a zone on the edge of chaos:

> How can one reduce the great peril, the great danger with which fiction threatens our world? The answer is one can reduce it with the author. The author allows a limitation of the cancerous and dangerous proliferation of significations within a world where one is thrifty not only with one's resources and riches but also with one's discourses and significations. (p. 118)

In this profoundly enlightening passage, Foucault, locating subjective and meaningful phenomena primarily in discourse and relations of power, argues that the novel developments in human thought arise, *in potentia* as it were, among the complex conflicts inherent in the domain of signification. The author, in touch with that domain but anchored in an actual world of lived subjectivity, 'limits, excludes, and chooses' (1984, p. 119) from the promiscuous interplay of meanings to which a human subject can relate. But the author can only serve this function as long as he holds together and imposes some form upon what he is doing from a source of integration for his own subjectivity. Once the author fragments, psychically, he is isolated and insight is obliterated; in this way, madness undermines the function of the author. That is evident in the epigram for Chapter 5 or, indeed, other excerpts from the same work.

> Whatever the reason, we all felt an Injackelating Quiver Giver coming on. The band crowded around me and wanted to know what to expect. I received some revelations. Slowly, I spoke: 'I went through a holocaust and brought World War Three down on my own head. I am the Holy Ghost. This is the last psychological war. I'll tell you a little story. It began when I was seven, when I was playing Runner Across, a game we played at school. I fell over and scraped my knees on the asphalt and when I went to the nuns for treatment

they noticed blood on my ankle and when they pulled down my sock they found a four-inch gash that required six stitches. Then years later while scavenging in a rubbish dump, I fell over and cut my wrist. See, on my forehead you can see the scars of crucifixion. I have all the scars of crucifixion. The stone that the builders rejected has become the cornerstone of the temple. I am the Holy Spirit. The Lamb that was slain since the beginning of the world.'

(Gates & Hammond, 1993, p. 95)

Foucault argues that an artist can only serve the function of creativity as long as she (or he) keeps herself (or himself) together, in a sense on behalf of all mankind, making of the significations at play in her (or his) mind something meaningful for her (or his) fellows.

Madness is the absolute break with the world of art; it forms the constitutive moment of abolition, which dissolves in time the truth of a work of art; it draws the exterior edge, the line of dissolution, the contour against the void. (1973, p. 287)

BD is important for creativity, a condition in which the hinge point between madness and meaning is repeatedly met as the subject cycles in and out of mania and melancholia traversing passages of subjectivity during which the mind is fertile, unconstrained, so that signifiers and significations are in exciting play. These are the ingredients par excellence for the authorial or creative function. The patient with BD may have extended periods of normal functioning as a well-loved and appreciated being-among-others, even if there is a (highly variable) progressive deterioration of cognitive function marked by the very process loosening and motivating the many novel connections between signifiers. BD therefore provides us with subjective narratives that make available the fruits arising in the 'borderland' between the everyday bustling market-place of significations and their law-like interactions on the one side and the chaos of unconstrained cognitive activity on the other. This fragile domain where 'the line of dissolution' has not yet been crossed is seen in the hypomanic creativity of Schumann, Shelley, and Byron, and in the schizoid melancholy of Dostoevsky or Kafka.

The moment when, together, the work of art and madness are born and fulfilled is the beginning of the time when the world finds itself arraigned by that work of art and respon- sible before it for what it is.

(Foucault, 1973, p. 289)

Foucault lays before us the responsibility created by the work of art that is inseparable from the fact that the border of madness (and therefore abjection) may be the niche in which it arises. The relation between madness and creativity noted by Jamison, psychological theories of creativity, and many clinical observations of mood disorders and their sufferers therefore raise in a forceful way important ethical questions about the treatment of mood disorders.

The lethal effects of BD do not spare the artistic sufferers of the disorder (such as Sylvia Plath) and a comprehensive catalogue of case studies, family histories, and empirical series demonstrate the association between BD and suicide (Jamison, 1993). What is more, confinement to psychiatric institutions or (historically) lunatic asylums, alcohol and drug abuse and dependency, and bouts of severe physical and social dysfunction are all stigmata of the disease. Despite this frightening morbidity, there is marked ambivalence about psychopharmacological therapy, and particularly, the 'normalizing' effects of maintenance treatments.

> Many artists and writers believe that turmoil, suffering, and extremes in emotional experience are integral not only to the human condition but also to their abilities as artists. They fear that psychiatric treatment will transform them into normal, well-adjusted, dampened, and bloodless souls—unable or unmotivated to write, paint, or compose.
>
> (Jamison, 1993, p. 241)

From a study of creative women writers, Ludwig concludes: 'The high rates of certain emotional disorders in female writers suggested a direct relationship between creativity and psychopathology' (1994, p. 1650). Other researchers concur (Andreason, 1987; Hershman & Lieb, 1988), making the debate about treatment quite pressing.

> Affective illnesses themselves are not something to romanticize. They bring pain and suffering and in their most severe form tragedy and suicide . . . Those that suffer them deserve the best that modern medicine can provide. But how do powerful psychotropic agents influence the generative process; might 'therapeutic' intervention and modulation of mood also threaten the essential creativity of the artist? Or will the muse blossom, freed from the constraints of serious pathology?
>
> (Whybrow, 1994, p. 477)

Numerous subjective reports describe lithium as a 'brake' on creativity but, even though these (subjective or anecdotal) impressions are not always supported by systematic investigations (Jamison, 1993, p. 245ff), the therapeutic imperative must be obeyed with great caution. Schou (1979), a Danish psychiatrist with an early involvement in the use of lithium as prophylaxis in BD, found mixed results in a small group of 24 artists: some reported increased creativity, some decreased output, and some no change (as assessed both objectively and subjectively and in terms of quantity and quality). Those with increased creativity reported that 'treatment had led to stabilization of their working ability, to better emotional control, greater maturity, and stricter artistic discipline' (p. 101). The patients with reduced productivity commented: 'I have the urge, but ideas do not come as readily as before' and 'I have the idea, but not the drive to put it on paper' (Schou, 1979, p. 101). The consensus seems to be that creative activity is not necessarily reduced or lessened although it may be less violent, extreme, and chaotic, suggesting that one should negotiate treatment with the particular patient concerned in the light of their responses and their aesthetic values (Andreasen & Glick, 1988).

But the problems directly related to creativity are only part of the complex ethical picture.

> Overall, there appears to be little evidence that lithium is effective for three of its commonly recommended uses: treatment of acute mania, prophylaxis of bipolar disorder, and augmentation of treatment in resistant depression. In addition, naturalistic follow-up studies fail to reveal any beneficial effect of lithium on the course of bipolar disorder.
>
> (Moncrieff, 1997, p. 117)

This uncertainty, combined with the very real risks of long-term lithium treatment and the subjective problems some patients experience, implies that patient refusal is ethically defensible and a therapeutic partnership between the health-care team and patient is essential. We ought to notice that drugs for maladies of the soul might be analogous to fast food as a response to hunger, and no substitute for the deep nourishment (of body, soul, and spirit) needed by the sufferer (usually received from family and friends, a circle of love). When we consider the importance of epigenetics for gene expression, we strike a further ethical problem that arises in relation to every heritable disorder.

Once we isolate and learn to detect genetic abnormalities predisposing an individual to a genetically mediated disorder, certain choices arise (Gillett, 2005). Should we try to select embryos that do not have the genetic defect? Should we try to modify the genetic material of affected individuals so that they develop with a more 'normal' genetic constitution? These ethical issues are pressing as a result of the human genome project and its promises in terms of our understanding of the genetic resources of the human race. BD is a test case for those issues that touch our lives and values.

6.4 **Two ethical problems**

Jamison (1993) notes that '[m]anic depressive illness appears to convey its advantages not only through its relation to the artistic temperament and imagination, but through its influence on many eminent scientists as well as business, religious, military, and political leaders' (p. 252), a remark recalling Winston Churchill and his black dog. Andreason (1987), reflecting on her prevalence studies among creative individuals, remarks 'affective disorder may produce some cultural advantages for society as a whole, in spite of the individual pain and suffering that it also causes. Affective disorder may be both a "hereditary taint" and a hereditary gift' (p. 292). Two ethical problems therefore arise: the first is *the unwitting sacrifice problem* and *the second the stigmatization of difference problem*.

6.4.1 **The unwitting sacrifice problem**

The significant morbidity and mortality of BD means that bringing a child into the world who is likely to develop it deliberately exposes an innocent and unconsenting human being to a risk of suffering. The suffering may, however, be offset by the gains that the rest of us may obtain from that person's life; but is it right to create unwitting sacrifices in this way? Imagine putting the problem to the embryo with the relevant genetic alteration.

> 'We are going to continue your life because, although you do not know it and have not chosen it, you are likely to bring certain advantages to us. The price you pay is that you will be affected by a somewhat unpredictable disease that may make you insane from time to time, cause you to go through periods of black despair and personal suffering, predispose you to become addicted to noxious substances, and perhaps even cause you to take your own life in an attempt to escape your torment. We could modify the genes carrying that risk but we have chosen not to. WE ARE NOT GOING TO ASK FOR YOUR ASSENT TO THIS CHOICE WE ARE MAKING.'

The ethical problems are quite evident and perhaps the embryo ought to say, 'If you do this, pray to God to give you strength to surround me with the love, support, and care I will need to stay alive and be healed as part of our victory over the genetic dangers that threaten me.' In any event, we need to ask whether we are justified in imposing this unwelcome choice.

6.4.2 **The stigmatization of difference problem**

A number of disabled people and groups have argued that selection against a genetic disorder seriously devalues the lives of those born with that disorder by conveying the message that it would have been better if they had not been born. The argument applies both to selecting against and to genetically modifying individuals carrying a genetic risk of BD. We seem implicitly to be saying, 'To live as a person like you is a bad thing and to eradicate people like you is a good and compassionate thing.' The motivation, although compassionate, arguably seems to 'compromise the respect we should feel for their differentness, independence, strength of mind, and individuality' (Jamison, 1993, p. 259), which sounds like a bad thing to do.

So, we now turn to other philosophical and ethical problems posed by BD and affective disorders.

6.5 **Mild mania and well-being**

Theories in moral philosophy often take *well-being* to be an important feature of any account of goodness and badness. But what is well-being? A neo-Aristotelian answer to this question is that human well-being is a state of excellence of functioning of a rational and social being (*eudaimoneia*) and that this is an ultimate value in any good moral theory (Barnes, 1982). The answer assumes that well-being goes along with normal function; so, why would a person with BD remark that she is best when she is mildly manic (Jamison, 1996, p. 92). The problem is thrown into sharp relief by the case of Mr M (Moore *et al.*, 1994).

> Mr. M was a teacher, and a married man with two daughters. He was referred to a psychiatrist at the age of forty-three, having been hospitalized and given electroconvulsive therapy (ECT) following a severe depressive episode. His psychiatrist found that Mr. M had experienced a similar episode seven years previously, and in the light of this, pre-scribed lithium as prophylaxis against further depressive relapses. (p. 166)

Mr. M begins, on occasion, to experiment with periods off the drug.

> [W]hen he was not taking lithium, he felt full of energy. He found his wife and family boring and claimed that his marriage had never been good. During his six-month period off lithium, he began an affair with a female colleague, openly expressing his intention to leave his wife and to marry his girlfriend . . . Some of his colleagues actually found him more stimulating when he was not taking lithium. Mr. M himself felt more creative during these periods: he composed songs, and his colleagues described him as full of ideas. During the periods when he was taking lithium, Mr. M described his relationship with his girl-friend as superficial and unimportant, and he stopped seeing her. He said that he wanted to stay with his wife and family, and he insisted that this had always been important to

him. He was less-stimulating company, but more reliable, and in terms of written output and effective teaching, he was more productive. (p. 167)

The authors ask what is best regarded as well-being for Mr. M and consider several theories including hedonism, desire-fulfilment theory, and objectivism.

Hedonism, in simple terms, is the theory that underlies the popular slogan: *If it feels good, do it.* It is usually taken to mean that the value most important in human lives is something like happiness or pleasure. On that basis, we might say to Mr. M, 'Do what makes you happier.' But that is problematic for two reasons. First, he might be happy off lithium in a different way from the way that he is happy on lithium—for instance, as (*inter alia*) a rake and a gypsy romantic rather than a father and husband. Alternatively, he might say that he could never be satisfied with himself if he settled for something as superficial as happiness or pleasure as the determinant of the value of his life. The second source of unease captures our intuitive sense that hedonist values are shallow and miss what we consider worthwhile about a human life. Think, for instance, of someone to whom the struggle to save academic standards in the universities is very important even though, comfortable as the person is and secure in her own job as a senior and well-respected professor, she sacrifices a lot of enjoyable and relaxing recreation in service of that cause. Whatever one thinks about her values, they are admirable and one can appreciate her dedication. But the value prevailing here is not contentment, happiness, or any other (plausibly biological) state of pleasure; it is something else.

That dissatisfaction does not, however, address Mr. M's first source of unease based on the very different kinds of good characterizing each of his two ways of being so that advice to do what he really desires (or whatever gives him most pleasure) misses the mark. He has two different sets of desires and it is unclear that there is any way of choosing between them or that either set of desires can be judged as likely to lead to a better life overall.

We are all beset by all kinds of desires all the time and some of them should not be satisfied in the light of who one is and the kind of life one values. Imagine, for instance, that Zoltan desires, among other things, to shatter the heads of perfect red rose (a desire with which Freudians would have a field day) and, furthermore, that sometimes this desire is so strong that it is hard to resist. Imagine that he also believes that such a desire is not only trivial but also faintly vicious and should not be indulged. Such a case implies that not all desires are equal and prompts some to invoke 'critical interests' (Dworkin) or 'second-order desires' (Frankfurt). In Zoltan's case, his desire to shatter red roses, though strong, is not one he endorses; so something apart from the relative strengths of a desire is significant in the value structure shaping his life (Taylor, 1991). Perhaps it is something like critical interests—interests with personal or narrative endorsement as integral to his life and psyche rather than disruptive to it (Smith, 1994; Taylor, 1989). Something of this kind is part of a good theory of well-being but does not meet the second worry—'Who does Mr. M want to be?'

The second worry persists and creates an impasse: 'In a sense, there are two selves in this case, and they have quite different sets of desires' (Moore *et al.*, 1994, p. 171). So which desire set should be endorsed and why? Can one make a clear judgement about the relative value of whole desire sets, when the person himself wavers between them? Is there an objective scale of values against which he and we can assess his whole life narrative?

Aristotle for one seemed to think that objectivism could be formulated in terms of the excellent functioning of a human being: a rational, social, animal (Megone, 1998). Some of the components are already at hand in the concept of *eudaimonea*—'a harmony of the lively demons' (those things which energize and motivate a person). Such a state might involve 'states of character, such as courage, humour, and integrity . . . relations between people . . . committed friendship, and love' (Moore *et al.*, 1994, p. 171). The question is, 'Where do we go from here?' We could direct Mr. M towards a life that maximally satisfies this general set of goods. But immediately we ask, 'Which particular set of general goods does one aim at in Mr. M's case?' We could just opt for one set of goods, but two problems arise. The first is paternalism. Do we have the right to tell him how to live his life? The second problem is relativism.

It is plausible that there are a range of possible sets of goods acceptable in response to the human problem of attaining well-being (Williams, 1981). Acknowledging this plurality, we could argue (with Nussbaum) that a plausible set of goods—desires and values—must be grounded 'in actual human experience' but be able to 'criticize local and traditional moralities in the name of a more inclusive account of the circumstances of human life and the needs for human functioning that those circumstances call forth' (Nussbaum, 1993, p. 250). It is then plausible that Mr-M-on-medication instances one set of desires and values and Mr-M-off-medication instances another. The problem recurs, 'Is there any principled way to choose which set of goods Mr. M should move towards?' Nussbaum (1993) considers that certain elements in the experiences of human groups are 'broadly and deeply shared' (p. 266). Arguably, these elements involve one's connectedness with others through structures of kinship and friendship (Gillett 2004, 2008), elements of which might be relatively enduring or relatively transient.

Moore *et al.* (1994) argue that theories such as hedonism, desire fulfilment theory, and hierarchies of objective goods do not resolve the issues in the case of Mr. M and consider other possible resolutions. Appeals to Mr. M's autonomous and authentic choice, his narrative identity, integration of life plans and projects, his rationality as distinct from the irrationality of mild mania, or the fact that mild mania is an illness all pose problems in that we seem to need the real Mr. M to stand forth—is he the free-wheeling, romantic, and expansive Mr. M or the solid, responsible, caring, respectable, and productive Mr. M, each with their own distinctive values? A rationality favouring boring solidity over 'a walk on the wild side' is suspect for aesthetic reasons (and also unfashionable). Invoking the illness is question-begging in that mania, similar to any other biological phenomenon, is only an illness because of the suffering and distress it causes and, for Mr. M, is not independent of the life-narrative problems it poses. To say that an illness is present when there is some disruption in the biological function of the individual concerned (Boorse) is problematic in that mild mania (of the type found in the case of Mr. M) is a disruption similar to religious conversions, radical changes of life values for other reasons, midlife identity crises, or falling in love, none of which are illnesses.

Moore *et al.* (1994) conclude 'that four prima facie alternative approaches to resolving this issue, involving respectively the notions of autonomy, personal identity, rationality, and illness, offer no straightforward solutions' (p. 174). Nordenfelt (1994), commenting on the case, considers classifying Mr. M's mania as an illness because of the fact that it interferes with his 'vital goals', which are 'the set of states that are necessary and together sufficient for A's minimal long-term happiness in life' (p. 180). But again, the two Mr. Ms have different routes to 'minimal long-term happiness', even though this constraint on pluralism excludes impulses and choices arising in scenarios where certain vital goals are threatened by disruptions from uncontrolled deteriorations in a person's illness.

Nordenfelt (1994) does classify mild mania as an illness because of facts such as the possibility of uncontrolled disruptions but cannot decide whether someone like Mr. M ought ever to be treated against his will, a question closely related to what Mr. M's case can tell us about a robust conception of well-being and, in part, addressed by Dawson (2007) in a recent discussion of facilitative freedom in community mental health orders.

Seedhouse (1994) also relies on a theory of health allowing an individual to 'achieve personal and group potentials' (p. 188) and 'to set people's creative potentials free' (p. 190). The appeal to the wider engagement of Mr. M with others implicitly relates well-being and connectedness to others, but Mr. M's case is problematic because, either way, somebody is going to get hurt—his wife and family on the one hand or his 'girlfriend' on the other. Seedhouse (1994) predicates treatment decisions on Mr. M's competence and claims with an air of *fait accompli*: 'All that is necessary is to ask Mr. M when he is competent what he would like to happen when he is not' (p. 191). The obvious objection is that there are two candidates for 'The competent Mr. M'.

Seedhouse (1994) does suggest that counselling may help Mr. M 'clarify his main purposes in life' (p. 191) and thereby gestures that the solution (in the case of Mr. M and often in clinical life) is not theoretical refinements of notions of health or well-being but a practical process of attaining wisdom, through 'argument' (in the sense that argument is to the soul what medicine is to the body), about well-being, or indeed health.

One could opt for a negotiated or pragmatic solution involving both treatment and psychotherapy whereby Mr. M is enabled to reflect on his life and the values he should realize within it. This may involve some constraints on medication and the criteria for using it in the light of his autobiography, personal relationships, satisfactions and dissatisfactions with career and relationship choices, moral commitments, and so on. A kind of authenticity can be deemed to attach to the emergent decision in virtue of the way that it has been arrived at rather than its content. If the process of making a clinical or personal decision is inextricably part of the goodness or badness of that decision and the goodness or otherwise of certain outcomes are less decidable in advance, we are left with a non-consequentialist theory of well-being and human good that is much more in keeping with the theory of individual health (Danzer *et al.*, 2002). What is more, discursive therapy and process-based solutions to problems such as those of Mr. M seem to support the autobiographical reflections of Kay Jamison on the role of psychotherapy in managing her two selves.

However, all of these 'solutions' to Mr. M's dilemma have the same deficiency. They are individualistic and blinkered, thriving on schizoid conversations and negotiations. In fact, this is a situation involving several people, all of whom have deep-seated interests in it and all of whom should be included openly in its resolution. Mr. M, his wife and family, and his girlfriend must, jointly with the therapist, produce the resolution and own it (or take responsibility for it) as something which connects them all to the truth (in the way Foucault suggests).

In a way, the same form of solution can be applied to the unwitting sacrifice problem in which those actually affected by BD and those who care for them need to negotiate a jointly acceptable response to the policy need in the face of increasing genetic knowledge.

6.6 Mood, mind, and intentionality

> Lithium prevents my seductive but disastrous highs, diminishes my depressions, clears out the wool and webbing from my disordered thinking, slows me down, gentles me out, keeps me from ruining my career and relationships, keeps me out of hospital, alive, and makes psychotherapy possible. But, ineffably, psychotherapy heals. It makes some sense of the confusion, reins in the terrifying thoughts and feelings, returns some control and hope and possibility of learning from it all. (Jamison, 1996, pp. 88–89)

If mental phenomena are such because of their intentionality (or aboutness) and moods do not have objects but rather affect one's whole way of thinking about the world, are moods mental states at all? Jamison (1996) would 'wake up in the morning with a profound sense of dread that I was going to have to somehow make it through another entire day'. Her work seemed 'pointless and painful' and she had an 'overwhelming sense of inadequacy and blackness' (p. 44), global changes in thought that seem not to be intentional (in Brentano's sense) and yet are usually regarded as states of mind and not merely of the body.

The claim that the essence of conscious mental acts is intentional falters if we concede that both moods are mental phenomena and yet not individuated by their objects or by being directed on anything; so perhaps, we should modify our theory of mind to accommodate that fact. But moods are not conscious mental acts similar to thoughts and seem, quintessentially, to reflect our psychosomatic unity as beings-in-the-world asking (value-laden or concerned) questions about our own being (Heidegger, Sartre). Two facts stand out about moods:

(1) A mood can only affect thoughts when it attaches to some intentional content or other.

(2) Moods can be changed by 'acts and inner determinations'. (Kant, 1789/1929, B574)

Imagine (*in re* of Fact 1) that I am feeling animated and positive; that state colours the contents of my consciousness in its own characteristic way so that it attaches to the relevant experience. If it was not attached to conscious experience, then it would be just a bodily state affecting me as would a tremor or a surge of nausea. A purely bodily phenomenon (a shiver or *nausea*) only becomes a mental state when it is incorporated into my mental life (by colouring my experience thus and so). Such a state therefore becomes a mental phenomenon through its attachment to, for instance, one's experience of the world today, thoughts about the meaning of life, or feelings about marriage and children. It is a mood because of this entanglement with a subject's intentional life (and may even be caused by what is going on there) and it affects (or is affected by) the meanings (and values) of the 'psychophysical ego' (Husserl, 1950/1999, p. 120) even though no particular content (or object-directedness) is part of its essence as the mood it is and any content will do as its locus of manifestation (much in the way that the soul is manifest in the body). We can now reconsider the phenomenological (Brentano's) claim in the light of a neo-Aristotelian theory of mind.

After Aristotle (1986), we regard mental acts as human functions that are part of the narrative activity of the subject whose *psyche* or soul is the sum total of those functions. Thus, bodily changes and states affect the *psyche* without necessarily being mental in their nature, origins, and effects, and moods have both bodily and intentional properties. What is more, this duality implies that any given mental phenomenon, although weighted towards one type of property rather than the other, dynamically reflects their combination (as implied by Fact 2—their being subject to acts and inner determinations).

That moods are sensitive to mental content and can be altered by mental acts is evident when we consider a directed mood such as being depressed about my exam result or the unsettled and uncomfortable melancholy that might result from a conviction that my family hates me. In such a case, the intentional focus of the mood is a route to its alteration as in cognitive behavioural therapy: I could persuade myself that the exam is not so important that it should have this impact on my life or that my family does not really hate me at all but that I have set them against me at the moment because of something I am doing. In either case, I have to do psychic work. I do not get the mood change for free once the cognitions change even though reflection might start it going and get me some of the way there. Things such as my friend's attitude towards the situation (e.g. if she said 'You have really blown it now with that exam result' or 'I'm sorry, but they really do hate you,' my mood may worsen), therapy, or 'transference work' on my 'stratified, isolated, and resistant interpretations' to give myself a 'new body' (Kristeva, 1995, p. 26) may affect me, because moods are embedded within the nexus of attitudes, beliefs, and values that characterize a psyche. But the phenomenon of non-directed mood—the free-floating variant that attaches to any psychic content that happens to be around—confirms the Aristotelian (and Lacanian) synthesis: a mood is a signification applied to the self on the basis of my actual (unsignified) state of being-in-the-world.

> I had a fabulous, bubbly, seductive, assured time. My psychiatrist, however, in talking with me about it much later, recollected it very differently. I was, he said, dressed in a remarkably provocative way, totally unlike the conservative manner in which he had seen me dressed over the preceding year. I had on much more makeup than usual, and seemed, to him, to be frenetic and far too talkative. He says he remembers having thought to himself, Kay looks manic. I, on the other hand, had thought I was splendid.
>
> (Jamison, 1996, p. 71)

The bodily aspects of moods allow them to colour indiscriminately a wide range of mental acts and, similar to all our subjective states of being, moods are by nature subject to physical factors such as biochemical changes and disruptions of the brain. For moods, non-directed, diffuse, vague, and haphazard relations to other mental events are the norm as for bodily or physiological changes. Consider, for example, the following possibility. 'My mind is in a state at the moment.' You respond, 'What are you concerned about?' The story can go two ways: (i) 'Well, it is about that building over there; I don't know how I feel about it' (this is not a mood but instead an inarticulate intentional state, such as fear, anger, curiosity, and wonder, or something else directed at the building); (ii) 'No, it's not like that I just feel something I find hard to express' (here, there is no intentional attitude and the state resembles a mood). Thus, a mood is a way that I am affected and is an undirected aspect of my psychosomatic being, whereas other mental acts are defined by their intentional content.

Our being is holistic, so the division is only rough and ready as further remarks indicate. The extent to which moods are intentional in nature is indicated by the characteristic way that we report them: 'I feel down, nothing is worth doing' (a mental state affecting the way I evaluate my activity) or 'I am so happy, my mind has been dominated by that exam for months' (a self-attribution linked to a specific object of thought). These are not reported as mere states of my body, and both examples demonstrate the entanglement of moods and thoughts. By contrast, 'I don't seem to have the energy to do anything' or 'Nothing can hold me down, my whole body is itching to move and dance and leap.' These are experienced as bodily states even though, were one to trace their origins, they may well have mental histories (e.g. 'I can hardly believe what I am hearing'; 'What he said has really got to me.')

Moods can cause attitudes to be shaped in a particular way as when depression shapes a person's interpretation of their life events, but events conceived or remembered (such as 'my exam' or 'what I am hearing') also causally influence moods. An achievement, an intellectual insight, or a gratifying message from a friend or acquaintance can elevate one's mood in an enduring way for days or weeks, perhaps beyond the point where one is actually remembering the source of that feeling.

The integration of moods into one's life narrative and thereby their conscious 'fame' (Dennett) as moods, along with the often-observed causal dependence of moods on thoughts (and meaningful relationships), therefore testify to the intentional features of moods even though in the classic sense of taking a discrete mental object they do not seem to be intentional at all.

6.7 **Philosophical puzzles**

We can now revisit our philosophical conundrums.

1. **If creativity involves focused and directed skills producing works of such quality that they are stand out from others, how can a disorder of the mind enhance that ability?**

The argument runs as follows:

(1) Creativity produces exceptionally fine works within an area of human endeavour.

(2) Exceptionally fine works are produced by excellent craftsmen.

(3) To be an excellent craftsman is to exemplify a human competence.

(4) A disorder is a malfunction of human competence.

(5) A person afflicted with a disorder cannot produce an exceptionally fine work.

If, however, there are two components to genuine artistic creativity—the controlled and refined technique constituted by a number of skills specific to a certain domain of creative endeavour; and a fertile stock of images, ideas, and associations falling outside of the bounds of those prescriptions—then the latter is characteristic of manic states. This twofold recipe is supplemented by Foucault's analysis in terms of the artistic work and the need for a human subject to render it accessibly meaningful. The argument fails in that 1 and 2 jointly embody a partial truth and 4 is, again, only a partial truth; thus one could argue:

(a) Creativity may sometimes occur without technical brilliance.

(b) Creativity requires more than just exceptionally fine work.

Therefore, 1 should read:

(1*) Creativity produces exceptional works that often display excellent craftsmanship but always display something more than just craftsmanship.

The 'more' that creativity requires gives a partial lie to 4 in that

(4a) Many disorders are extremes of unusual states.

(4b) In unusual states, experiences have effects beyond those in normal individuals. Then follows:

(5) A person, when actually being afflicted by a disorder, may not be able to produce a meaningful creative work but, as a result of (sometimes) being in an unusual state (such as melancholia or mild mania), can produce a fine and meaningful creative work. This seems (empirically) to be true of patients with BD.

2. If a person feels well and their life is more exciting and enjoyable than normal lives, then what justification do we have for altering their state of mind?

We could call this 'The Doctor Jekyll and Mr Hyde problem' because of its striking resonances with Stevenson's fictional scenario.

> There was something strange in my sensations, something indescribably new, and, from its very novelty, incredibly sweet. I felt younger, lighter, happier in body; within, I was conscious of a heady recklessness, a current of disordered sensual images running like a mill race in my fancy, a solution of the bonds of obligation, an unknown but not an innocent freedom of the soul.
>
> (Stevenson, 1886/1994, p. 44)

This elated state does not seem to be a state in which one would want to be medicated away but its dawning carries, as does the mania of bipolar illness, shadowy and sinister portents.

> I knew myself, at the first breath of this new life, to be more wicked, tenfold more wicked, sold a slave to my original evil, and the thought, in that moment, braced and delighted me like wine. I stretched out my hands, exulting in the freshness of these sensations, and in the act I was aware I had suddenly lost in stature.
>
> (Stevenson, 1886/1994, p. 44)

This passage brings to mind Foucault's 'enslavement of the mad to unconstrained passion'. Indeed, his pleasure at his new self does not last for the unfortunate Dr. Jekyll.

> When I came to myself at Lanyon's, the horror of my old friend affected me somewhat: I do not know; it was at least but a drop in the sea to the abhorrence with which I looked back on those hours. A change had come over me. It was no longer the fear of the gallows; it was the horror of being Hyde that racked me.

> (Stevenson, 1886/1994, p. 52)

This is the justification for treatment canvassed by Nordenfelt (1994), but the Jekyll and Hyde case has two components not found in the medicated and unmedicated selves of Mr. M. First, the unmedicated Mr. M is not horrendously depraved and evil as is Hyde, and second, the change is under his control (he can take or not take his medication). Indeed, Mr. M seems less like Dr. Jekyll than the two possible lives of Gauguin. In any event, whichever the more apt comparison, the process of resolution seems to be an important part of the correct resolution.

(1) An elevated state of mood is generally (and reasonably) valued.

(2) Drugs lessen the likelihood of one being in an elevated state.

(3) Drugs create disvalue and should not be used.

The counter-arguments interpose further premises between 2 and 3.

(2a) Drugs also stabilize one's mood and protect one from certain harms.

(2b) Drugs may allow one to act so as to bring about more favourable terms and conditions for important life projects and commitments (all things considered).

These premises problematize 3 and suggest a negotiated solution in which anindividual and those others intimately involved in the (moral) truth of his being-in-the-world-with-others are helped to reflect on and weigh the factors introduced by 2a and 2b.

3. If a person is gifted and can make a unique contribution to humankind even if that is at some risk, ought we to prevent that by using drugs or other means of changing their mood or, in the extreme, preventing them from being born?

This philosophical conundrum is at the core of *the unwitting sacrifice problem* and can only be resolved by a kind of imaginative identification, helped immeasurably by first-person accounts, with affected or potentially affected individuals. This argument goes as follows:

(1) The gifts of some gifted people go along with a risk of serious harm.

(2) The gifts benefit others.

(3) It is wrong to allow an unconsenting person to put herself at risk of harm to benefit others.

(4) BD patients can reduce their risk of harm by using medication.

(5) (Perhaps) We can also reduce the risk of BD and therefore harm by genetic intervention.

(6) We should not allow BD to go untreated and we should prevent it where possible by genetic intervention.

But imaginative identification and first-person reports suggest that some people with BD prefer the whole package (MDD + the gifts), feeling that overall, despite their sufferings and trials, their lives are worthwhile particularly when society listens to the reply of the embryo. Thus, the counter-argument attacks 2:

(2*) The gifts are valued despite the risk by those who have them and they also benefit others.

Then, 3 has to be modified to

(3*) It is wrong to allow an unconsenting person to receive a whole package including risks and benefits and also benefits to others which they might judge, overall, to be worthwhile.

This does not look nearly as persuasive as 3; in fact, it looks like what happens whenever we give birth to any human being (only in this case there are more extreme positive and negative aspects). It looks even less persuasive when we promise to help the individual stay alive and be healed by our support and care. Therefore, 5 does not unambiguously support 6.

4. If moods are biological, not directed on objects (i.e. not having intentional content), and can be chemically modified, then they are mental states that do not exhibit intentionality and a general doctrine of the intentionality of the mental is flawed.

The argument is best assessed in the following form:

(1) Mental states are intentional (in Brentano's sense) in that they have proper objects.

(2) Moods do not have proper objects.

(3) Moods are not mental states.

But we can relax the condition specified in 1, modifying it to

(1a) Mental states are either intentional in Brentano's sense or are inseparably conjoined with intentional acts directed at objects.

We can then add the following premises:

(1b) Moods are both perturbations of the body and mental phenomena.

(1c) It is essential to the identification of moods as mental phenomena that they attach to intentional states.

We can then accept 2 but reject 3 and substitute as follows:w

(3*) Moods are mental states in virtue of their attachment to intentional states.

Having discussed creativity and BD, we should perhaps note that biomedical science and the phenomena it embraces have other interesting interactions with creativity and particularly the disruptive and intrusive demands of creativity on an otherwise ordered life. A number of myths cluster in this area[1]. We can think of the way that the regularities of thought and the demands of a career in an established profession such as medicine could be thought to inhibit a creative life (cf. the Gauguin phenomenon). The myth receives some confirmation from the highly successful and creative careers in arts and letters that some doctors then go on to pursue when released from their duties of care. A prevailing myth also opposes reason and emotion (in much the way that Plato did). Thus, scientists can be seen as analytical and rational, lacking imagination and bound to highly ordered patterns of thinking. This is, to some extent, true in that careful analysis and cause–effect reasoning are essential in classical sciences but, increasingly, at the growing edge of science where chaos, immensity, and curious concepts such as *entanglement* roam wild and cannot easily be tamed, one needs almost to abandon the straitjacket of reason to begin to see the possibilities. If genius and madness are only separated by 'a whisker', then the whisker seems at times to belong to Schroedinger's cat.

The idea that artists and those with mental disorder are both emotionally gifted and touched by the gods has a long pedigree. Perhaps, the mind's new science and the shifting *mandala* that is the play of consciousness in the human brain, leaving quasi-stable traces and straining our attempts at ordering ourselves and our relations, should always be borne in mind as we deal with the fascinating profiles created by the psyche (as it lives, breathes, and examines itself in the mirror of culture, the source of those meanings that sustain it). It remains true that 'there's now't as queer as folk' and that it is sometimes the queerness of folk that reveals to us the contours of what passes as normal, particularly in its more tortured, or adventurous, forms. We ought also to beware of pathologizing the gifted and touched (by divine fire) because it is possible that in them the (creative) word can come among us uncomprehended but full of grace and truth.

We can now move on from the two forms of psychosis with an evident dependence on and explanation in terms of neurophysiological events to those where the association is more problematic. Despite the clear evidence of biological causes and the importance of biological treatments, the psychoses demonstrate the dual allegiance to biology and meaning that affects the human condition. We are creatures significantly formed by the mirror world and its images, symbols, and connections (both structural and associative), and just as the biological aspect of human subjectivity is fraught with vulnerabilities, so is our human entanglement with the techniques of power and discursive production.

We can first look at two disorders in which the brain as a whole is affected in ways that look like biological defects (affecting *psyche* through *soma*) more enduring and pervasive than any moods are but that interact closely with the discursive world.

---

[1] Brought to my attention by Richard Mullen, a valued colleague in philosophy and psychiatry.

Chapter 7

Fidgets

My sister was diagnosed as having Attention Deficit
Disorder without Hyperactivity when she was about
6 or 7. Soon after, she was put on a double-blinded trial
for the drug methylphenidate (brand name Ritalin),
a stimulant similar to the illegal substance commonly
known as speed. She's been on the drug ever since, and in
that time, we as a family have been able to accurately
monitor her drug intake by her behaviour. A common
phrase heard around our house is '[Barbara] have you
forgotten to take your pills?'
(Massarotto, 1996)

In keeping with its topic, this chapter is the shortest in the book. The syndrome known
as Attention Deficit Hyperactivity Disorder (ADHD) in children raises the question of
the medicalization of life in a pressing way in that some writers argue that ADHD is no
more than a range of undesirable and oppositional behaviours in children who fail to
develop socially validated conduct for any number of different reasons causing the
child to seek stimulation, interest, or escape.

ADHD is increasingly treated with amphetamine-like drugs, but is the treatment in
the best interests of the child or does it serve an agenda set by unrealistic parental
expectations and a school system that has failed the children concerned? This poses
questions about when a disorder is a disorder rather than being a variant of normal
behaviour medicalized by a clinical and pharmacological empire that sees every
departure from tightly bounded 'success' or socially legitimated behaviour as
a problem. The problems of medicalization and the binary construction of normality
and disorder are part of a cluster of problems rendering ADHD apt for philosophical
attention.

7.1 The phenomenology of ADHD

ADHD or *hyperkinetic syndrome*, defined as 'extreme restlessness, impulsiveness,
uncontrolled activity, and poor concentration' (Gelder et al., 1983, p. 657), is the most
common childhood disorder in North-American psychiatry (DSM IV prevalence rate
is 3–5%) but, 'in America, the diagnosis of hyperkinetic syndrome covers a much wider

group of overactive children. As a consequence, the diagnosis is made more frequently in the United States than in Britain' (Gelder et al., 1983, p. 657).

When diagnosed, ADHD is usually treated with Ritalin, a drug related to amphetamine. The difference in rates of diagnosis (up to 40 per 1000 children in the United States but only 1 per 1000 children in the United Kingdom [DSM IV; APA, 1994a, p. 82]) is striking given the treatment options. DSM IV defines ADHD as 'a persistent pattern of inattention and/or hyperactivity-impulsivity more frequent and severe than is typically observed in individuals at a comparable level of development' (p. 78) and the three main components—*inattention*, *impulsivity*, and *hyperactivity*—although distinct, are closely related.

Inattention

The DSM IV (APA, 1994a) lists several characteristics in the affected individual who

 (i) May 'fail to give close attention to details or may make careless mistakes in schoolwork or other tasks' (p. 78);

 (ii) May make 'frequent shifts from one uncompleted activity to another' (p. 78);

(iii) May 'avoid or have a strong dislike for activities that demand sustained self-application' (p. 78); and

(iv) Act in such a way that 'materials necessary for the task are often scattered, lost, or carelessly handled and damaged' (p. 79).

Hyperactivity

This is manifest in various ways:

 (i) 'Fidgetiness or squirming in one's seat' (p. 79);

 (ii) 'Running or climbing in situations where it is inappropriate' (p. 79); and

(iii) By appearing to always be 'on the go' or 'driven' or 'by talking excessively' (p. 79).

Impulsivity

The third feature usually 'manifests itself as impatience, difficulty in delaying responses, blurting out answers before questions have been completed . . . difficulty awaiting one's turn . . . and frequently interrupting or intruding on others' (p. 79).

The DSM requires the manifestations of ADHD to be of sufficient severity to cause 'clinically significant impairment in social, academic, or occupational functioning' and to be evident in more than one social context (p. 84). It also requires that the syndrome persists for more than six months and have been in evidence before the age of 7 (p. 84). Thus defined, ADHD is more common in boys than in girls (Sandberg, 1996, p. 11), with a peak age incidence of 6–9 years. The DSM IV remarks, 'it may be difficult to distinguish symptoms of [ADHD] from age-appropriate behaviours in active children' (p. 82). Gelder et al. (1983), noting the gross difference in prevalence between the United Kingdom and the United States, comment that the overlap between ADHD as defined and normal childhood exuberance (particularly among boys) is alarming and object to 'the wide definition' that is increasingly used.

First, if a wide definition of the hyperkinetic syndrome is used, the symptoms are very varied and do not correlate well with one another. Second, the same symptoms are common in conduct disorders. Third, no sharp dividing line can be drawn between the hyperkinetic syndrome, defined in this broad way, and active normal behaviour. (p. 657)

Their complaint is well motivated: we should be suspicious of any syndrome where the pathological basis is unclear and there is no typical core cluster of manifestations that almost invariably accompany one another. A genuine pathophysiological basis for any disorder is usually a matter of theory and conjecture rather than demonstration even though extensive research has examined the physiological and morphological markers of most mental disorders. Thus, as we have noted, a stereotypical pattern of behaviour, cognition, and affect is often 'as good as it gets'. Therefore, if ADHD is extended to cover a wide range of childhood behaviours, it is a further case in which the objections of the anti-therapists are well-grounded because there is no underlying disorder that the individual can properly be regarded as suffering. Second, the overlap between conduct disorder and entities such as oppositional defiance disorder, mathematics disorder, and the more dubious cognitive and affective disorders of childhood blurs data about age of onset, neuropsychological abnormalities, and response to therapy, thereby confounding a reasoned approach to diagnosis and treatment because of the unclarity and indistinctness of what is being discussed. Third, the spectrum of hyperactivity, constituting a behavioural dimension rather than a distinct clinical finding (Sandberg, 1996), fudges the line between children who are suffering ADHD and normal children who, for various reasons, are having difficulty adjusting to their contexts of life (or disruptions in them). This again is likely to confound good clinical and research work on ADHD.

Weiss (1985) argues that genuine disorders have postdictive validity, concurrent validity, and predictive validity, defined as follows:

Postdictive validity looks at the precursors of a condition such as ADHD and so brings into sharp focus a constellation of distinctive aetiological or historical factors found in it.

Concurrent validity looks at the extent to which the group of children diagnosed with ADHD at the time of presentation are distinctive from their fellows or other groups.

Predictive validity addresses the question of prognosis, in terms of the adolescent and adult lives of those diagnosed as having ADHD in childhood.

Each is problematic, partly in the way that Weiss applies them. Postdictive validity is sufficient to identify a disorder (or related spectrum of problems) but in many conditions no set of typical precursors or (biological) aetiology is known (anorexia, for instance) despite it being well established in clinical taxonomy. Weiss (1985) mentions hypertension, a genuine clinical entity but which, similar to ADHD, is probably best thought of as 'the final common pathway of a variety of antecedent variables including both biologic and psychosocial factors' (p. 740).

Several studies indicate the importance of psychosocial factors. Rutter and co-workers (1975) examined children in both rural and urban populations and found a number of familial and environmental factors important in mental disorder including severe marital discord, low social class, large family size, paternal criminality, maternal mental disorder, and foster family placement. Such factors were additive, in that 'as the number of adverse conditions accumulates, the risk for impaired outcome in the child increases proportionally' (Biederman et al., 1995, p. 466). The same researchers found 'a positive association between Rutter's index of adversity and ADHD' (p. 467), and the correlation between disorder and environment held even when they controlled for family history and despite the problems of multiple pathologies (particularly evident in the North-American cases).

Weiss's (1985) concurrent validity pulls together the heterogeneous group of symptoms that are associated with ADHD. However, those with a typical or core set of manifestations may be a bit similar to asthmatics where the typical syndrome (quite apart from the company it keeps and its diverse contributing causes) is sufficient for the diagnosis whereas a wide definition needs support from something else (such as concurrent validity).

> If a child is diagnosed to be pervasively hyperactive, he is more likely to have concomitant (1) cognitive defects (including lower IQ); (2) reading retardation; (3) more severe other psychiatric problems; (4) neurodevelopmental difficulties, for example, signs and symptoms of MBD [Minimal Brain Damage]; (5) symptoms of the syndrome that are likely to endure.
>
> (Weiss, 1985, p. 741)

This litany is produced by those using a wide definition of ADHD whereas the British practice of focusing on typical and obvious hyperactivity and attention deficit as the central problem yields validity from the stereotyped pattern of behaviour and the fairly reliable response to stimulants (to which we shall come). The further point concerning the 'low level of agreement among teachers, parents, and clinicians about which child is hyperactive' (Weiss, 1985, p. 742) is attributed to two possible sources of confusion quite apart from diversity in the syndrome itself: 'inter-observer reliability is poor . . . or . . . that the child's hyperactive symptoms are situation-specific' (p. 742). Both problems are worrying in that if 'two people looking at the same identical child do not agree on what they see' (Weiss, 1985, p. 742), doubt is cast on the recognizability of ADHD as a distinct phenomenon (less likely if we accept the more restricted British diagnostic practice). And the worry about situation-specific hyperactivity is that we are mistaking a feature of the relationship between the context and the individual for an individual disorder. That worry is lessened if (as is not the case) pervasive hyperactivity is an essential part of a stringent diagnostic process.

> There have been additional interpretive changes to the diagnosis. One need not demonstrate symptoms in every situation. Rather, one need only display symptoms in at least two environments. Similarly, one may concentrate satisfactorily at a number of tasks, perhaps even overfocus, yet still meet criteria for diagnosis if concentration and focus are problems for important tasks (for example, 'selective inattention' or 'attentional inconsistency').
>
> (Diller, 1996, p. 13)

This is truly alarming in that it suggests that diagnostic criteria might be relaxed to the point that many normal children would, on occasion, fulfil them, a further argument for tightening criteria rather than calling in question the diagnostic category as a whole.

THE PHENOMENOLOGY OF ADHD | 173

The point is strengthened when we note the difference in prevalence between Britain and the United States, and the clinical and epidemiological overlap with conduct disorder.

Despite the fact that a single child may be diagnosed with ADHD and a variety of other co-morbid disorders, Milberger et al. (1995) remark: 'analysis indicates that ADHD was not an artefact of symptoms shared with other psychiatric disorders . . . [and] that the co-morbid conditions themselves were not an artefact of symptoms overlapping with those of ADHD' (p. 1797). This is mildly, but only mildly, reassuring that diagnoses are not being multiplied on the basis of a diffuse presentation that does not fit any well-characterized syndrome.

Predictive validity has two aspects: outcome in adolescence and adulthood for those diagnosed as having ADHD, and therapeutic response to pharmacologic agents.

Weiss (1985) discusses her own five-year follow-up study of 91 hyperactive adolescents, noting that 'they were found to be immature, have difficulty maintaining goals, and became sad during the interview. They had poor self-image' . . . Low self esteem, poor school performance, and poor peer relationships characterized adolescent outcome in most studies (pp. 746–747). That finding suggests that there may be other, discursive, elements unattended to here. We should ask whether the group is more than just a wide range of children with poor upbringing and social circumstances, bad school records, disturbed peer relationships, and general maladjustment from a variety of unrelated causes, in which case we would not need to look beyond the selection criteria for the outcomes. Weiss (1985) lists the clinical outcomes for children diagnosed as having ADHD: 'the majority continue as young adults to have various continued symptoms of the hyperactive child syndrome. For example, impulsivity, lower educational achievement, poorer social skills, lower self-esteem than controls, and restlessness continued to be present' (p. 750). But the same reservations apply in that selection criteria that ground the diagnosis may turn out to be isomorphic with the precursors of the adolescent and adult problems, whether or not the individuals actually had ADHD (as a separately diagnosable or associated problem).

There is further evidence about the natural history of ADHD suggesting an exponential decline of diagnosable ADHD with age: 'the rate of ADHD in a given age group appears to decline by 50% approximately every 5 years' (Hill & Schoener, 1996, p. 1143). This trend 'suggests that virtually all patients who experience ADHD as children will improve over a predictable course of time' (p. 1146), an observation consistent with the low rate of ADHD in adulthood (Shaffer, 1994). It is worth noting that co-morbid syndromes such as antisocial personality disorder, borderline personality disorder, and similar psychosocial problems are more likely in post-ADHD adults, suggesting that the malaise here is of general adjustment not (at least not in all the wider group) a discreet diagnosable condition. However, a response to psychostimulants in adults is more likely if there is a clear history of childhood ADHD and inconsistent otherwise (Shaffer, 1994, p. 636) despite the fact that the diagnosis in ADHD in adults is especially problematic.

> Adult ADHD has now become the foremost *self-diagnosed* condition in my practice. I fear that the condition allows a patient to find a biological cause, which is not always

reasonable, for job failure, divorce, poor motivation, lack of success, and chronic mild depression.

(Shaffer, 1994, p. 637)

In the face of the many good reasons for scepticism, the pharmacology of ADHD is suasive. Most children with ADHD respond well to stimulants such as methylphenidate or dextroamphetamine (Greenhill, 1992; Klein, 1995; Sandberg, 1996; Wilens & Biederman, 1992) and there is a remarkable effect of tranquillizers and hypnosedatives.

> Phenobarbitone and benzodiazepines should not be used because they can have the paradoxical effect of increasing overactivity.

(Gelder et al., 1983, p. 659)

The age-related decline in incidence, when examined, also affects psychostimulant use in all the groups studied (Hill & Schoener, 1996, p. 1144); in adults, where the concurrent validity provided by stereotypy of presentation and symptom complex is least, the response to psychostimulants is quite unclear. What is more, methylphenidate seems to be effective in ameliorating symptoms of conduct disorder even where ADHD treatment effects have been statistically discounted (Klein et al., 1997).

Where the symptoms are well developed and the child is a typical case with the three main characteristics of hyperactivity, attention deficit, and impulsivity pervasive across a number of situations, the role of stimulants seems well established. Klein (1995) remarks:

> In addition to having the cardinal features of their disorder eliminated, appropriately medicated children experience improvement in other important functional domains, such as social interactions with parents, teachers, and peers, in academic performance, and in self-esteem. (p. 429)

> The medication's effects appear to be independent of age: amelioration of the signs of motor drivenness, restlessness, inability to attend, non-compliance, and aggressiveness are reduced in controlled studies of preschool and school-aged children, and more recently, in adolescents.

(Greenhill, 1992, p. 11)

Their success has made methylphenidate (and related drugs) the most popular drug in the therapeutic armamentarium of child psychiatry.

> Psychostimulant medication has emerged as the most widely used treatment modality for . . . ADHD . . . in the United States, given to as many as 750 000 children per day. The popularity of this treatment may be related to the frequency with which the ADHD diagnosis is made, the low cost of the medications, the medication[']s proven efficacy in suppressing the core signs of ADHD, their safety, lack of diagnostic specificity, and their wide range of tolerated doses.

(Greenhill, 1992, p. 1)

Optimal treatment seems to combine drugs and psychosocial factors (Greenhill, 1992, p. 24; Jensen et al., 2001; Martin et al., 1997, p. 54; Wilens & Biederman, 1992, p. 216). Drug treatment seems to facilitate all other interventions: 'improvements have been shown in measures of cognition, vigilance, and reaction time . . . short-term memory and learning of verbal and non-verbal material . . . improvements in measures of inattention and distractibility' (Wilens & Biederman, 1992, p. 198). Stimulants, for instance, 'curtail the impulsive behaviours that interfere with school performance, enhance accident proneness, and worsen peer difficulties' (p. 199) and they also 'improve mother–child and overall family interactions' (p. 199). 'Compared with stimulant non-responders, there was increased maternal warmth, decreased maternal criticism, greater frequency of maternal contact, and fewer negative encounters with siblings among responders' (p. 199).

Despite the fact that stimulants seem to be part of the most effective treatment regimes, the proportion of those taking them who go on taking them decreases over time for various reasons. That decreased use is not associated with a deterioration in the problems attributed to ADHD, suggesting that long-term medication does not confer significant benefits even though some of those diagnosed with ADHD in childhood go on to have serious social and behavioural problems (Jensen et al., 2007). I have noted that there is an overlap between ADHD and other patterns of disruption and maladaptation in children so that one might expect that, even in a well-ordered study of treatment (such as the National Institutes of Mental Health Multi-modal Treatment study of ADHD [NIMA MTA]) some of the findings may be difficult to evaluate.

Apart from the problems associated with overdiagnosis of ADHD, caution seems to be required in that the response to medication may not be specific to the core set of cases of typical ADHD. The problem with overlapping symptom sets between ADHD and other syndromes is well illustrated by the following case history.

Jeremy is six years old and lives with his mother, a teacher. He is the only child to his mother's second partner, his parents having separated when he was four years old . . . Over the previous year, Jeremy had been treated for attention deficit disorder by his paediatrician with both dexamphetamine and imipramine. His mother had been told that his case was 'severe'. At times, Jeremy appeared to respond to medication but such improvements were short-lived and inconsistent . . . Battling to get him to school, Jeremy's mother reported that he acted aggressively towards his peers (both at home and in school), was making poor progress with his school work (although he appeared bright), demonstrated oppositional behaviour, had erratic eating patterns, and had occasionally lit fires . . . Jeremy's father was also thought to have ADHD, being described as 'impulsive' and 'aggressive at times'. Between the ages of two and four years, Jeremy had witnessed domestic violence (verbal and physical abuse) towards his mother by his father. In addition, his mother described the household at this time as 'chaotic'.

Jeremy presented as a rather dishevelled, barefoot boy, avoiding direct contact with the therapist. He was not overactive, nor distractable when left to his own devices, but became oppositional and agitated when asked to interact or cooperate. At the beginning of his assessment and brief therapy, links were made between both Jeremy's mother's and Jeremy's past experiences (especially the family violence), and questions were raised about the effect of these on both his mother's parenting and on Jeremy's mastery of developmental tasks . . . Psychological assessment during this time found Jeremy to be of average intelligence with fluctuating attention mainly dependent on his interest in and motivation for a task.

(Martin, et al., 1997, p. 47)

The authors argue that in Jeremy's case 'the original diagnosis was made somewhat precipitously on inadequate criteria' (p. 47), highlighting the ease with which a child like Jeremy can be started on psychostimulants. Jeremy and other children like him (where Rutter's adversity factors are prominent) clearly need a thorough assessment in terms of familial and contextual risk factors so that their psychosocial needs are not overlooked and they become victims of a quasi-psychiatric medicalization of everyday life. There is a real concern that the diagnosis of ADHD and the use of Ritalin are increasingly subjecting (particularly American) children to 'the medical destruction of childhood' when the real explanations for many phenomena treated as individual abnormalities are the artificial pressures of an increasingly stressful and success-oriented culture.

7.2 The problem of boundaries and the medicalization of childhood

Recent newspaper reports have described a teenage boy who gets into trouble in school. He won't turn in his homework, he won't answer questions in class, and he often simply leaves school in the middle of the day to go hang out at a local bowling alley. The school authorities call in his mother, who is divorced and trying to earn enough money to support herself and her son. She says she cannot do anything with him because he suffers from Obedience Defiance Disorder (ODD). Anything she requests, he refuses. Any rule she imposes, he breaks. He automatically defies any authority. She says the boy's psychologist has identified this behaviour as caused by ODD and that he is being treated for it.

(Donley, 1997)

ODD appears in the DSM IV along with 'Conduct Disorder', diagnosed on the basis of aggression to people or animals, destruction of property, deceitfulness or theft, serious violations of rules (APA, 1994a, pp. 90–91), and other uncomfortably similar categories. A number of common problems in academic attainment are now DSM numbered disorders such as mathematics disorder (315.1), disorder of written expression (315.2), developmental coordination disorder (315.4), and expressive language disorder (315.31) all of which (surprise, surprise) have familial patterns. To many of us, this seems like categorization gone mad if categorization is supposed to track indications for therapeutic intervention.

In the ordinary civilized world, children are allowed to be bad at maths without having *mathematics disorder* particularly in kindergarten or first grade. I would guess that mathematics disorder responds to corrective one-on-one coaching or remedial teaching in the same way that behaviours identical to reading disorder (315.00) do in places such as the United Kingdom and New Zealand. What is more, a subtle pattern of neurological disorder associated with these so-called syndromes does not justify the medicalizing move. In all countries, there are children who are not well coordinated at sport and who are accident prone, who 'fall, bump into things, or knock things over' (DSM IV; APA, 1994a, p. 54), and it is extremely implausible to believe that these problems have nothing to do with their neural networks, but that is a poor reason to label the problem as a disorder, particularly given that there is not specific treatment for these problems apart from what commonsense would recommend in any event.

Diller (1996) is quite critical of this tendency to make disorders out of relatively modest deviations from what, in some cases, are parental and social ideals and expectations.

> The line between children with 'normal' variations of temperament, lively or spontaneous children who are sensitive to stimuli and those who have a 'disorder' has become increasingly blurred . . . Now children who sit quietly and perform well in social situations or in one-on-one psychometric testing can still be candidates for the diagnosis and treatment of ADHD if their parents or teachers report poor performance in completing tasks at school or home. (p. 13)

That children can be labelled and treated for a medical disorder on the basis that they do not fully satisfy the expectations of their parents and educators is extremely worrying and suggests that we ought to realize that the psyche is fundamentally relational in that it connects or attunes the subject to the world, an interaction that should be centre stage when we examine maladjustment or a breakdown in individual adaptation.

7.3 **ADHD and the anti-medication voices**

> When presented with a potentially complex child behavioural problem, the physician may be attracted to the option of prescribing a medication rather than addressing the thornier and more time-consuming issues of emotions, family relationships, or school environment. (Diller, 1996, p. 14)

The case of Jeremy is telling, and the difference in prevalence between the United Kingdom and the United States suggests that there is a tendency to use ADHD to justify the use of stimulants in an attempt to 'cosmetically' medicate children into a more acceptable social profile. What is more, the fact that 'Ritalin improves the focus and performance of those who do not meet ADHD criteria' (Diller, 1996, p. 15) means that cosmetic use may be difficult to contain:

> The increasing availability and use of Ritalin to enhance performance also raise questions of subtle coercion and fairness. As more children and adults use Ritalin to work more efficiently at school or in the office, will those who are also struggling to perform feel pressured to consider medication? (p. 16)

A crucial ingredient in the ethical problem is the competitive and success-orientated attitudes prevalent right from the earliest years of childhood ('Little Miss Sunshine' step forward). In this connection, we do well to remember how much of children's learning has nothing to do with measurable academic attainment and is about living in the real world to achieve long-term social adjustment, a balanced adult life, and sustained, balanced career development. An artificial 'success'-driven childhood, in which even the informal exploratory play of infancy is turned into pre-academic attainment and natural cognitive functions are a target for chemical enhancement, may well predispose to later misuse of the same (pharmacological) recourse, dysfunction, and loss of enjoyment in life.

Even where they help, designer drugs might be used with poor indications to provide a semblance of normality in what is otherwise a disordered life. The 'double whammy' of inappropriate medication and inattention to the fundamental psychosocial problems is malignant mix, bringing us to the justification for treatment in ADHD.

7.4 Why treat ADHD?

The obvious justification for treatment in ADHD is that it makes some children better. But the question must be asked 'Better, in whose terms?' If the benefits are defined by a distorted set of social mores, then there is a real issue about the use of drugs. If in the child's own terms or according to an objective reading of 'best interests of the child' the medication is beneficial, then it is justified. We are therefore influenced by 'personal and affecting testimonies of dramatic improvements after using Ritalin have been reported on national television broadcasts and many syndicated talk shows' (Diller, 1996, p. 15). Often, the benefits affect cognition, temperament, social adjustment, conduct at school and home, impulsivity, and aggression.

> Double-blind ratings by parents, teachers, and professionals report improvement in three fourths of the children treated . . . When given MPH [methylphenidate] at 0.6 mg/kg, ADHD boys obtain more frequent nominations for being 'cooperative', 'fun to be with', and acting like 'best friends'.
>
> (Greenhill, 1992, p. 11)

These measures suggest that psychostimulants have a beneficial role in the treatment of ADHD, but data from the first-person point of view is not so unequivocal.

A study of the feelings of children on psychostimulants about their treatment does not fully support the confident pronouncements of 'objective' scientific reports (Sleator et al., 1982). Children diagnosed as hyperactive and treated with psychostimulants were asked about their treatment:

(1) Only 42% stated that they thought that the drugs clearly helped them; (p. 475)

(2) Another 42% of the children disliked or hated their medication; (p. 476)

(3) And 65% of the children had at one stage or another tried to avoid their medication. (p. 477)

Those who found their treatment helpful made remarks such as 'If I forget, I go get it fast, otherwise I'm in trouble' (Sleator et al., 1982, p. 475), but the authors go on to note that 'In contrast, his file showed he had used every device to avoid medication. He fought taking it daily and often deceived his mother into thinking he had taken it when he had not.' Discrepancies of this kind were common, casting doubt on the basis of the first-person reports of benefit. The child's public face seems to conform to the expectations of others regarding treatment, despite the private opposition and non-compliance (a finding which might be expected given Donaldson's [1979] work on infant interview behaviour). The authors note that, in other studies, 'stated compliance was greater than that determined by other methods' (Sleator et al., 1982,

p. 478), a discrepancy (in tolerability, compliance, and subjective appreciation) that problematizes best-interest judgements about medication.

> Above all else, we found a pervasive dislike among hyperactive children for taking stimulants . . . The intensity of dislike of many hyperactive children for taking stimulants is a troubling phenomenon. The problem is made more difficult by the fact that many of the most vigorous objectors, according to all observers, are benefited by medication in school achievement, in freedom from the open disapproval of elders at home and at school, and in improved peer and sibling relationships.
>
> (Sleator et al., 1982, pp. 478–479)

These findings pose the ethical problem of a treatment widely thought beneficial but to which the patients themselves have mixed attitudes. Debates about the reality and prevalence of the syndrome being treated and the possibility that it is, in part, an artefact of unreal expectations on normal children accentuate that worry: 'twenty-five years ago, three- and four-year old children were not expected to know the alphabet and numbers' (Diller, 1996, p. 13). What are we doing to these children?

Despite these concerns, we ought to notice that the divergence between first-person and third-person avowals is not unique to ADHD but is a more widespread phenomenon in psychiatry. It is a common feature of compulsory treatment for some patients with a disorder of mind sufficient to cloud their judgements about their own best interests, and in diverse areas (e.g. the lack of insight often found in psychosis, in the inability of psychopaths to appreciate their true problem, and the ambivalence of some people with bipolar disorder about the treatment of their hypomania), we are guided by a balance of objective judgements and first-person testimony. Discounting first-person testimony is, however, most defensible when the therapeutic benefit seems clear and in accordance with the life-goals (or critical interests [Dworkin]) of the person concerned who, at the time of treatment, does not seem to appreciate what must be done to safeguard those interests (Dawson, 2007).

One could argue that ADHD is such a case in that children and young people suffering the disorder do have a problem making balanced evaluative judgements and long-term assessments about their best interests. What is more, patients tend to endorse their treatment (Sleator et al., 1982), but one might wonder whether that is because they have been socialized into the accepted view of their conduct or because their disordered childhood experiences have been recast so as to see them in a 'better' light (as in the plasticity of memory). Given that we do not have the in-depth qualitative and discursive data needed to appreciate the subtlety of the feelings in question, we ought to be agnostic about the issue.

There is, however, a further significant concern in the current climate of health care: 'Because stimulants "work" more quickly, they are more attractive not only to families and physicians but also to managed-care companies and financially strapped educational systems.' (Diller, 1996, p. 14)

Most health-care funding bodies do not like psychiatric care, where chronicity is the rule and definitive interventions are often not to be found. In the area of child psychiatry in particular, many problems have complex psychosocial causes and require extended intervention attentive to the needs of child, family, and community.

'Quick-fixes' are not the rule and, therefore, the need for care is not easily quantified in the terms beloved of economists and accountants. But to allow a generation to be overmedicated with (who knows what) long-term social consequences because of policies designed to allow some parties to make more money is just evil.

7.5 **Philosophical problems raised by ADHD**

The subjective and objective goods problem

The divergence between subjective and objective assessments of treatment creates a situation in which children are potentially coerced against their best interests on the basis of role expectations to which they ought not be subject. The argument runs as follows:

(1) Treatment is generally used to make people better.

(2) Some treatment is unpleasant.

(3) The justification for unpleasant treatment is that overall there is a net gain in well-being for the individual concerned.

(4) The principal measure of well-being is first-person and subjective.

(5) In ADHD, the loss of well-being and the consequent benefit are predominantly from a third-person perspective.

(6) First-person assessment of psychostimulants implies that they have negative effects on well-being.

(7) There is no justification for treatment in the face of dubious objective and negative subjective assessments of the effect of treatment on well-being.

We can, however, challenge the conjunction of 3 and 4 and argue that, as elsewhere in psychiatry, the individual may not be the best judge of the effectiveness and benefit of treatment. It is plausible that a person with a condition such as ADHD is not clear about what is conducive to well-being in the medium to long term so that, arguably, we should not abandon them to their own deficient assessments (and self-assessments) but rather be guided by systematic medium- to long-term assessments of benefit.

The medicalization of childhood problem

Many of the behaviours included in a wide definition of ADHD are fairly typical of normal childhood. To treat these by using powerful psychostimulants is, some would claim, to rob children of the important aspects of childhood experience: in particular, spontaneity, a high level of activity, excited curiosity, exploratory fervour, frantic creativity, and the turmoil of youthful ideas. If that were true, then psychostimulant use (in the context of a regimented and achievement-oriented society and education system) is of serious concern, and we should examine the effects of psychostimulants on tests of children's creativity and spontaneity, such as those used in studies of creative intelligence (Wallace & Kogan, 1972). It may emerge that performance on such tests is, in fact, facilitated by psychostimulant medication of children diagnosed with ADHD. It is plausible that their thinking is better when not disrupted by a deficient attention setting mechanism, but it ain't necessarily so.

The therapeutic creep problem

(1) Children with ADHD are improved in their cognitive and behavioural functions by psychostimulants.

(2) Children who show some features of ADHD are also improved.

(3) The functions concerned are conducive to academic and career success.

(4) Those who wish for such success might be induced to try the medications.

(5) It may become difficult for doctors and educators to not provide such medications even where the target individuals seem normal on most assessments.

The danger is created by the (unholy) narrowing of the concept of well-being to focus on the functions referred to in premise 3. If childhood well-being is equated to social mores linked to success, then this is worrying. But it is not the use of psychostimulants per se that is the problem, rather the milieu in which certain (reductive) social values are legitimated that makes them potentially dangerous.

In fact, leaving aside all consideration of medicating childhood, the narrowing of gaze in assessing the *eudaimonia* of a child is a pervasive problem. We have sanitized childhood and tried to regiment it in a whole raft of areas: we must have safe (and boring) playgrounds; we must introduce academic skills earlier and earlier; we must make children's play 'educative' (often as defined by pedagogues and politicians with stunted imaginations); we must make children use their time productively (as defined by a society riddled with social problems due to its narrow conception of productivity); and above all, we must *do* childhood better (without ever really reflecting on what counts as 'better'), all problems that obviously go far beyond methylphenidate and ADHD.

The therapeutic response as indicator of a genuine psychiatric category

I have noted the (not so) subtle role played by pharmacology in psychiatric nosology. Psychostimulants are a great example.

(1) Psychostimulants correct the cognitive defects of ADHD.

(2) If you are cognitively improved by psychostimulants, you must be suffering from some form of ADHD.

(3) Many more people are improved by psychostimulants than those falling under a restrictive definition of ADHD.

(4) The definition of ADHD should be widened.

(5) ADHD, similar to most psychiatric disorders, is clearly a chemical imbalance in the brain.

The transparently false move here is in the transition from 1 to 2 in that to make this transition you need the following premise:

1a. Only ADHD and conditions similar to it respond to psychostimulants.

This premise is false. Cognitive studies have shown that psychostimulants affect normal people in somewhat the same ways as patients with ADHD when used in focused tasks and circumscribed areas of cognitive achievement (Rapoport et al., 1980).

The last statement (5) is the byword of the reductive slide of psychiatry into biological psychiatry (Diller 1996, pp. 16–17), a serious consideration in an age of managed care and tightly controlled budgets for psychiatric treatment (Eisenberg, 1995). The philosophical credentials of the reductive slide are found wanting in the present work, but political or functional pragmatism, rationalism, and the demands of the economic order, rather than intellectual purity, often seem to rule clinical behaviour and prevail in social policy (Gillett, 2008; see especially Chapter 9 of that work).

Chapter 8

I and the other robots

Bye-Child by Seamus Heaney

He was discovered in the henhouse where she had confined him. He was incapable of saying anything.

When the lamp glowed,
A yolk of light
In their back window,
The child in the outhouse
Put his eye to the chink

Little henhouse boy,
Sharp-faced as new moons
Remembered, your photo still
Glimpsed like a rodent
On the floor of my mind,

Little moon man,
Kennelled and faithful
At the foot of the yard,
Your frail shape, luminous,
Weightless, is stirring the dust,

The cobwebs, old droppings
Under the roosts
And dry smells from scraps
She put through your trapdoor
Morning and evening.

After those footsteps, silence;
Vigils, solitudes, fasts,
Unchristened tears,
A puzzled love of the light.
But now you speak at last

With a remote mime
Of something beyond patience,
Your gaping wordless proof
Of lunar distances
Travelled beyond love.

The 'bye child' is neglected, cut off from human contact by being shut from birth in a henhouse. One can only wonder at the person who would condemn a child to such a fate, but there are many other children cut off by infantile autism from the natural human contact most of us enjoy although they exist in the midst of comparative plenty.

Autism raises a number of questions about the human mind that reveal why autistic children and those caring for them revert to robotic imagery when describing it and it throws new light on philosophical questions about machine consciousness, the foundations of human knowledge, and the existence of other minds.

The experience of autism, from the perspective of those who suffer it and those who care for them, introduces one of the most 'alien' of the discontents of the mind and offers support for a phenomenological stance towards human subjectivity whereby intersubjectivity is actually the foundation of all human knowledge and a human being truly does exist through and with others. This has profound implications for epistemology and the problem of other minds.

8.1 **The autistic world**

> I never thought about how I might fit in with other people when I was very young because I was not able to pick people out as being different from objects. Then, when I did realize that people were supposed to be more important than objects and became more generally aware, things began to take on a new and more difficult light.
>
> Objects are frightening. Moving objects are harder to cope with because of the added complexity of movement. Moving objects which also make noise are even harder to cope with because you have to try and take in the sight, movement, and further added complexity of the noise. Human beings are the hardest of all to understand because not only do you have to cope with the problem of just seeing them, they move about when you are not expecting them to, they make various noises, and along with this, they place all different kinds of demands on you which are just impossible to understand.
>
> (Joliffe *et al.*, 1993, p. 16)

This testimony by an autistic person who, as an adult, is still under psychiatric care speaks of a process that is normally completed before children can articulate their own experiences and vividly illustrates the differences between a literate, verbally competent, and relatively well-adapted autistic person and others.

> People do not appreciate how unbearably difficult it is for me to look at a person. It disturbs my quietness and is terribly frightening. (Joliffe et al., 1993, p. 14)
>
> Reality to an autistic person is a confusing interacting mass of events, people, places, sounds, and sights. There seem to be no clear boundaries, order, or meaning to anything. A large part of my life is spent just trying to work out the pattern behind everything. Set routines, times, particular routes, and rituals all help to get order into an unbearably chaotic life. (p. 16)
>
> Trying to keep everything the same reduces some of the terrible fear. Fear has dominated my life. (p. 16)
>
> When somebody starts to speak to me, I have nearly always lost the first few words before I realize that I am actually being spoken to. (p. 17)

Kanner (1943), who first identified autism, noted four features: a pattern of onset in the first two years of life and an 'autistic triad' of *autistic aloneness, speech and language disorder,* and *obsessive desire for sameness* (Gelder et al., 1983). Affected children are more frequently found in upper socio-economic classes and may initially seem to be developing normally.

Autistic aloneness involves poor interpersonal communication, lack of emotional expression, absence of normal eye-to-eye contact with other human beings, and lack of responsiveness (to parents as distinct from other human beings, and to human beings in general as distinct from other objects). The alienation means that 'autism goes deeper than language and culture; autistic people are foreigners in any society' (Sinclair, 1993, p. 156).

'I look like Frankenstein.'

(Cesaroni & Garber, 1991, p. 310)

Normal people, finding themselves on a planet with alien creatures on it, would probably feel frightened, would not know how to fit in, and would certainly have difficulty in understanding what the aliens were thinking feeling and wanting, and how to respond correctly to these things. That's what autism is like.

(Joliffe *et al.*, 1993)

Autistic people link their alienation to their fear of stimulation and especially novel stimulation.

I didn't like to be around noise, confusion, new environments, or new people. I spent most of my time hiding from all the stimulation, and when that didn't work, I sometimes banged my head, spun myself and jar lids, or lined up objects.

(Landry, 1989)

This first aspect of the Kanner's triad is hard to describe from the outside: 'aloneness' does not convey 'the inside story' (a feature common to many mental disorders).

The second aspect is *speech and language disorder*, a severe cognitive defect:

A relative (not absolute) lack of what are otherwise ubiquitous propensities and abilities among children—especially the capacities for non-verbal communication and affective contact with others, for intimate relationships, for creative symbolic play, and for flexible context-sensitive thinking and language.

(Hobson, 1991)

It emerges that these pervasive defects are best unified and explained by the centrality of intersubjectivity in the cognitive development of the infant and in normal human experience. Hobson (1991), in fact, notes that it is difficult, in the mental development of a child, to separate cognitive, affective, and social aspects of unfolding mental capacities and observes that 'a distinctive feature of autism is characteristic sparing of non-verbal, non-meaningful, and non-social cognitive functions relative to impairment in other intellectual abilities' (p. 7).

The centrality of intersubjectivity in the world of meaning is a recurring theme in phenomenology endorsed by many writers on cognitive development (Bruner, 1990; Donaldson, 1979; Trevarthen, 1979). Temple Grandin gives us an insider's view.

'I couldn't figure out what I was doing wrong. I had an odd lack of awareness that I was different. I thought the other kids were different. I could never figure out why I didn't fit in.'

Something was going on between the other kids, something swift, subtle, constantly changing, an exchange of meanings, a negotiation, a swiftness of understanding so remarkable
that sometimes she wondered if they were all telepathic. She is now aware of the existence
of these social signals. She can infer them, she says, but she herself cannot perceive them,
cannot participate in the magical communication directly, or conceive the many-levelled
kaleidoscopic states of mind behind it.

(Sacks, 1995, p. 260)

The philosophical implications of intersubjectivity as a foundation of human experience (made vivid by the cognitive impairments in autism) are radical for traditional
(Empiricist Representational Theory [ERT] of mind) epistemology.

Kanner's description noted a third feature—*the obsessive desire for sameness*—manifest as a desire for the same food, the same clothes, stereotypical behaviour patterns,
and reluctance to deviate from well-practised daily routines. Autistic people are well
aware of the phenomena.

When I read about the high-functioning autistics who travel, I am reminded of my inability
to tolerate the slightest change in routine. Unlike their flexibility which improved, mine
took the opposite direction. Everything from changing seasons, changes in my mental
health professionals' schedules, to changes in my mealtime routines disturb me. During
certain times of the year when changes are more frequent, I'm so miserable I want to crawl
into my bed and sleep.

(Comm, 1994)

If 'the world is a bewildering, alien, and frightening place' to an autistic person, many
of these symptoms are understandable. But as well as representing a retreat to well-
practised and therefore reassuring sameness, stereotyped behaviours seem to arise
automatically at certain times of excitement, with some autistic people reporting their
spontaneous occurrence when they are not attending to their bodies. The stereotypies
seem, therefore, to evince both *withdrawal* and a need to express or *discharge activity*.
'It was like my brain was running at 200 miles an hour instead of 60 miles an hour'
(Grandin, 1992, p. 111). She mentions that being firmly but gently held by a 'squeeze
machine' would calm her but that vigorous exercise or fixating on an intense activity,
or withdrawing into oneself and minimizing outside stimulation, can also decrease
stereotyped and disruptive behaviour. The desire for sameness can therefore be seen
as a way of regularizing the world and staying within well-worn strategies so that stereotypy and fixation on simple stimuli such as spinning tops are ways of shutting out a
disturbing and frenzied world. But the relation of repetitive and stereotypical behaviour to emotional tone indicates a further feature to do with a drive towards rhythmic
physical activity.

Autism is not only a debilitating disorder of childhood but also a disorder from
which 60% of the sufferers do not improve (Gelder et al., 1983), and there are obvious
contrasts with other conditions severely affecting cognition and learning (for instance,
autistic individuals can learn complex and highly structured material in a favoured
area such as art or mathematics). Disorders of language and communication such as
dyslexia are much more circumscribed in their impact on the child than autism.
A dyslexic person does not seem alien or other in the same way as an autistic child.

Such specific language disorders are not marked by poor play, lack of imagination and creativity, echolalia, and stereotypy or by the distress and fearfulness always haunting the behaviour of the autistic child. Having said this, some circumscribed differences, such as congenital blindness and deafness, also cut the child off, to some extent, from interpersonal communication. But one might predict that blindness and deafness would cause 'autistic-like clinical features such as personal pronoun difficulties, echolalia, impairments in symbolic play, lack of interest in stories, and more general role-taking disabilities' (Hobson, 1991, p. 12), explained by the child's inability to make full use of the auditory and visual clues and signals that serve intersubjectivity and our common activity in a shared world (Husserl, 1950/1999).

Asperger's (1944/1991) original paper on 'Autistic Psychopathy in Childhood' contains some striking observations:

> Autism refers to a fundamental disturbance of contact . . . Human beings normally live in constant interaction with their environment, and react to it continuously . . . the autistic is only himself . . . and is not an active member of a greater organism which he is influenced by and which he influences constantly. (p. 38)
>
> He was never able to swing with the rhythm of the group. (p. 57)
>
> Normal children acquire the necessary social habits without being consciously aware of them: they learn instinctively. It is these instinctive reactions that are disturbed in autistic children. To put it bluntly, these children are intelligent automata. (p. 58)
>
> Autistic children have a paucity of facial and gestural expression. In ordinary two-way interaction, they are unable to act as a proper counterpart to their opposite number, and hence, they have no use for facial expression as a contact-creating device. (p. 69)
>
> Autistic children are able to produce original ideas. Indeed they can only be original . . . They are simply not set to assimilate and learn an adult's knowledge. (p. 70)
>
> The fundamental disorder of autistic individuals is the limitation of their social relationships. The whole personality of these children is determined by this limitation . . . Their behaviour in the social group is the clearest sign of their disorder and the source of conflicts . . . especially pronounced . . . within the family [where] the interplay of feeling between parents and children . . . [is met] with incomprehension and even rejection. (p. 77)

Autism presents a striking contrast to Down's syndrome, another pervasive developmental disorder, in which the child is affectionate and sometimes overly demonstrative. There are many things about the world that a child with Down's syndrome does not seem fully to understand, but they do not affect his or her ability to form emotional bonds and respond to others in a warm and engaging way. This striking difference supports and emphasizes intersubjectivity as the key defect in autism rather than any other cognitive problem affecting a theory of mind (or some other) 'module' with circumscribed cognitive functions (Trevarthen, 1979; Zahavi, 2005).

Temple Grandin, in her autobiography, discusses the 'squeeze machine', a casket the walls of which can be controlled by her to exert a firm but gentle pressure on her body.

> When she was a little girl, she said, she had longed to be hugged but had at the same time been terrified of all contact. When she was hugged, especially by a favourite (but vast) aunt, she felt overwhelmed, overcome by sensation; she had a sense of peacefulness and pleasure, but also of terror and engulfment.

(Sacks, 1995, p. 251)

This conflicted phenomenology, focused on interpersonal activity, is as intriguing for the observer as it is distressing for autistic children and those who care for them and is almost certainly related to the failure of the 'mirror neurone system' serving primary intersubjectivity, part of the natural bedrock of experience for a normal child allowing 'the enactment of direct intersubjective perception' (Gallagher, 2005, p. 223). Autism, a 'severe disruption in their experience of interpersonal relations as interpersonal' (Hobson, 1991, p. 10), therefore offers important clues (overlooked in post-Cartesian accounts) of the shaping of mind and personality. Putting intersubjectivity in such a central place in the human psyche that disrupting it leads to a 'pervasive developmental disorder of childhood' is quite alien to the dominant empiricist view, the problem of other minds to which it gives rise, and the embedded conception of human children as 'scientists in the crib' (Bruner, 2000).

The problem in autistic children is manifest by their marked impairment, compared to normal children with similar intellectual capabilities, when they are given a *false belief* task.

> The original false-belief task involved a character, Maxi, who places some chocolate in a particular location and then leaves the room; in his absence, the chocolate is then moved to another location. The child is then asked where Maxi will look for the chocolate on his return.
>
> (Carruthers & Smith, 1996, p. 2)

Normal children succeed at this task fairly consistently from the ages of 4–5 years onward, but autistic children (with similar or greater intellectual capacities on other tasks) do not, a failure generally attributed to the inability of autistic children to realize (the fact) that other people have minds.

The knowledge of other minds is regarded by post-empiricist philosophers as one variety of understanding of complex objects and, as such, is prone to certain sceptical doubts about 'complex ideas' and inferences. But a philosophical examination of autism displaces this view in favour of a more engaged, existential-phenomenological view of the psyche as our mode of becoming attuned to meaning (or significance) in a shared world.

8.2 Two views of the epistemology of human beings

Traditional empiricist theories of mind have the individual thinker building a picture of the world from sensory impressions and the regularities she or he discerns in them so as to arrive at thoughts that can be expressed to others. Thus, the child is like a 'scientist in the crib'. Neo-empiricist theories have the thinker borrowing procedural rules, models, and interpretive frameworks from the social milieu to apply to his or her egocentric data and generating representations of the world more or less modelled on the idea of truth-assessable hypotheses about the way things are (Bolton & Hill; Davidson; Heil). In such hypotheses, people figure as complex objects doing things as a result of internal processes aimed at achieving certain ends or satisfying certain needs. Their behaviour is apprehensible in terms of complex patterns of physical stimuli and knowledge of their mental lives is constructed by inference to the best explanation for that behaviour (in terms of the rules and regularities operating 'around here'), a posit remarkably reminiscent of the worldview of an autistic person.

The alternative (phenomenological, hermeneutic) view sees human beings as co-inhabitants of a shared life-world, reading significance into what is going on according to a horizon of meaning that structures that world. On this account, the presence of others is a basic or primordial feature of the life world that is evident whenever we act or look around us, and evident in the gestures, cooperative activity, and artefacts created by them (Heidegger, Sartre, Wittgenstein). The *psyche* is our way of mapping the patterns of meaning incarnate in that world. We are, on this view, creatures of a cross-categorical world (Armstrong, 2004) in which truth, meaning, and value (and their fused horizons) structure who we are and what we do. In Lacan's terms, we are creatures in whom the mirror of the world (language) comes into focus in the contingencies of nature, changing it in ways that make it habitable.

Neo-empiricist theories and a *Verstehen*-based or phenomenological view both give a central place to knowledge of the behaviour of others (which an autistic child finds difficult). However, the theorists concerned are not offering an account of the actual development of natural language despite their view that the attainment of shared meaning or an appreciation of the meaningful connections lying behind utterances is dependent on an individually elaborated theory adequate to the data confronting a person (as in an IBE, or theory-theory, type of view). By contrast, an interactive view (along with Bruner, Vygotsky, and the phenomenology of Husserl and Merleau-Ponty) is that the individual is helped to make sense of the world by other persons. The contrast emerges clearly in Sacks' (1995) conversation with Temple Grandin.

> But what about children, I asked her. Were they not intermediate between animals and adults? On the contrary, Temple said, she had great difficulties with children—trying to talk to them, to join in their games (she could not even play peek-a-boo with a baby she said, because she would get the timing all wrong)—as she had such difficulties herself as a child. Children, she feels, are already far advanced, by the age of three or four, along a path that she, as an autistic person, has never advanced far on. Little children, she feels, already understand other human beings in a way she can never hope to. (pp. 257–258)

Children use many cues to understand the ordinary interactions between people including an intuitive or natural ability to 'fit into' these on the basis of interpersonal pragmatics, characterized as *second-person* embodied interactions with other persons perceived as others like me (Gallagher, 2005, p. 224). The relevant skills not only describe and predict the behaviour of others but are also part of 'a shared engagement in the common world' through 'our way of being together and understanding each other' (Zahavi, 2005, p. 165). Our mutual participation in doing things to and with each other aided by words conveys both relationship skills and the means of self-understanding (Zahavi, 2005, p. 166), and the discourse producing this result is grounded in a natural congruence between human beings such that patterns of behaving interactively are as natural to us all as the perceptual ability to track moving objects.

However, the natural capacities of the autistic are startlingly different: they do not seem to have the equipment to engage in these formative interchanges. Wittgenstein uses the term 'bedrock' to refer to that natural equipment (based, no doubt, on biological propensities underpinning human forms of life). The relevant capacities enable us to adapt to human discourse (whatever particular version of it we are exposed to) so that our lives are informed (in-formed) by the terms of that discourse, Lacan's 'imperative of the word as law' (demands, appeals, messages, evaluations). Some features of the 'second nature' that results are universal for creatures extensively nurtured by other human beings and others have distinctive features in different cultures as diverse cultural norms are 'inscribed' in their subjective bodies.

The arguments from training (Kant) and intersubjectivity suggest that the language informing the psyche, as all language, is essentially shared, allowing a human individual to make use of communal resources to shape an *imago*—a lived-in reflection of self derived from one's interactions with others and articulated by discourse. Language provides a set of tools usable both individually and interactively to organize behaviour and understand the self, so psychological congruence, in the normal case, is an a priori result of the interactive milieu that produces a human being as an essentially discursive creature. The defect in autism is a failure to develop that nature because of the lack of intersubjectivity, the bedrock of human life.

Currie (1996) rehearses other worries about both theory-theory and simulation theory:

(i) Whereas theory-theory-based accounts imply that autistics cannot form meta-representations, 25% of the autistic people can meta-represent on false belief tasks.

(ii) Autistic people perform well on false map and false photograph tasks compared with false belief tasks whereas normal children are the reverse (Leslie & Thaiss, 1992).

(iii) A defect of theory of mind does not account for autistic deficiency and lack of interest in pretend play.

Things are not much better for simulation theory:

(i) Autistic children do well on visual perspectival tasks, whereas they should not be able to simulate the visual position of others.

(ii) Simulation theory does not account for executive failures in task performance and the autistic desire for sameness.

(iii) Simulation theory does not seem to account for defects in pretend play or in remaining on task the way that normal children do. (Currie [1996] suggests that the lack of imaginative ability in autistics might cause them not to enjoy activity in which the crucial elements are imaginative or to miss the imaginative identification of a goal required for sustained application to a task.)

He also suggests that the problem with novelty and unpredictability might reveal a defect in the imaginative rehearsal of response to novelty. But Grandin's 'squeeze box' suggests a different interpretation: autistic children have a sense of insecurity because their lack of attunement to others makes the actions of other people random, alien, and threatening rather than reassuring, familiar, and intuitively fitting to a shared situation.

The inadequacies of explanation, both philosophical and empirical, tell against currently popular theories about the defect in autism and our knowledge of other minds and direct us back to accounts of interpersonal experience as 'a form of embodied practice' (Gallagher, 2005, p. 208). These recent theorists, in fact, recall Bruner's claim that a child is not a Cartesian epistemic individualist but an intersubjective being from the beginning who elaborates forms of self and other knowledge according to the mirror world she or he is always already located in.

8.3 The psychological foundations of knowledge

The child is a being in the process of becoming an ego-agency or subject through a symbolic or discursive matrix enacted in 'a dialectic of identification' (Lacan, 1977, p. 2). In fact, even the earliest activities of infants are thoroughly interpersonal in nature: a newborn child imitates facial expressions from a few minutes after birth (no doubt through the mirror neurone system), implicitly reacting as a self (albeit relatively inchoate) among others (Gallagher, 2005, p. 65ff).

> There is evidence that even 10-month-olds have some awareness of the subjective life of others, for they seem to share experiences by showing things and pointing things out to others, they request things of others, and they manifest a variety of related interpersonal accomplishments.
>
> (Hobson, 1990, p. 203)

Hobson (1990) notes the primacy of relatedness in the epistemic world of children: 'certain perceptual properties of people bring out "natural" patterns of affective-conative response in infants and the patterns of response are part and parcel of the infants' perception of people as a special class of object' (p. 205). These 'modes of relatedness to people' are similar to Gibson's 'affordances' forming a series of 'biologically prepared mechanisms for establishing commonality across individuals' (p. 207). 'If an infant can imitate or affectively "resonate" to bodily expressions, then already the infant might sense something of the conative affective "personal life" such expressions express' (p. 208).

We are now increasingly realizing the extent of the perceptual, action-based, emotional, and relational links between young children and adults that engage a child in the human life-world. The infant's growing capacities for coordinated action in shared space have two components:

(i) Even very young babies may enter into a communication network with others through comprehension of an adults direction of gaze; communication is not solely dependent upon the greater cognitive sophistication of the adult.

(ii) The phenomenon of joint visual attention presupposes a world of objects, albeit seen from different points of view, existing in a common space. (Butterworth, 1991, p. 70)

Looking where someone else is looking and discovering there an object whose features capture one's attention seems to serve as an epistemic foundation for shared or cooperative action (and coreference) even though 'none of these mechanisms require the infant to have a theory that others have minds' (Butterworth, 1991, p. 55). Rather than it being a theoretical attainment based on an extrapolation of self-knowledge, the infant's intersubjectivity (and thus, the knowledge of other minds) is a primitive given, elaborated during encounters with others, reflected in the mirror of language or discourse (as one might expect from Husserl and Lacan).

The emerging picture recalls Kant's (1789/1929) discussion of cognitive development. He argues that one is trained by others to use concepts and is confident of (or convinced about) the objective validity of a judgement about the world when simulating the verdict of an ideal other in the conditions in which one finds oneself endorses that judgement.

> The touchstone whereby we decide whether our holding a thing to be true is conviction is therefore external, namely, the possibility of communicating it and finding it to be valid for all human reason. (B848)

Both arguments suggest that a human being thinks of himself or herself (a priori) as inhabiting a shared or public space of mutually accessible objects (allowing a cognitive map to be built on intersubjective norms). The fundamental role Kant gives to the of the other in a human being's idea of truth paves the way for later philosophical accounts of a 'sphere of … intersubjective or intersubjectively communalized experience' (Husserl, 1950/1999, p. 107).

The scope of the primitively formative extends beyond the cognitive to the emotional components of interpersonal life through 'primary intersubjectivity'—the psychological connectedness between the infant and others that arises as early as 2–3 months of age.

> In film and television recordings of face-to-face interactions of mothers and their infants aged one to three months, my students and I have observed extremely complex behaviours that have led us to accept the idea that human beings are equipped at birth with a mechanism of personality which is sensitive to persons and expresses itself as a person does.
>
> (Trevarthen, 1979, p. 321)

Infants act as if they are in the presence of responsive conscious beings in all their interactions with the world and, within the context of that (a priori) attitude, develop modes of thinking, feeling, and acting that are appropriate to persons: 'in the second month after birth, their reactions to things and persons are so different that we must conclude that these two classes of object are distinct in the infant's awareness' (Trevarthen, 1979, p. 322).

Trevarthen (1979) uses the word 'rhythm', thereby strengthening the case against inappropriate attempts to intellectualize or use propositional content (beliefs and theories) to explain what is going on: 'We find that a close integration of rhythm of mother and baby is one of the clearest features to emerge from microanalysis of happy communications between two-month-olds and their mothers' (p. 334). The mutuality of the mother–child dyad is primitive or biological and it initiates, is inseparable from, and develops within the primary discursive reality of persons in communication, as if infants echoed in their behaviour Wittgenstein's (1953) remarks on the interpersonal realm of experience—'My attitude towards him is an attitude towards a soul. I am not of the opinion that he has a soul' (p. 178e).

Trevarthen (1979) focuses on the child's underlying 'attitude' (thereby indicating a non-propositional mental act) that she or he is in contact with other souls or subjects because the cues given out and registered by the infant to and from others are inelimimably subjective:

> Acts that make subjective processes overt include the following: focusing attention on things, handling and exploring objects with interest in the consequences, orienting or avoiding while anticipating the course of events, and meeting or evading them. (p. 322)

These acts recall Wittgenstein's (1969) emphasis on the foundations of knowledge being in 'the deed': 'it is our acting which lies at the bottom of the language-game' (¶ 204).

> Our findings with infants two or three months of age lead us to conclude that a complex form of mutual understanding develops even at this age. It is both naturally accepted and strongly regulated by the infant. Two-month-olds exhibit many different expressions, some highly emotional, and they make a variety of attempts to gain the lead in an exchange with another person. They are also sensitive to subtle differences in the mother's expression.

> (Trevarthen, 1979, p. 346)

These observations reinforce phenomenological warnings about overintellectualizing intersubjectivity; a human child is naturally disposed to act in certain ways rather than cognitively 'thematizing' what is going on with self and others (Zahavi, 2005, p. 165). The natural mutuality (or being-in-the-world-with-others) in evidence shapes the psychological concepts one learns to use and 'sheets them home' to a pragmatic and affective context engaging the developing thinker with others as subject or agent . Many of the interactions occurring there (through the words and expressions they make meaningful) articulate the child's growing awareness of self as a psychological being such that the cumulative weight of multiple and varied encounters with others both predate and infect one's knowledge of self through the 'dialectic of identification' that makes one into somebody (a human being with an identity).

Wittgenstein (1953), reflecting on our personal being, notes the 'imponderability' of the grounds of 'attitudes to souls'; 'Imponderable evidence includes subtleties of glance, of gesture, of tone' (p. 228e), and he concludes that much of our knowledge of others does not proceed by evidence and inference (and other theoretical or ratiocinative) processes but in other ways.

> I may recognize a genuine loving look, distinguish it from a pretended one (and here there can, of course, be a 'ponderable' confirmation of my judgement). But I may be quite incapable of describing the difference. (p. 228e)

Bruner (1990) also argues that early mutuality or intersubjectivity is a primary biological adaptation towards communication and sets the stage, as it were, for the learning of language by the child (p. 67ff). Once learnt, as I have suggested, the language itself informs experience, the organization of behaviour, and the development of self-knowledge.

The early communicative and interactive behaviour of young children casts doubt on the idea that one has a derivative perception of others as analogous to oneself on the basis of analogy with introspective epistemic 'primitives', the foundations of empiricist philosophy, but also corrects the simulation view of other-minds knowledge.

Theory-theory is a *cold theory* ('inference from one set of beliefs to another'), but simulation is a *hot theory* based on 'motivational and emotional resources and one's own capacity for practical reasoning'. But, it does not tell us how the child begins to conceive that there are other subjectivities around (nor does it avoid the private language problem) despite its instructive points of resonance with intersubjective theory.

Gordon (1996) claims that a child 'ascends' from asking the question 'Is P true?' to the assertion (provided certain constraints are met) using an 'ascent routine'. The result is a set of beliefs that facts and feelings are held or experienced at certain subjective locations (so that the child can attribute e.g. *pain* here/there and *belief that P* here/there, where 'here' and 'there' are points of subjectivity) so that knowing what others are thinking and feeling is based on the child's own feelings, reactions, and dispositions to believe thus and so in certain conditions (thus a 'hot' theory) relying on introspective knowledge. However, such an account does not provide an account of how the child learns the content of those attributions, a question that drives us into the arms of Kant (training in judgement), Wittgenstein (learning rules), or the phenomenologists.

Discursive theory argues that the ability to understand others may involve imitation of others but is, at heart, a way of framing myself against the discourse of others through the way they interact with me and the words they direct at me (in teaching) and use of me. It builds on the primary knowledge that I am among other minded creatures, a fundamental feature of my being and not a secondary development on my epistemic journey (Husserl, Bruner, Hobson, Zahavi). Competence on the false-belief task requires the skill of mapping oneself on the meaning structure of intentional life (or subjectivity) and also the ability to go beyond basic congruence to take account of diverse positions in the human life-world. Even for a normal child, those are non-obvious skills, but an autistic child has profound problems because the failure of primary intersubjectivity undermines the secondary skills that are built upon it as part of adaptation to the shared human life-world.

8.4 The phenomenological foundations of knowledge

Phenomenology offers a radical alternative to traditional empiricist epistemology in that it 'begins with the study of human consciousness; it is an attempt to define the structures that are essential to any and every possible experience' (Solomon, 1989, p. 159). Connections with Descartes and Kant are obvious in that it suspends belief in overarching presuppositions and appeals to first-person experience to investigate the structure of experience on the basis of what is implicit within it (when critically examined).

Husserl approached human thought by arguing that we must suspend the 'natural' or realistic attitude that the world exists independent of us and has a certain physical form and begin by examining our experience and what it implies (without any presuppositions). In particular, we must refuse to predicate an account of human knowledge on a scientific theory about human beings such as that found in Cartesian materialism and also in Millikan, Dretske, Sober, and Pinker. We cannot allow metaphysical assumptions about the foundations of human knowledge or understanding lying within the psychophysics of the sensory receptors of the individual to overrule the primary data of our being-in-the-world-with-others, always already aware of them as subjects and engaged with them through intersubjective relations. We are, as is evident, belatedly discovering the empirical data (about infant development and mirror neurons, and so on) that add suasion to the phenomenological and anti-individualist arguments against the 'scientist in the crib' view.

When we interrogate experience and experiment about the foundations of human knowledge ('heterophenomenologically' [Dennett]) without Cartesian (or methodologically solipsist) assumptions, we see that the origins of knowledge and adaptation are interpersonal or intersubjective rather than a function of the cognitive individual. Thus, other human beings, their resonance with me, and their 'dealings with the world' (Heidegger) are basic and salient in our experience of the world in ways that Husserl (the world of shared accessibility and the intersubjective life-world of embodied subjects), Sartre (the look), Levinas (the face and the enigma of other subjectivities), and Lacan (the mirror stage that forms the I) have explored.

> This relation which I call 'being-seen-by-another', far from being merely one of the relations signified by the word *man*, represents an irreducible fact which cannot be deduced either from the essence of the other-as-object or from my being-as-subject.
>
> (Sartre, 1958, p. 257)

The look places the other subject as a fundamental conditioning feature of any situation as is evident when one is aware of being seen, of being an object for the other (an experience that is heightened and made threatening in psychosis and the ontological uncertainty or vulnerability at the centre of psychotic alienation and depersonalization).

> The look which the eyes manifest, no matter what kind of eyes they are, is a pure reference to myself. What I apprehend immediately when I hear the branches crackling behind me is not that *there is someone there*; it is that I am vulnerable, that I have a body that can be hurt, that I occupy a place, and that I cannot in any case escape from the space in which I am without defense—in short, that I am *seen*. (Sartre, 1958, p. 259)

Shorn of its existential *angst*, this primal feature is centrally significant in human experience—the experience of being observed or in the presence of another rather than being alone. Individual history and the (implicit) imperatives (or reactive attitudes) accompanying the mirroring of self in the subjectivity of others attach positive or negative affective weight to this aspect of one's being-in-the-world so that *value* is a mode of being that comes naturally to us.

The phenomenological exploration of experiential basicness recalls Wittgenstein's later thought in which language comprises the tools used for relating to others in a shared action space. Such a reading of human understanding and meaning reinforces the idea that the psyche is structured by informal rules mediating cooperative activity, a practical mutuality underpinning Wittgenstein's use of *Im anfang war die tat* ('In the beginning was the deed' [Goethe]). We are primarily beings who do things with each other and our knowledge grows out of that practical acquaintance (dealings) with the world.

The a priori congruence between self and others is part of a normal child's starting position in understanding the world.

> Well before the child can understand the spoken words of his teacher, even in early infancy, he learns to comply. He complies with and responds to the glance of the mother, the tone of her voice, the look of her face, and to her gestures rather than the words themselves. In short, he learns to respond to the infinitely rich display of human expressive phenomena.
>
> It is not the content of words that make a child comply with requests, by processing them intellectually. It is, above all, the affect of the caregiver which speaks through the words.
>
> (Asperger, 1944/1991, p. 47)

Strawson (1959) argues that our language about our thoughts and ourselves as subjects logically entails that one is aware of being a person among other persons whose use of psychological terms to understand themselves articulates their mental lives in (essentially) shared terms. He subsequently relates this to the reactive attitudes at the heart of moral and forensic thought in a way that makes intersubjective evaluations a basic feature of human reason and intentional activity (Strawson, 1974).

Human beings are, we could say, primarily communicators—beings who know themselves to be in touch with other minded and subjective beings. When we incorporate that orientation into our epistemology, it restructures our view of the foundations of human knowledge in a way that is reinforced by examining situations that contrast with both normal development and the most prevalent kinds of autism. The first of these involves the defects shown by feral and severely neglected children, and the second the cognitive attainments of autistic 'savants'.

8.5 The wolf-children

In 1920, a missionary called the Reverend Joseph Singh went out into the jungles of Bengal on a 'ghost' hunt; he found the 'ghosts' in a den of wolves.

> Close after the cubs, came the 'ghost'—a hideous looking being, hand, foot, and body like a human being, but the head was a big ball of something covering the shoulders and the upper portion of the bust leaving only the sharp contour of the face visible. Close at its heels, there came another awful creature exactly like the first, but smaller in size. Their eyes were bright and piercing unlike human eyes.
>
> (Maclean, 1977, pp. 60–61)

The den, an old termite mound, was opened, the mother wolf killed, and the 'ghosts' and the other cubs captured.

> The two cubs and the other two hideous beings were there in one corner, all four clutching together in a monkey-ball. It was really a task to separate them from one another. The ghosts were more ferocious than the cubs, making faces, showing teeth, making for us when too much disturbed, and running back to reform the monkey-ball.
>
> (Maclean, 1977, p. 66)

The 'ghosts' were two children, aged about three and six years—Amala and Kamala. Rev. Singh took them back to his mission, but surprises were in store as the wolf-children began to explore their new surroundings.

Astonished by the way the dogs seemed to recognize the child as one of them, as much by the eagerness and complete lack of inhibition she displayed in going among them, Singh watched as the girl, on bandaged knees and elbows, darting glances askance at her new companions milling around her, lowered her face to the dog bowl, seized her food, and bolted it with convulsive shakes of her upper body, keeping her head close to the ground. She secured a large bone and carried it off to a corner of the yard away from the others, where she soon settled down, holding it under her hands as if they were paws, and began to gnaw at it, occasionally rubbing it along the ground to help separate the meat from the bone.

(Maclean, 1977, p. 79)

We have seen in the case of autistic children that, without the distinctive cueing of a well-tried set of world-related techniques, the world can be both bewildering and alarming. Children are designed to latch on to the intentional (world-related) and intersubjective practices of their caregivers; so, in the case of the wolf-children, we see a wolf-like pattern of learnt attunement to the environment (including distinctive patterns of such basic actions as food swallowing).

The narrative reveals the deeply disruptive effects of a schism in the attuning environment brought about by a change in caregivers.

Fear registered chiefly in their eyes, which during the day were always heavy as if with sleep, often half-lidded; at night, when they became generally more active, their eyes would be open wide, alert, and piercingly bright.

(Maclean, 1977, p. 85)

Even two months after their capture, Amala and Kamala's reaction to human beings was 'a threatening display or else to hide away in a corner of their cage and refuse to look around' (Maclean, 1977, p. 90). Their first contacts with their human caregivers were tentative, cautious, and hesitant. 'At first, only Amala could bring herself to look at Mrs. Singh, but by and by Kamala commenced to look at her, at first stealthily by side looks and then slowly by looking straight and meeting her eyes as she looked' (p. 117).

Gradually, the wolf-children began to accept their human caregivers although they were still quite 'alien', uneasy, or uncomfortable in the presence of humans. Unfortunately, Amala, the three-year-old, died of what was thought to be kidney disease some 11 months after her capture without ever readjusting to her schismatic autobiography. Kamala finally learned to seek the company of other children but never developed the 'natural' relationships that normal children seem to develop so easily. She did, however, become quite attached to the missionary's wife, Mrs. Singh.

The contrast between the children's early wolf-like habits and their discomfort in the presence of human beings, and the later attempts by Kamala to 'fit in' with her human 'pack' can be seen in two excerpts.

Like wolves, the children at first were nocturnal, displaced aliens in the human world. After midnight, the children never slept and were constantly on the move, prowling around, pacing to and fro . . . sometimes at night they howled. (p. 87)

Later, after Amala had died, there was a poignant episode where Kamala was left outside the house while the others went in. She sat beside the door, got restless, ran from door to door, and finally 'she heard someone talking inside and she gave a shrill cry. . . After a while, another cry and an abrupt push on the door. At last the door was opened and she crawled in quietly.'

(Maclean, 1977, p. 165)

On one occasion, after Mrs. Singh had been away for a few days and Kamala heard that she had returned, there was a genuine indication that she had bonded to her foster human mother and had begun to adopt the ways of a human child.

Kamala's face suddenly brightened . . . She left the room on all fours and ran out into the garden to meet her, welcoming her with the words 'Ma Elo' (Mama come). Catching hold of Mrs. Singh's hand, she stood up and walked with her very slowly on two feet down the drive, refusing to let any of the other children come near and jabbering excitedly as if trying to recount everything that had happened in her absence.

(Maclean, 1977, p. 183)

Despite the fact that she lived with the Singhs for nearly nine years, Kamala never really adapted to human skills and expectations and she died aged about 15.

The story of the wolf-children suggests that human infants are primed to catch the acculturation and adaptations of their caregivers and that they assimilate these into their own patterns of responding. That orientation normally allows a child to acquire the techniques of human discourse, but it cannot do so if the narrative context is too abnormal.

8.6 **The lonely children**

Seamus Heaney's haunting poem about a boy kept in a henhouse and fed through a flap in the door, and the wolf-girls change from their wolf mode of existence into a more human one recall other stories that teach the same lessons.

Victor, the wild boy of Aveyron, was discovered naked on a tanner's doorstep in post-revolutionary France of 1800. The enlightenment was in full cry, and human reason and language were the focus of intense interest. Reason and communication, universal attainments, seemed to speak to the innate distinction between humanity and other beasts. Victor and later Genie (discovered in 1970 in California) both problematized the ideology of nativism, the latter when the language-cognition debate raged between Chomsky and Skinner.

Genie was confined to a small bedroom harnessed to an infant's potty seat. . . . Genie was left to sit, tied up, hour after hour, often into the night, day after day, month after month, year after year.

(Rymer, 1994, p. 19)

Genie, harnessed by day and constrained in a sleeping bag by night, was not spoken to by her parents and if she made a noise she was beaten. Genie's mother complied with this regime but was herself blind and 'felt helpless to do anything' (Rymer, 1994, p. 21). Genie was finally discovered at 13 years of age when her mother left her husband, took Genie with her, and went to seek medical help for her blindness but, by mistake, walked into a social security office.

Both children initially showed a marked indifference to other human beings, but Genie, unlike Victor, had a rudimentary vocabulary.

> Her vocabulary comprised only a few words—probably fewer than twenty. She understood 'red', 'blue', 'green', and 'brown'; 'Mother' and some other names; the verbs 'walk' and 'go'; and assorted nouns, among them 'door', 'jewellery box', and 'bunny'. Her productive vocabulary—those words she could utter—was even more limited. She seemed able to say only 'Stopit' and 'Nomore', and a couple of shorter negatives.
>
> (Rymer, 1994, pp. 10–11)

Both children were exposed to intensive language rehabilitation with marked initial success.

> For a while, the boy was off on a rocket ride of comprehension. He learned not only to find an object if he was presented with its written name but also to write the name when he was shown the object. And not just objects: he learned adjectives and verbs as well, with which he could both comprehend and concoct written sentences. Interestingly, even this little bit of language seemed to open up new ways of thinking for him. The boy who had been completely adrift could concentrate. Chores he had performed mechanically were suddenly imbued with spontaneity and imagination.
>
> (Rymer, 1994, p. 76)

In both cases, the rapid attainment tailed off, and although the children developed some language skills, their linguistic abilities in social interaction were permanently stunted.

> That Genie's language seemed motivated by social strivings contained a pathetic irony, because she was especially incompetent at. . . the interactions essential to social discourse.
>
> (Rymer, 1994, p. 127)

Both children failed; Victor, the wild boy of Aveyron, lived until he was forty years old.

> The Wild Boy never spoke. The Wild Boy was abandoned. The Wild Boy was put in a small house near here and eventually forgotten.
>
> (Rymer, 1994, p. 79)

Genie's fate is equally pathetic. She was returned to her mother's custody when 21 years old.

> I saw her again when she was twenty-nine, and she still looked miserable. She looked to me like a chronically institutionalized person. It was heart-rending.
>
> (Rymer, 1994, p. 219)

The plight of human children raised without the normal intersubjective resonance, nurture, and communication emphasizes the importance of love in the development of language and cognition. The implications of phenomenological analysis, developmental psychology, poetry, and anecdote are now confirmed by the evidence of brain scans of Rumanian orphans. The human mind or brain needs to develop on a diet of interpersonal commitment and care, and one of Genie's teachers remarked as follows:

> Genie's problem was seen too much as a pedagogical one, not an emotional one. . . Our advancements take place in a relationship. In order for an infant to learn anything—and this takes you back to Victor, the Wild Boy of Aveyron—there has to be a relationship in which the child gets enough nurturance to proceed. Affective attachment plays the primary role. It is not an intellectual process. Intellect rides on the back of affective bonding. And affection's not easy to come by.
>
> (Rymer, 1994, pp. 221–222)

Those most concerned with Genie are eloquent on the theme of the soul's need for intersubjectivity and a loving climate in which a human being is inscribed with ways of being: 'This is soul sickness. . . There is no medical explanation for her decline into what appears to be organic, biological dementia' (Rymer, 1994, p. 219).

These final words underscore the holistic interaction between the world of meaning (and therefore of interpersonal relationships) and our human flesh, an understanding that should inform the medical ethos and our studies of the human mind. The human psyche exists through engagements, and Genie's fate is appropriately called 'soul sickness'.

8.7 **The idiot savant**

The lack of interpersonality or intersubjectivity as a fundamental defect in cognition (that is almost certainly very demanding in terms of cognitive megabytes) seems to have the effect of enhancing other kinds of cognitive skill (which may be truly outstanding and idiosyncratic) as in the case of autistic 'savants' or gifted children with 'Asperger's syndrome'.

The *Diagnostic and Statistical Manual of Mental Disorders IV* (DSM IV; APA, 1994a) characterizes Asperger's syndrome as comprising

(A) 'Severe and sustained impairment in social interaction'; and

(B) 'The development of restricted, repetitive patterns of behaviour, interests, and activities' (p. 75).

Asperger's syndrome is generally less severe than autism and may not be distinct from the problems of other high-functioning autistic children. Such children vary a great deal but often show severe social impairments, 'such as literalness, poor social comprehension, lack of empathy, lack of reciprocity, inappropriate social behaviour, failure to appreciate subtle humour, and restricted behavioural repertoires' (Rumsey, 1992). Others echo Asperger's original report of autistic 'loss of contact': 'they cannot modify their social behaviour to the demands of the environment. They are always "out of context"' (Szatmari, 1991, p. 83).

Szatmari (1991) also notes the obsessive interests that can be developed by such children.

> These can often take an unusual or bizarre form. For example, children with Asperger's syndrome may develop an extreme interest in subjects such as astronomy, meteorology, subways, bus timetables, or certain addresses. (p. 83)

The obsessive activities can shade into the preoccupations of normal children but, if considered in isolation and assimilated to normal cognitive abilities, these obsessive tendencies can obscure the truly outstanding mental feats that may be in evidence.

One mother, whose son was a high-functioning autistic child, remarked, 'Joseph can multiply four-digit numbers in his head almost as quickly as you can punch buttons on a calculator' (Sullivan, 1992, p. 244). A remarkable anecdote tells of this ability. Joseph visited his uncle who was impressed by the fact that his new computer could answer 'such questions as what number times what number will give the answer of 1,234,567,890'.

> Just about then, Joseph walked into the room.
> 'Joseph, what number times what number will give you 1,2,3,4,5,6,7,8,9,0?'
> As quickly as you could say your own telephone number, Joseph said '9 times 137,174,210'.
>
> (Sullivan, 1992, p. 244)

Joseph in fact showed quite amazing cognitive powers at quite a young age.

> One day when he was about 4, we were alone in the station wagon. The almost-always-silent Joseph threw off the blanket he had wrapped around his head, popped his thumb out of his mouth, and said—to no one in particular—'Dangerous Intersection, 21 letters', then went back to his reverie.
>
> (Sullivan, 1992)

Such feats demonstrate just how computationally complex the operations of autistic children can be, as is seen in *Rain Man* when the autistic brother counts 147 toothpicks as they drop to the floor from a waitress' tray (based on a real-life event in which autistic twins instantly counted 111 matches that had fallen from a table before they hit the ground).

The strangeness of the high-functioning autistic is evident even in the most ordinary situations; one commentator describes it as autistic eccentricity and comments on his friend Jack.

> We were sharing a garden melon when he commented, 'Sally did not like muskmelon. Then she tried some and found out that she liked it after all.' I pondered this, and asked him to tell me who Sally is. 'Dick and Jane's little sister', he replied. After an interlude of 35 years, he was making this casual reference to a character in a preprimer.
>
> (Dewey, 1992, pp. 285–286)

A further story illustrates how socially dislocated the responses of an autistic to everyday interpersonal situations can be. The incident concerned Michael, a friend of the author, who had come to visit and was served a casserole for lunch.

> When Michael saw the casserole. . . he left the table to look in the refrigerator for something more to his liking. I asked, 'Does your mother ever tell you to try things she has prepared before you decide you do not like them?' 'Oh yes', Michael conceded cheerfully. 'She always wants me to do that.' I told Michael that I happened to feel like his mother. Thereupon he put a generous serving of the casserole on his plate.

> Michael next asked for a pepper mill. We watched first in fascination, then in horror, as his steady grinding continued. Finally I said, 'That's a lot of pepper, Michael. It will burn your mouth.' No problem. He explained that he wanted to hide the taste of the food. His plate resembled a mound of fireplace ashes, completely grey. And he ate it all.
>
> (Dewey, 1992, p. 287)

This is a strange solution to the social problem, but not at all surprising for an autistic person.

It is tempting to think of the 'savant knowledge' of high-functioning autistics as a domain of methodical, logical, and number-crunching roboticism exclusive to humans whose cognitive structure is inflexible and not attuned to patterns evident to the rest of us. But some artistic attainments of 'savants' cast doubt on the 'intelligent automaton' (Asperger) conception.

> I had never before properly recognized the cognitive structure of savant talents. I had, by and large, taken them to be an expression of rote memory and little else. Martin, indeed, had a prodigious memory, but it was clear that this memory, in relation to Bach, was structural or categorical (and specifically architectonic)—he understood how the music went together, how this variation was an inversion of that, how different voices could take up a line and combine them in a canon or fugue, and he could construct a simple fugue himself. He knew, for at least a few bars ahead, how a line would go. He could not formulate this, it was not explicit or conscious, but there was a remarkable implicit understanding of musical form.
>
> (Sacks, 1995, p. 212)

This intriguing set of observations does not portray a stilted and mechanical intelligence but someone with a graceful and sensitive grasp of a cognitive field in which human lyricism and creativity are exemplified a fortiori. His command of that field suggests that the defect in autism is localized to the realm of the interpersonal and is only (secondarily) pervasive because of the pervasive role of interpersonally developed discursive skills in human thought and activity. The pervasive defect is not apparent in those who focus on 'theory of mind' or simulation in relation to other minds, but the 'interaction theory' (Gallagher, 2004) or discursive view is radically different from both and motivates a restructuring of the foundations of epistemology.

8.8 Restructuring the foundations

The study of autism dramatically endorses the primacy in human knowledge of intentionality as related to objects and significant others in the environment (or being-in-the-world-with-others). The actions of human beings in situations where language is taught and learnt give meaning or significance to the things that children encounter as in Temple Grandin's case.

> Somehow the school and the speech therapist got through to Temple, rescued her (she came to feel) from the abyss, and started her on her slow emergence. She now remained clearly autistic, but her new powers of language and communication now gave her an anchor, some ability to master what had been total chaos before. Her sensory system, with its violent oscillations of oversensitivity and undersensitivity, started to stabilize a little.
>
> (Sacks, 1995, p. 259)

The comparison between autistic and normal children supports the phenomenologists' claim that the foundations of knowledge are interpersonal or intersubjective. Human intentionality is mapped out in a context of relatedness to very special beings—human beings. Sometimes, these subjective objects are nurturing, warm, welcoming, and responsive, and at other times or in other cases, they are condemning, rejecting, and critical. Genie suffered profound damage when the abusive and rejecting elements of interpersonal interaction occluded any other features. But what normally happens when a child learns to think about the world?

First, there is the establishment of congruence with other human beings that becomes full-bodied on the basis of a natural predisposition towards intersubjectivity. The increasing growth of congruence cues the child's perceptual processes onto those bits of the world worth thinking about and begins to cement in place knowledge of objects and properties that human beings have found useful around here. This happens in an atmosphere of care encouraging exploration and defining limits to the child's engagement with her context through a 'mirror' of evaluative responses: 'Good girl,' 'That's not nice,' 'Aren't you clever,' and so on.

The atmosphere of (inherently intersubjective) cognitive engagement with a shared world lays the groundwork for thought by marking those things significant to others and marked in language. Thus, the interpersonal comes naturally to the normal child, but what is more difficult are the interwoven and theory-laden groupings and categorizations (secondarily) constructed on the basis of the primitive intersubjective resonance that shapes cognition.

Why is the autistic child so globally impaired except in areas of savant knowledge? A clear answer now emerges: the autistic child cannot use the scaffolding provided by intersubjectivity as a basis on which to erect his or her knowledge of the world. One adult autistic patient gives a telling testimony to this impoverishment in relation to emotion and knowing his own psyche.

> And through all this condescending concern about feelings and emotional issues, no one ever bothered to explain to me what the words meant! No one ever told me that they expected to *see* feelings on my face, or that it confused them when I used words without showing corresponding expressions. No one explained what the signals were or how to use them. They simply assumed that if *they* could not *see* my feelings I could not *feel* them. I think this shows a serious lack of perspective taking!

> (Sinclair, 1992, p. 297)

Here we see the breakdown of intersubjectivity and the inability of an autistic person to develop the discursive skills needed to express and develop his emotional life. It suggests, especially in the light of the creative savant skills of Martin the musician, that the autistic person is not a cognitive robot but rather a complex cognitive being who cannot use the primary trick of human evolution—the trick of intersubjectivity allowing one to become attuned to the world of others and latch on to their adaptive tricks in knowing both the world and oneself as a being-with-others-in-the-world who instances the same properties as they do.

The autistic, deprived of intersubjective access to a shared world, is faced by a problem that is fiendishly difficult: it concerns human beings and is best expressed as 'How does this complex machine work?' That this problem has kept generations of scientists busy since the beginning of human history explains why so many autistics fall at the first hurdle and cannot achieve a coherent and developed cognitive system. It should also allow us to address some philosophical issues forming the backdrop to the present discussion.

8.9 Philosophical problems

I have argued that a child learns to understand the world by using his or her natural propensities to fit into a discursive milieu of human intersubjectivity. The intersubjective nature of experience and the child's biological predisposition to develop on that basis mean that an internal or external defect in intersubjectivity creates pervasive developmental problems. Either a breakdown of the natural resonance, rhythm, and facility of intersubjectivity in autism or a contextual breakdown in cases such as Genie and the wolf-children can give rise to debilitating defects in the foundations of human knowledge, a problem with dramatic implications for traditional approaches to epistemology.

The argument from perceptual basicness

(1) The mind is a set of functions realized in the nervous system.

[(1a) The hierarchy of functions in the mind reflects the hierarchy of function in the brain.]

(2) Perception involves gathering information through the sensory systems.

(3) Perceiving begins with the simple impingements on the sensory receptors—simple impressions.

(4) Perceiving complex things proceeds by the combination of simple impressions according to induction, conjecture, custom, and so forth.

(5) Objects in the external world are complex things not simple impressions. Therefore,

(6) My knowledge of external things is less certain than my knowledge of simple impressions.

Personal knowledge corollary

(7) People and their behaviour are complex objects.

(8) Our knowledge of other people as thinking, acting beings is derived from and more tenuous than our knowledge of objects.

(9) Our knowledge of other minds is much more tenuous than our knowledge of simple impressions.

(10) Our knowledge of other minds is a complex intellectual attainment.

The contrast between autistic and normal children has shown us that 10 is false and thus prompts a re-evaluation of the supporting premises. That reveals that the combination involving 1a, 2, and 3 is false and therefore 6, 7, 8, 9, and 10 are all mistaken. 1a, 2, and

3 are false because the mind does not start with the primitive inputs amenable to investigation of the sensory systems considered in isolation. Infants are inherently intersubjective beings, preprogrammed to latch on to the techniques of others such that two primitive dispositions or attitudes underpin all cognitive development:

(A) *I am surrounded by others just like me.*

(B) *These others already know what the world we share is like.*

These two attitudes are the foundations of human knowledge and only a misguided deference to the physical sciences and physiology in particular has blinded empiricist epistemologists to that fact. Given that the starting point of much epistemology (and Western psychology) is mistaken, it is no wonder that we have got ourselves into such a mess not only about other minds but also about language and thought, and about facts and values.

The 'other minds' conclusion expressed in 10 and the scepticism flowing from it actually 'gets the cart before the horse'. The 'go-cart' of human cognition is, as Kant claims, real-world examples in association with which other people, cognitively speaking, take my hand. The autistic child is the individualist, empiricist cognitive explorer (the 'scientist in the crib') and his epistemic task is so fiendishly difficult that it is no wonder that only a minority of autistic people ever achieve anything similar to normal human adaptation to the world around them.

The distinctness of facts and values

(1) Facts are states of affairs that exist in the world.

(2) Values are attitudes towards states of affairs based on evaluative judgements.

(3) We learn to detect states of affairs first and then secondarily we make evaluative judgements about them based on our own feelings and those that others communicate to us.

(4) Our evaluative attitudes are based on our emotions and the evaluative responses of others both to states of affairs and to ourselves.

(5) Our appreciations of fact are prior to and independent of appreciations of value.

The crucial mistake here is in premise 3. It is false because we learn to detect and respond to states of affairs in the world based on the evaluative responses of others to our fledgling discursive efforts in a shared environment (the mirror of our infant lives). Thus, our knowledge of facts is secondary to evaluative exchanges between ourselves and others such that, to some extent, evaluations affect all human knowledge (as postmodernists claim).

Consciousness and machines

(1) Consciousness is a matter of complex cognitive operations.

(2) Cognition involves detecting and processing information from the world.

(3) Machines can detect and process information from the world in ways that are as complex as we can.

(4) Machines can be conscious.

The problem here is not consciousness but the complex intersubjectivity and fluid resonance between human beings (and some animals) that results in the complex conative-cognitive processes we call sensing, feeling, being responsive to, and thinking about the things around you (and therefore grounds our attributions of those states and processes to others). Our brief glance at the autistic world has suggested that we attribute mental states to others and ourselves partly on the basis of the feeling quality we discern in the responses and reactions of others so that the judgement that something or someone is conscious embeds such discernment. That is why we are more ready to attribute consciousness to animals who can feel bodily pain than to machines who cannot (whatever their cognitive attainments). If we made machines that flinched and cried, then perhaps our attitudes would change because, as Wittgenstein (1953) notes, our attitudes are basic in knowing that another being is or is not a conscious soul (p. 178e).

This, in fact, is a good point to turn our attention to the problem of psychopathy because in that condition it seems that many cognitive structures remain intact apart from features of cognition crucially centred on the moral appreciation of the feelings and vulnerabilities of others.

Chapter 9

Moral insanity and evil

For the I of the basic word I-You is different from that in the basic word I-It.
Basic words do not state something that might exist outside them; by being spoken, they establish a mode of existence.
The basic word I-You can only be spoken with one's whole being.

(Buber, 1970, pp. 53–54)

Section A: **Psychopaths**

9.1 **Introduction: a picture of psychopathy**

David E. is 23. He is in police custody because he inflicted injuries leading to severe brain damage in a 29-year-old woman. He met the woman at a dance where he had gone with some friends. He danced with her a few times, bought one or two drinks, and agreed to take her somewhere quieter for coffee. He asked his friend if he could have the keys of his car, giving the impression, it was later said, that he only wanted them for a moment or so. He took the woman in the car to a fairly isolated spot near the city and there raped her, becoming angry when she protested. She was later found having been raped and also having suffered severe head injuries including extensive skull fractures produced by a spanner from the car. When found by the police, David readily admitted that he had had sex with the woman and roughed her up a bit. His remarks throughout the interview took the form of self-justification. He didn't think his friend should cause a fuss about his taking the car because, after all, 'That's what friends are for.' He said that the woman obviously wanted sex because she was 'carrying on with him' at the dance. He said that he got annoyed when she began screaming because she was going to cause trouble if she carried on and so he 'gave her a bit of what for to teach her not to be such a silly bitch'.

David, for whom this is just one of a series of violent episodes beginning in his teenage years, has been labelled as a psychopath. The two major criteria characterizing those diagnosed as psychopathic (*antisocial personality disorder* or *sociopathic disorder*) are their callous and inconsiderate treatment of others and a recurring pattern of antisocial and destructive behaviour. Popular imagination often links this term to the serial killer or mad gunman whose behaviour is both violent and incomprehensible causing others to talk about 'evil incarnate' or 'animal', overlooking the fact that animals are rarely violent unless they live by predation or are cornered and desperate (perhaps a clue to the more extreme cases discussed in this chapter).

The *Diagnostic and Statistical Manual of Mental Disorders IV* (DSM IV; APA, 1994a), profiling antisocial personality disorder (ASPD), mentions 'a pervasive pattern of disregard for and violation of the rights of others occurring since age 15' (p. 649) and DSM III included 'markedly impaired capacity to sustain lasting, close, warm, and responsible relationships with family, friends, or sexual partners' (pp. 317–318). These characteristics also motivate the now outmoded term *moral insanity*. Prichard originally provided descriptions of cases showing 'morbid perversion' of emotion and action coexisting with 'an apparently unimpaired state of the intellectual faculties' (Whitlock, 1967, p. 73). His cases were, in fact, a mixed bunch, but the appeal of the name and the striking lack of intellectual impairment meant that the term was available for later use (Cleckley, 1941/1976). The category was at odds with the M'Naghten rules and other legal attempts to characterize exculpatory insanity (Berrios, 1993) because although the person's intellect was usually unimpaired (although perhaps not well developed), their 'moral sense' was grossly deficient as is evident from psychological studies in prison populations (Eysenck, 1965). That fact alone does not distinguish between the bad and the mad although the impression that there is something seriously wrong (some soul sickness) with psychopaths and the relation between personality disorders and what we commonly call 'defects of character' or even 'character traits' requires careful scrutiny (Berrios, 1993).

Berrios rehearses a history of poorly characterized behavioural problems under the loose terms 'psychopathic inferiority' and 'personality disorder' associated with 'degenerative deficiency of the mind' or 'psychic and moral constitution'. The uncomfortable similarity between these symptoms and general 'antisocial activity or asocial nature' of diverse types has made many commentators suspicious of the idea that psychopathy is a 'true illness' (Berrios, 1993; Blackburn, 1988).

The insanity of the psychopaths is often related to the fact that the destructive effects of their behaviour are not confined to the lives of others but also tends to undermine their own long-term interests (Cleckley, 1941/1976). Their impulsivity, violence, shallowness, and lack of consideration, taken together with the adverse effects on their own lives, suggest that these individuals have severe defects in practical reasoning or volition even though their alleged mental disorder appears to be very strange in that they may be able to converse about their actions with apparent reasonableness and see why they have offended others, or even use a fairly developed knowledge of the moral and emotional effect of their acts on others to refine the cruelty and impact of those acts. Indeed, when we see the actions that some psychopaths commit, we are struck by their bizarre violence or perversity and the thought that anybody who could do something like that must be mad. Thus, psychopaths, both individually and as a group, inhabit the border zone between madness and badness and problematize both categories:

First, when is bad behaviour properly regarded as due to a psychiatric disorder?

Second, what is volition or the will and how can it be pathological in its operation?

Third, is there such a thing as freedom of the will (and moral responsibility)?

Fourth, what is morality and what does it mean for an agent to have moral sense?

Fifth, are there people who are 'radically evil' so that 'evil becomes their good'?

The first question covers ground traversed already but sharpens the focus on the relation between brain dysfunction and mental disorder in that obvious and widely disruptive cognitive disorders of the acute psychoses are not in evidence and cognition, narrowly construed, seems to be intact. The next questions take us into the philosophy (and neurophilosophy) of volition and are relevant to the issue of moral responsibility for one's actions. The last question has vexed philosophers for centuries and is raised by cases such as Sutcliffe (the Yorkshire Ripper), and the Boston strangler. So, what can philosophy say about this condition variously called *Antisocial Personality Disorder, Sociopathy, Psychopathy*, or *Moral Insanity*?

9.2 Insanity and moral insanity: theories of psychopathy

What are psychopaths like, and why should one think they are suffering from a single disorder? Many psychological and other experiments on psychopaths recruit their samples from populations of criminal offenders currently in prison (Blackburn, 1975). We ought first to contrast psychopaths with psychotic (or clearly criminally insane) patients.

> A man who is sane by the standards of psychiatry, aware of all the facts which we ourselves recognize, and free from delusions but who conducts himself in a way quite as absurd as . . . the psychotic becomes another problem altogether . . . I find it necessary first of all to postulate that the psychopath has a genuine and very serious disability, or disorder, or deviation.
>
> (Cleckley, 1941/1976, pp. 403–404)

The phrase 'quite as absurd as the psychotic' conceals a very real difference: psychotic thought is disordered whereas the psychopath seems to be 'calling the shots' in an unbalanced way despite the fact that his trains of thought are often coherent and self-interestedly rational much as those of you or I. The DSM IV criteria for ASPD include 'failure to conform to social norms . . . deceitfulness . . . or conning others for personal profit or pleasure . . . impulsivity . . . irritability or aggressiveness . . . reckless disregard for the safety of self or others . . . consistent irresponsibility . . . lack of remorse' (APA, 1994a, pp. 649–650).

Miller (1987) fills out the profile.

> Psychopaths are described as being impulsive, self-centered, and aggressively opportunistic. They appear easily bored and restless, evidence a low tolerance for frustration, seem to act impetuously, and cannot delay—let alone forego—prospects for immediate gratification. They are unable to endure the tedium of routine or to persist at the day-to-day responsibilities of school, job, or interpersonal relationships. Many seem to enjoy taking chances, thrill-seeking, and other forms of dangerous stimulation, and there is a tendency to jump from one exciting and momentarily gratifying escapade to another, with little or no care for potentially detrimental consequences. When things go their way, they are capable of acting in a gracious or cheerful manner, but even when slightly frustrated in their pursuit of gratification, they quickly become furious and vindictive, easily provoked to attack, their first inclination is to demean and to dominate. (pp. 119–120)

Miller does not mention the ultimately self-destructive nature of psychopathic behaviour so that, as it stands, his description reminds one of too many professional, business, and personal acquaintances neither diagnosed nor diagnosable as having a mental disorder.

The diagnosis of psychopathy (or ASPD) is based on a life story deviating so markedly from our norms of reasonableness and rectitude that the term 'moral insanity' seems apt. The austere ASPD is, however, almost vacuous in that it can suggest a pattern of petty misdemeanours all too common in the 'normal' population. A subset of offenders who persist in offending beyond the 'normal' offending trajectory, and who are responsible for a disproportionate amount of the total crime committed by the criminal population (particularly at the heinous end), show a more dramatic combination of lack of moral sensitivity and commonsensical prudential reasoning.

> Tom looks and is in robust physical health. His manner and appearance are pleasing. In his face a prospective employer would be likely to see strong indications of character as well as high incentive and ability.

(Cleckley, 1941/1976, p. 64)

We find that Tom (from a comfortably off, middle-class family) has a long history of maladjustment, including fecklessness—'he could never be counted upon to keep at any task', stealing, aimless petty destructive acts, deceit; 'he lied so plausibly . . . that for many years his real career was poorly estimated', forgery, petty fraud, minor violence and misdemeanors, defecation into a relative's grand piano, and so on. On each occasion, he demonstrated apparently genuine penitence and intentions to change but a particularly telling episode with a friend of the family who tried to help Tom mend his ways shows that those promises are meaningless.

> The conversation, once begun, developed amazingly. The younger man not only promised to behave from now on in an exemplary fashion but analyzed and discussed his past in such a way that the older found there was little that could be added . . . He was so impressed by points this young man had brought out and by his apparent earnestness and resolution that he felt himself wiser from this experience.

(Cleckley, 1941/1976, p. 69)

After this conversation, Tom left his would-be mentor at the front gate, and was not heard of for a week; 'news then came of his being in jail again at a nearby town where he had forged, stolen trifles, run up debts, and carried out other behaviour familiar to all who knew him.'

Tom is quite unlike David, but both show a 'disorder of volition' in that each seems to have an inability to bring his life in line with values he quite openly acknowledges and may even discuss, avows, reason about, or even defend. So is this just deceit and insincerity or is it a disorder of volition? Answering that question is likely to have profound implications for more general concepts of morality, rationality, and intention and our understanding of the psyche linked to older analyses of moral judgement, character, and responsibility, those of Aristotle, Kant, and Nietzsche.

David E.'s violent rape justifiably attracts a harsh judgement but, if he is suffering a mental disorder, should we not have compassion and treat him for his problem? The difficulty in a shift towards the therapeutic attitude lies in understanding the nature of the defect and integrating it into an explanation of behaviour that justifies treating the person concerned differently from many other individuals who seem, by any criteria, just plain bad. I have noted that many studies of psychopaths select their samples from prison populations of male offenders who practice systematic violence on others, show little or no remorse for their actions, and for whom there is little if any hope of correction. In fact, the prisons of any developed nation contain any number of individuals who fit the accepted diagnostic criteria for psychopathy and who are (recidivist) criminals known and feared in urban ghettos and other dangerous areas of society.

Some are highly sceptical about psychopathy as a psychiatric category, claiming that it is a 'moral judgement masquerading as a clinical diagnosis' (Blackburn, 1988), but that question demands a detailed examination of volition or the will and the neuro-philosophy of psychopathy.

Cleckley (1941/1976) goes beyond the alternatives of moral insanity or disaffected scepticism about psychopathy to develop an unifying thesis about the psychopathology involved. He argues that the psychopath has intact cognition (thus ethical reasoning seems fine) but 'a persistent lack of the ability to become aware of what the most important experiences of life mean to others' (p. 407). He links the moral defect to 'the common substance of emotion or purpose . . . from which the various loyalties, goals, fidelities, commitments, and concepts of honour and responsibility' arise, and uses the metaphor of *superficiality* and *depth* to characterize this lack.

> Let us assume that this dimension of experience which gives to all experience its substance or reality is one into which the psychopath does not enter. Or, to be more accurate, let us say he enters, but only so superficially that his reality is thin or insubstantial to the point of being insignificant. (p. 407)

The reality under discussion here is 'what in social or personal life means something' (Williams, 1985, p. 201) and the psychopath's deficient grasp of that domain of human experience is a main feature of the disorder and the close connection between inter-personal dynamics and moral judgement indicates a fundamental moral defect in the core cases of psychopathy.

9.3 Hare and other believers

Hare (1970), deeply influenced by Cleckley, investigated the personality configurations underlying the vexed category of psychopathic disorder. He claims that a social or operational definition of psychopathy in terms of antisocial behaviour neglects the underlying personality factors suggesting a particular dynamic genesis of that behaviour. His *Psychopathy Checklist* (PCL) has two factors: one focused on personality and one on lifestyle (Hare, 1980, 1983; Harpur et al., 1989). The former comprises 'selfish, remorseless, and exploitative use of others' (Harpur et al., 1989, p. 6), 'lack of empathy', 'pathological lying and deception', 'grandiose sense of self-worth', 'lack of sincerity', 'lack of affect and emotional depth', and 'glibness/superficial charm' (p. 7). The second factor includes 'proneness to boredom/low frustration tolerance', parasitic lifestyle', 'poor behaviour controls', 'impulsivity', 'lack of realistic long-term plans', 'irresponsible behaviour as a parent', and juvenile antisocial behaviour (p. 7). He believes that the underlying personality disorder reflected by Factor 1 is expressed in the behaviours clustered under Factor 2. Current work supports that claim: the superficiality and lack of empathy of 'Factor 1' seem to cause a lack of self-control or practical wisdom evident in the ('Factor 2') manifestations as a result of deficient processes in the development of 'second nature' (Aristotle, 1925; Curzer, 2002).

Hare uses standard psychometric instruments to measure states and traits in psychopaths and notes 'a robust negative relationship between anxiety and Factor 1' (p. 11) confirming the belief, held by many, that the components of Factor 1 do reflect a lack of conflict about interpersonally abusive actions and attitudes (Fowles, 1993). Hare also notes that, whereas Factor 1 is related to narcissism, it is not correlated with 'social class, family background, or educational achievement' as Factor 2 is. He also notes a curious finding about language and Factor 1.

> When asked to judge whether a string of letters formed a word, non-psychopathic crimi-
> nals responded faster when a word was emotional than when it was neutral. This is the
> pattern shown by normal non-incarcerated subjects. Psychopaths, however, failed to
> show this Reaction Time (RT) facilitation.
>
> (Harpur *et al.*, 1989 , p. 13)

The neural network model (discussed in Appendix A) explains the ability of the brain to react to emotive words faster by invoking the convergence of several possible paths of excitation on such words. Raine's (2002) systematic review identifies crucial limbic interconnections involved in 'the mechanisms underlying psychopathy' (Hare, 1970, p. 14). Hare's view that there are underlying and measurable abnormalities in the psychological functions of the psychopath differentiating him from other incarcerated criminals and that help to explain his criminality tells against more sceptical views but does not answer the philosophical question about the will and moral responsibility.

Bursten (1972), a clinician, analyzes psychopathy in terms of a manipulative personality that is 'driven to manipulate primarily by his inner dynamic position—his character structure' (p. 319); 'the manipulative personality has an intense but fragile narcissism. Any depreciation or threat of depreciation leads to compensatory reactions designed to support the person's inflated image of himself' (p. 320). He adds two ingredients to the emerging picture: narcissism and 'the exhilaration of putting something over on the other' (p. 319); 'it is the hallmark of the manipulative personality that he will attain his goals by manipulation, rather then by other means, because he is constantly engaged in the unconscious struggle to shore up his narcissistic self-image.' (p. 320)

The 'hallmark' rings true in many cases and explains the savagery and the sinister aspect of some psychopathic behaviour. David, for instance, seems to have a fragile and defensive self-centered ego that erupts into violence readily and without inhibition.

Vaillant (1975) focuses on drug addicts (substance abuse is correlated with psychopathy) and identifies 'ego processes' that are deficient because they have failed to deal constructively with frustrations such as postponement of gratification, the need to discipline themselves to pursue clear and lasting goals, and the anxiety and hurts that can arise from close relationships. His explanation of this lack of formation of stable 'ego processes' is, predictably, dynamic.

> All had lacked a benevolent, sustained relationship with the same-sexed parent. All were afraid of intimacy and of assuming responsibility for it. None could believe that others could tolerate their anxiety, and all devoutly feared responsibility for achieving success by open competition. They could neither identify with authority nor accept its criticism. (p. 181)

His explanation focuses on the lack of a parental model for self-control (cf. Aristotle) and the lack of an interpersonal context in which inadequate and immature aspects of self can be explored and developed (and so resonates with phenomenology and Wittgenstein). I will argue (following Aristotle) that the building of inhibitory and socially mediated controls on behaviour is a crucial factor in the genesis of psychopathy.

The two strands of explanation—neurobiological or learning theoretic and psycho-dynamic—are, in fact, mutually consistent despite the deep theoretical contrasts between them; both identify fundamental abnormalities in the psychopathic psyche that explain the antisocial behaviour and both suggest defects in a sceptical view of the problem.

9.4 Blackburn: the sceptical view

Blackburn (1975) has developed sophisticated measures of the differences between the various subgroups of individuals labelled as psychopaths. He is motivated by the (essentialist and individualist) worry that there may be no distinct reference class for the concept *psychopathy* so that individuals labelled as psychopaths have in common 'only a history of antisocial behaviour' (they are 'bad' not 'mad'). His worry, shared by others (Holmes, 1991), persists despite recognition that there seem to be two significant groups.

> One group is in general terms socially outgoing, relatively free from tendencies to feel anxious or depressed . . . This group seems to represent the primary psychopath. The other, characterized by high levels of social withdrawal and emotional disturbance, appears to correspond to the category of secondary or neurotic psychopath.

> (Blackburn & Lee-Evans, 1985, p. 93)

Blackburn's (1975) early research used the Minnesota Multiphasic Personality Inventory (MMPI) and the Wechsler Adult Intelligence Scale (WAIS) and isolated four profiles in non-psychotic male offenders admitted to a security hospital. All groups had high scores on the Psychopathic Deviate (PD) scale . He found a group who corresponded to the Cleckley stereotypes in which he identified undersocialization, impulsivity, aggressivity, a lack of anxiety, and extraversion. Another group, showing high anxiety and social avoidance along with hostility, impulsivity, and aggression, he called 'secondary psychopaths' (p. 459). A third group evinced denial and a high degree of control and a fourth mainly social shyness, introversion, and depression. He concluded that the concept of psychopathy was vindicated in the type 1 case and that impulsivity was probably a pervasive feature across all groups.

His classification into *primary* and *secondary* psychopathic types was tested by investigating readiness to respond in anger-evoking situations (Blackburn & Lee-Evans, 1985). He found that both groups tended to react strongly in terms of aggression and anger but that primary psychopaths 'exhibit lower somatic arousal . . . similar to that of sociable non-psychopaths' (p. 98). However, he also invoked 'a cognitive bias to perceive threat from others' and suggested that psychopaths might be 'hypervigilant for any violation of their personal domain, and hence more likely to interpret the behaviour of others as unwarranted attack' (p. 99). That 'paranoid' or 'suspicious' attitude to others fits with the narcissism, self-centredness, and discounting of the feelings of others that, in some psychopaths, forms an explosive combination with violent impulsivity.

Blackburn argues that, despite his two-category classification, 'none of these has been shown to identify a homogeneous class uniquely associated with antisocial deviance' (1988, p. 511).

> It must be concluded that the current concept of psychopathic or antisocial personality remains 'a mythical entity'. The taxonomic error of confounding different universes of discourse has resulted in a diagnostic category that embraces a variety of deviant personalities. Such a category is not a meaningful focus for theory or research nor can it facilitate clinical communication and prediction . . . Such a concept is little more than a moral judgement masquerading as a clinical diagnosis. (p. 511)

Blackburn contends that the idea of psychopathy arises from confusion between our need to explain certain kinds of behaviour which we morally condemn and our wish to classify and treat personal and social deviants according to a structured body of scientific knowledge. But his scepticism about psychopathy as an identifiable psychiatric disorder runs counter to recent discoveries about the underlying neurobiological mechanisms that seem to give rise to enduring patterns of antisocial behaviour.

He notes a philosophical problem: 'The contribution of personality characteristics to antisocial behaviour is an empirical question that can only be answered if the two are identified independently' (Blackburn, 1988, p. 507). That worry is not completely offset by the identification of a personality type that may or may not cause psychopathy depending on the social context of a person's development (Raine, 2002) because there remain problems in relating insights into the underlying neural correlates and phenomenology of the disorder to an ethical appraisal of our treatment of psychopaths. Despite statistical analyses and positivist measurements (of workers such as Eysenck and more recent neuroethical accounts), an analysis of life history and the discursive skills of the individual concerned may reveal factors, beyond the control of the individual, that an informed moral judgement should take into account (Maden, 2007).

9.5 Mullen: an account informed by philosophy

Mullen (1992) combines moral theory and psychiatric knowledge in his understanding of psychopathy, arguing that the psychopath has 'a developmental disorder of ethical action'. He discusses a group that, in his opinion, show characteristics of either antisocial or borderline personality disorder and remarks that we tend to label them as 'mad' because of 'their unpredictability, their self-destructive behaviour, and their odd and often frightening outbursts' (p. 235). His arguments are of interest in trying to understand the genesis of psychopathy and are highly relevant to serial killers in that these individuals are significantly different from other offenders in 'the erratic nature of the offending, the impulsivity, the self-destructiveness, and the difficulty in understanding the motives which are, on occasion, as inexplicable to the offender as they are to observers' (p. 238). Such individuals have a long history in which experiences produce a highly dysfunctional outcome and Mullen identifies

(1) Broken and disrupted homes,

(2) Violent and abusive relationships as children,

(3) Fostering and institutionalization,

(4) School problems,

(5) Peer relationships with 'other behaviourally disordered youngsters',

(6) Unstable emotional and sexual relationships, and

(7) Alcohol and substance abuse.

Many of these factors are common among young offenders, but he argues that a constitutional vulnerability, now becoming evident (Raine, 2002) from other studies, is common to the individuals in his sample. He also claims that 'the gentler emotions of sadness and guilt are rarely obvious, but self-loathing is not infrequently present alongside anger at the world' (p. 237).

He explains the developmental disorder by drawing on both Aristotle and Bakhtin and makes a connection between a sense of personal integrity, responsibility for your own actions, and 'a habit of virtue' acquired through learning by doing (p. 241). Recent developmental work confirms his emphasis, invoking not only training in virtue but also affective empathy and the need for children to model their behaviour on that of consistent caregivers (p. 242).

Mullen's group includes, as he notes, individuals diagnosed with borderline personality disorder (as in the DSM IV) involving identity disturbance, 'a pattern of unstable and intense interpersonal relationships . . . alternating between extremes of idealization and devaluation', emptiness, self-destructiveness, and paranoia (DSM IV; APA, 1994a, p. 654). He comments on the 'fragility of their own identity', drawing our attention to the relationship between moral character and personal identity (Taylor, 1989) that will figure prominently in connection with dissociative conditions (such as Multiple Personality Disorder). When these thoughts about development and its disruption are combined with work on the development of action and emotion through intersubjectivity and the mirror that makes one's *imago* a good (-making) production (Lacan), we begin to discern the link between a disorder of volition and the moral self (a being who is well integrated into the human life-world). That link is illuminated by the neurophilosophy of action, self-control, the nature of the will, and the neural abnormalities found in psychopathy.

Section B: **The neurophilosophy of volition**

Neurophilosophy, a philosophical approach using theory and data from neuroscience, is a valuable tool in linking psychopathy, the will, and moral responsibility.

9.6 **Moral sense and moral action**

An action is a human intervention in the world to produce a desired effect and people can be more or less skilled in bringing about such effects. The relevant skills have a mental component, in that what to do needs to be envisaged (as Sartre notes), and a further component, the ability to translate that conception into action (as Aristotle, Nietzsche, and Davidson argue), where lies the difference between a strong and a weak will (see Appendix F). Aristotle offers an account of moral development and moral action whereby the ability to do the right thing is similar to any other technique in that it develops over time and training in actual life situations.

> The things we have to learn before we can do them, we learn by doing them, e.g. men become builders by building, and lyre players by playing the lyre; so too we become just by doing just acts, temperate by doing temperate acts, brave by doing brave acts.

> (Aristotle, 1925)

Thus, one learns to be good by acting well in a wide range of situations, thereby cultivating the habit of goodness. To try and teach virtue by loading a person with precepts and injunctions (in the manner of Polonius) is to do too little and too much. Morality, or virtue, is not absorbed as a set of rules or thoughts adequate for all the varied challenges of life but through *hexes* developed in *praxis* (as the case of Tom shows). One is exposed to an interpersonal situation containing a moral challenge; one is aware of certain general maxims and, perhaps, of the specific demands of the situation; one determines what to do to meet the requirements of virtue in the specific situation and, through practice, becomes accustomed to acting that way.

For instance, imagine I am visiting an academic friend who has a propensity to gossip and recount incidents showing the weaknesses and failures of his colleagues. I could join in this type of conversation or keep my own counsel (no doubt somewhat disappointing him). I go along with him, quietly indulging in a bit of envy and general pulling down of the mighty (especially those who think they are mighty but are not). Afterwards, talking to a friend who has a more generous spirit, I might regret the mean and somewhat petty thoughts, the disaffected conversation, and my demeaning myself through my part in it and resolve to react differently in future. The self-evaluation is a result of my interaction with my more virtuous friend and helps to form me so that it becomes natural for me to act virtuously. Through many such experiences, doing virtuous things (for their own sake) becomes 'second nature' to me (Burnyeat, 1980, p. 73). Sartre also notes that I can choose how to behave and that I am the product of my lived experiences in that *I am* what *I do* and not what I think of doing so that I am informed by the 'habits of the heart' that I enact, themselves shaped in the discourses influencing my values and self-conception (Lovibond, 2002).

Burnyeat (1980) notes that it is important, in developing a 'second nature', 'to learn to enjoy doing it, take pleasure—the appropriate pleasure—in doing it' (p. 77). This enjoyment in what is good and the complementary pain at doing anything ignoble or unjust make a young person 'receptive to the kind of moral education which will set his judgement straight and develop the intellectual capacities (practical wisdom) which will enable him to avoid such errors' (p. 79).

From all this, it follows not only that for a long time moral development must be a less than fully rational process but also, what is less often acknowledged, that a mature morality must in large part continue to be what it originally was, a matter of responses deriving from sources other than reflective reason. These being the fabric of moral character, in the fully developed man of virtue and practical wisdom they have become integrated with, indeed they are infused and corrected by, his reasoned scheme of values.

(Burnyeat, 1980, p. 80)

Curzer (2002) stresses the pain of moral education and the need for discipline by others (largely conveyed through their emotive and caregiving interactions with oneself that are part of training in virtue, thereby touching a point that is central in understanding the volition of a psychopath). Tobin (1989), elaborating the Aristotelian position, notes three components in moral character:

(1) Perception or sensitivity

(2) Disposition or the tendency to act rightly

(3) Reflection on a situated morally relevant act

She grounds a moral response in an *awareness* of the morally relevant features of a situation, a kind of 'emotional sensitivity and responsiveness' (p. 195) that lets one know what is at stake morally (for instance, who stands to be hurt and what kind of hurt might be involved). To do this, one must detect where others are particularly vulnerable or needy and act so as to take due account of those facts (in a way that virtu-ously reflects the action's probable effects on others). One might sense where a person would be gratified, amused, or encouraged by a given action and act accordingly. The relevant sensitivities are the stuff of moral perception without which moral action is 'blind' and prone to miss the mark, and as in any other area of perception, they are developed and refined through experience in (or attunement to) the human life-world and others within it. In a natural domain, a critter is attuned to the patterns conveying the affordances of a situation (Gibson, 1966) and the moral domain is full of affor-dances reflecting 'what in personal and social life means something' (Williams, 1985). Variations and nuances of interpersonal experience are cued and detected, usually at the 'knee' of a skilled moral judge who holds a mirror of acting well with others to one's experiences and teaches one resonance with their affective aspects (Schore, 1998). An intelligent learner fills in many details over and above what is conveyed to him or her by mentors, but the discursive terms (and their affective accompaniments) provide an essential scaffolding for the structure of moral signifi-cance inherent in human experience.

The awareness of what is at stake in an interpersonal situation does not by itself guarantee a virtuous response; indeed, as we have seen, it may merely be used to further the efficacy of Machiavellian intelligence in serving the will to power as it structures human action.

The ability and *inclination* to make an informed morally sensitive response must also be learnt and comes more or less naturally to most of us through the intersubjec-tive resonances of infancy and childhood whereby we are attuned to and feel with the feelings of others (Gilligan & Wiggins, 1988). The knowledge of what is fitting to do or say can therefore be learnt superficially or deeply depending on the extent to which evaluations informed by the feelings of others are an intrinsic part of them. Superficial learning results in successful but limited behavioural strategies, furthering the demands of the self-centered individual who is uninformed by proper engagement in meaningful interpersonal encounters. 'Deeper' moral learning structures the maxims on which one acts in the light of a developing appreciation of the significance of the situation to others. This inscribes the agent with the traces of the other (Levinas) so that the effects of one's actions on the other affect one's own feelings. This depth of seeing allows a more organic response (as the I of I-You) to the interpersonal demands of life based on emotional engagement or identification with others. As these habits and techniques of responding are increasingly refined, the person begins to achieve genuine practical wisdom (or virtue) rather than mere cleverness (Aristotle, 1925, p. 156).

Tobin's third component is *reflection* on the material of moral perception and response. The reasoning involved informs both action and self-formation articulating it with one's evolving trajectory of dealings with others. Reflection allows one to learn from the results of acting thus and so and the skills involved embrace the situation, one's response to it, and the results of one's action engaging that complex whole with the 'mirror world' of the reactions of others. In thought, one evaluates alternative responses and imagination is called upon to suggest other ways of construing the situation and acting within it in the light of one's inherent appreciation of and attunement to 'reactive attitudes'. The reflection *names* what one has done and thereby articulates it within ramifying networks of interpersonal significance. Thus, moral reflection disciplines and structures the soul by inscribing one with the realities of the human (intersubjective) life-world so as to create genuine practical wisdom. The result of this process frames moral knowledge in a distinctly Aristotelian way. Fields (1996) argues that the understanding of moral principles involves three factors:

(i) To be motivated to act in accordance with it;

(ii) To take it as supplying the basis of a justifying reason for action that ought to have high priority over non-moral reasons for action;

(iii) To be disposed to experience certain emotions and to have certain attitudes in certain situations. (p. 268)

At this point, abstract rules or 'moral beliefs' look irrelevant and the psychological reality is reminiscent of contemporary work in virtue theory (Baier, 1985; Nussbaum, 1990). The complex 'developmental disorder' (Mullen, 1992) is now beginning to emerge. The psychopath constructs action *schemata* that sit curiously with the intersubjectively mediated techniques articulating social and personal life to give it meaning. The psychopath's grasp of such techniques is shallow, lacking a commitment informed by an engagement with the other and the disposition to be moved by its effect on one (as in the Aristotelian and developmental accounts discussed earlier). Self and the relevance to one's own ego (considered narrowly) is all for the psychopath (who considers everybody else, despite their apparent virtue, to be the same—so that they are either dissembling or stupid and naïve). The neurophilosophy of psychopathy confirms this view in startling and dramatic ways.

9.7 **The neurophilosophy of psychopathy**

When we try and define where, in the process of moral development, the disorder shown by psychopaths ought conceptually to be located, it is interesting to examine the abnormal psychophysiological characteristics that illuminate the cognitive processes underlying action and where they go wrong in the psychopath (Blair, 2003). That study yields insights not only into the mental function of the psychopath but also into the nature of the will and intentional action.

Recall that actions are not perspicuously individuated in terms of bodily movements but in terms of operations on identified and, as Sartre has it, *signified* features or objects in the subject's environment. The idea that the objects have to be signified warns us against a 'bare' reading of the intentionality of action as mere object-directedness. This defect in the 'bare' reading is also evident when we note that automatisms (stereotyped sequences of behaviour resulting from temporal lobe epilepsy) relate to items in the environment but do not qualify as conscious or intentional actions. An adequate characterization of intentional action begins by noting that 'people have in mind a certain idea of what they are doing or want to do and use this prepotent identity as a frame of reference for implementing the action, monitoring its occurrence, and reflecting on its attainment' (Vallacher & Wegner, 1987). Thus, 'the immediate precursor to action is a mental representation of what one is doing' (Vallacher & Wegner, 1987, p. 8); but the implicit theory of action in play here is overly causal and a better account portrays an action as the enactment of a decision by an agent to endorse (and commit himself or herself to acting on) certain reasons (Gillett, 1993b, 2008). The preferred account has three main features: (i) reasons (the beliefs, desires, perceptions, values, and so on that structure the action); (ii) the evaluation of those reasons; and (iii) the skill to act on the reasoned evaluation guiding the action.

Any action has a structure: for example, 'He is going outside to smoke his pipe.' There is the action to be performed—going outside, some 'props'—his pipe, and an aim or end—his smoking his pipe. The conceptual content of an action (such as <I will smoke my pipe>) depends, *inter alia*, on the agent grasping the concepts <smoke> and <pipe> (as discussed in Chapter 1); it thereby engages the subject in the symbolic mediation of his or her activity in the actual world. Thus, Luria (1973) remarks, in discussing goal-directed behaviours, 'at the level of a complex conscious action . . . they are dictated by intentions which are formed with the close participation of speech' (p. 37). He notes the role of the highest levels of the neocortex in the control of action, particularly the frontal lobes, 'an apparatus with the function of forming stable plans and intentions capable of controlling the subject's subsequent conscious behaviour' (p. 198). The 'close participation of speech' again implicates the frontal lobes of the brain in which shared and socially imparted norms are intimately tied to complex rule-following and 'social behaviour as a distinct specialization' (Miller, 1987, p. 132), forming 'self-schemas'—'knowledge structures about the self that derive from past experience and that organize and guide the self-relevant information contained in the individual's social experiences . . . They function as interpretive frameworks for the reflective understanding of this behaviour' (p. 132).

Miller directs our attention to the complex cognitive work that goes into the development of socially adaptive behaviour patterns and the way that activity shapes one's narrative as a being-among-others, highly relevant because the frontal areas of the brain show interesting patterns of events preceding actions, some of which are quite distinctive in aggressive psychopaths.

The Contingent Negative Variation (CNV) 'is a slow negative potential change . . . which occurs in the cerebral cortex when a subject is preparing to respond to a stimulus' (Howard et al., 1984). It is a measure of readiness to emit a motor response which has previously been conditioned to a cue stimulus. The most simple paradigm uses a paired click and flash with the latter following two seconds after the former. Just prior to the flash, the subject's electroencephalogram (EEG) is sampled and an averaged recording made so that the characteristic variation emerges (statistically) from the background activity (some imaging studies use similar averaging techniques). Variations of the same methodology allow one to show the effects of different response–condition contingencies. The paradigm of particular relevance to psychopathy requires the subject to react differently according to the nature of the warning and imperative stimuli. In one condition, the subject must respond and in another he or she must refrain from responding. This is called a Go–No Go task and successful performance (in the experiments we are discussing) occasions non-punishment.

The CNV patterns are disrupted in psychopaths in ways directly relevant to an understanding of their defect in volition. Psychopaths, as we have noted, can be classified into two groups: 'a secondary type, characterized by social withdrawal and emotional disturbance, and a primary type, characterized by a high degree of sociability and a lack of emotional disturbance'. Primary psychopaths show low anxiety on many tasks and are 'less troubled by emotional problems' (Blackburn, 1988); they are therefore closest to the type of psychopath so graphically described by Cleckley, who seem to regard life as a win-win game for their own pleasure. Their CNVs in the standard Click–Flash paradigm are more pronounced than normal or secondary psychopaths (Howard et al., 1984). An interesting qualitative observation is that when primary psychopaths are asked about their experience in the boring and repetitive Click–Flash paradigm, they report that they tend to fantasize, often about gunfights or 'being fast on the draw' or something similar. However, in the Go–No Go paradigm, where the situation is not win-win and may involve punishment, their CNVs are deficient, resembling those of the secondary group more than those of normal controls (Howard et al., 1982). The secondary group show high anxiety and seem to regard life as a series of no-win situations. They have a strong anticipation of punishment but their CNVs are poorly formed under both paradigms. Both groups are impulsive, show the antisocial behaviours characteristic of all psychopaths, and exhibit a lack of warmth or depth in their relationships and social behaviour.

For the purposes of the present study, the simple behaviour control required in these tasks can be thought of as follows. The subject can only make successful responses by using two abilities:

(i) Attention to the relevant cues

(ii) The adaptation of response to contingencies of reward or punishment

The second of these factors can be simple or complex in that response sets might be monovalent, always react as fast as possible, or bivalent, react sometimes not others.

Control over actions is vulnerable to poor attention and to lack of well-differentiated patterns of responding to negative and positive contextual cues. The dependence on attention assumes some importance in that psychopaths have 'low cortical arousal as indexed by EEG signs' (it is also affected in schizophrenia). Thus, psychopaths are deficient in the ability to adapt and control their behaviour so as to make maximal use of environmental and especially social and interpersonal cues to inhibit inappropriate response tendencies. Normally, the inhibition of inappropriate behaviour is required for actions conditioned by 'all-things-considered-best-judgements' and low impulsivity, and both psychopaths and patients with frontal lobe dysfunction find these difficult (a finding which recalls the painful path of virtue outlined by neo-Aristotelian writers).

Patients with frontal lobe damage tend to show 'a generalized disinhibition and gross changes in affective processes, characterized by a lack of self-control, violent emotional outbursts, and gross changes in character' (Devonshire et al., 1988, p. 339). Their impulsivity and emotional blunting is unimportant in the simple Click-Flash paradigm, because they can form well-developed responses to simple and univalent cue–outcome contingencies. A win-win cognitive set is fine for such situations and (cerebral) preparation or readiness is likely to be well developed or salient (for instance, 'spiced up' by the excitement of drawing a pistol in a fantasized gunfight).

Secondary psychopaths, similar to primary psychopaths, lack the deeper level of processing required to deal with complex situations and contingencies (such as those involved in moral and prudential considerations) and have quite different response tendencies. Their undifferentiated no-win anticipation causes poor responses even to simple contingencies on the basis of a chronic and maladaptive anticipation of bad outcomes. One would expect that the anger and frustration of such subjects brought about by constant failures and poor life skills would combine, under certain conditions, to cause tragic and violent effects as a result of immoderated reactive aggression (which the psychopath has never learnt to deal with). In fact, the pathetic desperation resulting from such a maladaptive and no-win history is one of the more common ingredients of that brand of evil seen in a serial killer or mass murderer (Mullen, 2004).

9.8 A neurophilosophically informed account of action

The present analysis implies that human action involves the higher control and modulation of motor activity in accordance with certain regularities of outcome found in the human life-world. Human beings control or structure their behaviour on the basis of judgements as to their context and its possibilities, and the success or otherwise of their actions depends on their life skills—their ways of seeing the truth of their situation and acting on that knowledge. A (informed) 'will to power' is developed in a social and cultural setting, and makes one's behaviour deeply responsive to that reality (a mirror world of imperatives, permissions, and appeals). Thus, the analysis of human behaviour transcends basic need (or drive)-related dispositions to respond thus and so and embraces non-obvious and complex relations between cue stimuli and patterns of reward and punishment (multiplex montages of symbol and desire). In fact, one might conclude that the psychopath's impulsivity is the reflection of a fairly primitive behavioural control structure that cannot cope with the demands of a highly signified or discursive ecological setting embodying complex response contingencies. The psychopath is, one could say, an inexpert child who elevates the ego above its own reality (the truth of its situation) and disconnects it from the constraints of being-in-the-world-with-others.

The account can be synthesized by noting that the 'identity structures' mapping our activity onto the world we share with others (Vallacher & Wegner, 1987) are built on certain foundations:

First, there is a montage of impulses, drives, yearnings, symbolic strivings, and frustrations.

Second, there is our accumulated knowledge or experience of the domain of action and the contingencies operating within it.

Third, there are our habits of response.

Fourth, there are the results of reflection on the contingencies of past responses.

The first and second of these foundations are in a dynamic interplay with the third and fourth and some of the most complex contingencies, and the reasoning they produce, concern the impact of our actions on others. If one is to function successfully as a rational and social being, one must engage with other human beings upon whom one depends not only for certain imminent rewards and satisfactions but also to whom one bears more enduring relationships. This takes more than knowing how to get what you want (in terms of simple cleverness) and requires one to develop practical wisdom properly informed by the reactions and feelings of others, evident in the 'reactive attitudes' (Strawson, 1974) that shape reason and being. Personal responsibility follows responsivity and grounds our moral judgement, and the resulting interpersonal dynamic limns the 'sources of the self' (Taylor, 1989) and forms us as ethical beings of value or worth (Lovibond, 2002).

We could therefore regard the moral 'ought', and the sincere appreciation of it (which the psychopath seems to lack), as expressing and drawing content from the awareness of and readiness to be influenced by how things matter to others. The moral 'ought' reflects the points at which the needs and vulnerabilities of others should and do modify one's own dispositions, intentions, and emotive responses. Both the understanding and control of one's behaviour in the light of these complex interrelationships between events and people around us and their reactions and feelings are crucially dependent upon functions linked to the frontal lobes (and associated limbic areas). It is therefore highly significant that these capacities are noticeably deficient in psychopaths of both primary and secondary types.

Therefore, the defect evident in psychopathic behaviour begins to become clear; it is either

(i) An insensitivity to the normal emotive and moral force of the non-obvious, complex but highly important cues associated with adaptive patterns of interpersonal action; or

(ii) An inability to respond to that information in forming intentions and acting on them.

The first factor parallels the cognitive disruptions in the M'Naghten rules (governing insanity) and has been likened to an inability to appreciate the cruelty that would be involved if it turned out that plants were sentient and sensitive to injury (Levy, 2007). The second is a problem of practical reasoning in that the psychopath cannot construct adequately informed patterns to control his action in the light of its effects on others because they have no force for him. He has 'prefrontal dysfunction and a lack of inhibitory control over the antisocial violent behaviour' (Raine, 2002, p. 320), for which he requires 'multiple executive functions—sustained attention, behavioural flexibility to changing contingencies, working memory, self-regulation and inhibition, abstract decision making, planning, and organization'—despite the fact that, for a young offender, 'the prefrontal cortex is still maturing, with myelination . . . continuing into the twenties and beyond' (p. 321). That is the anatomy (or neurophilosophy) of a defect in volition (or lack of phronesis in Aristotle's terms).

In the case of the secondary psychopath, whose social background and educational attainment is generally poor and for whom life is a series of no-win situations, the defect is readily explained in terms of a failure of the social learning due to inconsistent and vicious (non-virtuous, or malignly defective) upbringing.

The primary psychopath is otherwise: he has a biological (genetic or acquired, dominantly right hemispheric, amygdalo-frontal) inability to sense aversive unconditioned stimuli such as the distress, fearfulness, or sadness of others (Blair, 2003) and a congenital lack of anxiety. These individuals are typically articulate and engaging; Cleckley obviously found them very attractive and their discursive or intellectual understanding of the interpersonal world may be plausible and well developed, but things do not affect them the way they affect other people. Their social backgrounds are unremarkable and, as far as one can tell, unmarked by psychological or physical abuse (if they are abused, the problems are intensified [Raine, 2002]). Yet, they do not develop the social and interpersonal sensitivities and habits of the heart that result in contingencies affecting us in a way that underpins moral sense. They therefore lack empathic response sets attuned to complex social and interpersonal cues. We can think of this quite simplistically in terms of the mechanisms governing Win-No Win situations, the most complex of which depend upon intersubjective cues, or we could use the language of *depth* to highlight the disconnection (in psychopathy) between the verbal or propositional understanding and emotive or conative grasp of moral demands that underpins normal empathy.

In situations requiring careful consideration of the impact of one's actions on others and a long-term view of the way in which contingencies may be connected, psychopaths fail to feel the force of the emotional impacts of what they do; therefore, they respond to what is salient or to what appeals as interesting and novel. Their defect lies in an inability to control and shape their own behaviour in the light of complex reasons entwined with the subjectivity of others rather than self-serving consequences (dominated by simple, shallow, and insensitive motives). The primary type of psychopath, at least at a superficial level, articulates and may master some fragments of moral discourse but misses its felt interpersonal and prudential imperatives that normally inscribe in one what matters to others, including the 'other' who is my removed self (in time or role). This, in a complex moral and interpersonal world, is a kind of irrationality or maladaptation relating to shared emotional aspects of the *sensus communis* (in both its integrative and social functions). Their alienation is thus different and more restricted than the fragmenting disruptions of psychosis.

9.9 **Freedom, volition, and psychopathy**

The essence of the psyche is rule following so that the soul, to use Foucault's (1984) expression, is the 'present correlative of a certain technology of power over the body' (p. 176). The rules embed shared norms (the stuff, *inter alia*, of morality). And in being trained to follow a rule, a subject is not causally compelled to do anything but is rather equipped with ways of forming and articulating his or her reasons for and powers to act on the basis of his or her skills of signification and the enactment of meaning. The rule gives a thinker a reason to signify things in a given way if he or she wants to appreciate the opportunities contingent upon the mastery of a technique that has an established compositional role in the structure of social adaptation within his or her human group. He or she may choose to use or not use such techniques for any one of a number of reasons (and any of those reasons might or might not be the kind of thing endorsed by most of those within his or her social context or discourse). He or she might, for instance, be non-conformist, contrary, or perverse (all forms of resistance to the dominant or legitimated power structures). For instance, 'She used the word "bastard" not just because she felt impelled but because she despised, hated, resented, and feared him and she felt protected or sheltered from the bad effects of saying it by the presence of the social worker.' Our explanation reveals phenomenological or experiential factors highly specific to the subject and his or her construction of the situation such that the idea of psychological or social causation is problematic.[1]

First, psychological or social causation is very different from ordinary (physical science or billiard-ball) causation. Social contexts inculcate the use of certain symbols that tend to structure the responses of individuals, but their use depends on the projects of those individuals themselves. A symbol mediates semantic responses to presentations in which the individual aims to be true to a practice located in a discourse in which he participates. The idea of *representation* suggests an entity distinct from reality, whereas *signification* emphasizes the entanglement of the social reality and the psychological subject or agent in structuring the human life-world. A human being actively structures the field of his or her own action according to the symbols available in a certain discourse (so that whether the action shapes the context or the context the action is a chicken-and-egg problem).

Second, discursive activity both makes certain responses available and constitutes some of those responses as dominant for the individual subjectivities who move within it. Therefore, it determines, in part at least, the way they relate to their world.

Third, the human agent cannot simply choose the context within which he or she is born and then lives. The agent's abilities of signification emerge in the practices and discourses he or she is inscribed by in a given historical, cultural, and interpersonal situation; they help to make him or her what he or she is and inform what he or she can become.

Fourth, and contrary to deterministic theses, the individual describes a trajectory reflecting his or her commitments and subjectivities (i.e. individual positions

---

[1] Appendix B discusses the causation—psychological, biological, and social—of action.

within discourses [Foucault]) so as to become a self armed with certain discursive tendencies but never just a pawn of them.

The psychopath has social, prudential, and moral disabilities related to the lack of caring and consistent moulding of a fledgling self as a being-among-others. That may reflect a kind of blindness: he may not discern, for constitutional reasons, what is at stake in the impact of events on others (the primary psychopath) or may have been subject to haphazard, unstructured, or even malevolent (the secondary psychopath) childhood influences. Either undermines practical wisdom and the reflective skills required to incorporate the needs of others sympathetically into one's own motivational structure. The primary psychopath can be clever about social and interpersonal life, but the results of reflective contemplation do not sympathetically shape crucial dispositions and deep intuitions that can guide his actions and form his moral character.

Michael Smith's (1994) analysis of action in terms of normative reasons focuses on the reasons generated when I believe that I ought to have, and therefore am motivated to develop, a maximally coherent set of beliefs and desires that takes account of all the relevant mental states that are part of my current character and life experience. Such reasons are complex and progressively shaped by moral commitments in the way that psychopathic thoughts are not.

The psychopath has a defect at two levels: one involves his ability to feel the relevant other-directed motivations and use them to shape prereflective dispositions to action; the other is his training in reflective self-control. He does not develop the prereflective dispositions to act more or less correctly in a wide range of situations because he does not have the feelings to motivate these dispositions and cannot develop them. He cannot refine his, already deficient, prereflective dispositions in the light of subsequent reflection and self-evaluation because he lacks the skills needed to do that (as more than a merely cognitive exercise). Our judgement on him must be that he is immature, undeveloped, or primitive in moral sense and character despite any impression to the contrary based on his verbal and pseudorational skills in the domain of moral discourse.

We can summarize and conclude the examination of volition and psychopathy by reconsidering the two kinds of exculpation of the M'Naghten insanity rules (a failure to comprehend the nature of the crime or its wrongness). Psychopaths may seem to be impaired in two ways: (i) they lack practical knowledge—the ability to construct a well-organized and adequately informed intentional structure for action through no fault of their own; and (ii) they seem to be unaware that what they are doing is wrong (moral knowledge). Levy likens the first to the defect in a talentless artist who we do not blame for her bad art and the second to our treatment of plants. The talentless artist has not got the ability to translate any aesthetic sense she might have into art no matter what she does. The second problem of the psychopath—the inability to feel the pain of others (as would be true of us if plants were sentient)—sees morality as convention and not anything more and discounts the actual wrongness of the crime. The arguments are given more force by the fact that psychopathy is a developmental disorder not in control of the agent because it affects the formation of character rather than (as a normal intentional action for which we hold a person responsible) reflecting the character of the agent.

The psychopath is morally and interpersonally shallow and may be quite cruel. It is debatable the extent to which he can ever develop moral competence on the basis of the muddled and poorly formed structures resulting from the impoverished primary experiences that have formed him. It seems, therefore, that he is no more responsible and blameworthy than a child but unfortunately he is also, to some extent, ineducable. What is more, he has the cognitive and physical powers of an adult and his lack of sympathy may mean his psyche is dominated by cruelty or the enjoyment of violence and excitement. That our society cannot adequately deal with him is evident from Eysenck's historical work on crime and delinquency and Mullen's (2007) reflections on the proper response of a caring society to these abject individuals.

9.10 Eysenck: biology and crime

The recent discoveries about the neurobiology of psychopathy revive issues originally raised by Eysenck in his work on personality and abnormal psychology from the sixties. Eysenck (1965) treats conscience as one might expect a behaviourist to do: 'There exist theoretical grounds for believing that conscience is in fact a conditioned response' (p. 267). By this, he means that conscience (the 'inner policeman' making us behave decently and in a civilized manner) is based on the association between punishing or secondarily punishing stimuli and the performance of forbidden acts. For Eysenck, acts are caused by drives based on unconditioned reinforcers and conscience is a secondary reinforcer moderating a disposition to act driven by an opposing primary impetus.

His account of personality, as I have noted, focuses on extraversion and introversion; the introvert is subject to a preponderance of higher-order inhibitory cortical activity designed to keep behaviour under strict controls, as illustrated by the Porteus maze test: 'This test consists of a series of printed mazes which have to be traced by the subject who is given a pencil and certain instructions such that he is not to lift his pencil to cross lines, or cut corners' (Eysenck, 1965, p. 269). The test generates a Q score based on 'various kinds of misdemeanour . . . behaviour which goes counter to the test instructions'. If the test is administered to young individuals who have fallen foul of recognized authorities, then 'the delinquents incur over twice as many penalties as do the non-delinquents' (p. 269).

This is hardly news in that picking people for their non-conformity to authority might be expected to select those with a tendency to transgress instructions on a test administered by establishment figures and Q scores may well indicate a greater ability among introverts and normally socialized people to follow the rules or fit in with the normative regularities governing human adaptation. The relation to well-developed rule-following abilities (and therefore, highly developed conceptual and reflective content in the control of behaviour) is obvious. It would support the claim that psychopaths, to the extent that they share characteristics with 'delinquents', do not have good inhibitory controls in the cortical pathways that normally structure behaviour. The rule-following considerations (and therefore, inhibitory effects in the articulated cortical information-processing networks serving conscious thought) provide a perspicuous philosophical analysis of that phenomenon and make the link to moral sense and moral action by invoking the complex interpersonal stimuli and intersubjective world that is the focus of moral reflection.

The complexities of social and psychological causation imply that there is no easy route from these observations to a reductive thesis about human action and the biological determination of behaviour, but Eysenck (1965) is not deterred:

> To the biologist, behaviour is a product of heredity and environment, the two combining to produce a particular state of motivation and a particular set of habits. The resulting behaviour is the outcome of this combination and, as such, must be supposed to be completely predetermined. (p. 288)

His mistake is to move from the common observation that there is a biological predisposition to act in certain ways in various kinds of social situation to the conclusion that each particular act performed by an agent is determined by antecedent conditions. But explaining a tendency or disposition does not explain the particular events that statistically contribute to it, and the argument that our actions are not consciously produced and therefore not subject to rational control is, as an approach to meaningful human action, quite ungrounded[2].

But, if freedom of action and self-control are skills inherent in and developed as a result of the (second) nature of a human being as a rule follower and autobiographical author of a conscious life experience (Gillett, 1993b, 2008), then human beings negotiate and construct a life story in and through relations with others and that activity forms the basis of the moral significance of our actions (Gillett, 1992). That is also the basis on which we appraise others, acknowledging that present actions have a (causal) history and that a developmental disorder may reflect a disordered development (Mullen, 2007). The psychopath has some understanding of moral discourse, even though he violates its norms, and it is clear (even to his blunted sensibilities) that his victims are not enjoying what is going on so that, as in every human action, the evil that his victims are telling him about is 'down to him' or his responsibility (as is his failure to treat them with any respect or consideration) although we might recognize that his sensitivities, skills, and dispositions are, in a number of ways, highly deficient. We therefore cannot totally excuse him especially when we consider the extremes of psychopathic behaviour.

Section C: **Evil**

9.11 **Evil incarnate**

We need to supplement our developing picture of psychopathy (per se) by a discussion of that species of criminals who most provoke the everyday use of the term. Serial killers are a breed apart from normal folk and the brutality and arbitrariness of their sickening and violent crimes seems to indicate that they must be suffering some disorder of the mind. Among those who attended the trial of Ian Brady and Myra Hindley, the 'Moors Murderers' who (between 1963 and 1965) raped and murdered five children on the Yorkshire Moors, was a novelist; he remarked, 'one of the most frightening

---

[2] See Appendices B and F.

things about the accused was their sheer ordinariness. They seemed unaware of the enormity of what they had done' (Wilson & Seaman, 1992, p. 19). A separate but in many ways related group are those who commit 'autogenetic massacre' (Mullen, 2004).

Byrne, a psychiatrist who examined 29-year-old Martin Bryant—the perpetrator of the Port Arthur massacre in Australia (shooting 35 people, some from point-blank range)—comments as follows:

> The great mystery to psychologists and psychiatrists is that as much as we try to begin to build a portrait of the kind of person who does this, we know that there are hundreds, perhaps thousands, of other young men in the community who fit that portrait perfectly well.

> (quoted by Montgomery, 1996)

Paul Mullen's brief pen-portrait has a familiar ring to those who study such cases.

> Almost all of them are men, almost all of them are young, the majority of them are people who are socially isolated and socially incompetent. They are often people with a really exaggerated sense of their own worth and ability, which is not shared by anyone around them; so they become increasingly angry and resentful at the world, increasingly distressed at their own failure and isolation.

> (Montgomery, 1996, A13)

The contrasting public perception of these people as 'monsters' and 'embodiments of evil' is easy to understand in that 'the perpetrators indiscriminately kill people in pursuit of a highly personal agenda' (Mullen, 2004) often related to 'psychological disabilities' such as 'suspiciousness, obsessional traits, and grandiosity' and an isolated and dysfunctional character. Consider the catalogue of crime amassed by the 'Yorkshire Ripper', Peter Sutcliffe:

> The first three attacks occurred in the second half of 1975. Two women were knocked unconscious by hammer blows dealt from behind: in the first case, the attacker had raised her dress and was about to plunge the knife into her stomach when he was interrupted and ran away; in the second, he made slashes on the woman's buttocks with a hacksaw blade. The third victim, a prostitute, was knocked unconscious with the hammer and then stabbed to death. She was the first of thirteen murder victims over the next five years. Some were prostitutes; some were simply women or girls who happened to be out walking in the dark. In most cases, the victim was stabbed and slashed repeatedly in the area of stomach and vagina, although the killer stopped short of actual disembowelment.

> (Wilson & Seaman, 1992, p. 27)

The violence is abominable, its subjective cause 'a brooding resentment about a prostitute who had cheated him . . . which had become (in the illogical manner of serial killers) a desire to punish all prostitutes' (Wilson & Seaman, 1992, p. 28). There was considerable debate about Sutcliffe's sanity, only resolved when he later became floridly psychotic, but as in many other cases, his initial assessment revealed a morose inadequate individual who takes violent revenge for a minor offence, insult, or slight against him. The moral insanity here borders on (and in some cases clearly overlaps with) genuine insanity, as is becoming increasingly clear in successive cases.

> In October 1975, Robert Poulin, an eighteen-year-old schoolboy, suddenly went berserk with a shotgun in Ottawa; he entered a classroom at his school and shot seven students, afterwards blowing out his own brains in the corridor. In the room where he lived—in the basement of his parent's home—fireman called to a blaze found the charred naked body of seventeen-year-old schoolgirl, Kim Rabat, who had been repeatedly raped and sodomized, then stabbed to death. (Wilson & Seaman, 1992, p. 149)

This young man lived in a basement, on the margins of society, even of his own family. He has no diagnosis of ASPD but rather the psychological profile of the serial killer, serial rapist, or sadistic sex killer, in its lonely, sick, sad outlines. The pathological features begin in childhood, often very young childhood, with a pattern of neglect, abuse, and rejection.

> The psychological damage resulting from such a deprived or miserable childhood all too often manifests itself in a number of recognizably aggressive traits . . . defiance of authority, theft, persistent lying, acts of willful destruction, arson, cruelty to animals and other children, with such symptoms accompanied by long periods of daydreaming.
>
> (Wilson & Seaman, 1992, p. 41)

Other features—immature and neurotic childhood behaviours such as enuresis and the explosive final outcome with its overt hostility to society—depart from Cleckley's paradigm cases but are similar to David E. Sex killers often have a preoccupation with pornography and the resulting power-sex fantasies, and tend to have a history of sexual inadequacy. 'That is their fantasy: to dominate and control, to inflict pain and suffering on the victim' (Wilson & Seaman, 1992, p. 43). The fantasy is acted out repeatedly on victims chosen capriciously on the basis of availability and opportunity, many of whom then lose their lives.

These 'monsters' and 'embodiments of evil' are paradoxical: they are so needy that 'the urge to self-esteem—to be liked and respected by others—was paramount in them (Wilson & Seaman, 1992, p. 186). They are inadequate and immature, they want the world to recognize them, they want to be powerful and in control, and (similar to the psychopath) they lack the moral checks and balances and social skills that open up a productive path for these to follow.

An Aristotelian approach to moral development both explains the defect and accounts for our reluctance to accept that a mental disorder is involved. The killer's needs are primordial, but their intensification and expression is socially produced in that they feed on images current in society, and their content and form arises from the life story of the individual concerned. The serial killer, lacking the moral sense that most of us develop as second nature, lacking skills to engage with others, hurt and impulsive, translates cruel pathetic thoughts and images into grotesque and violent acts cementing forever the individual's alienation from and resentment of the lives and feelings of those whom he destroys; somewhat like the mass murderers, 'they are inadequate, sad, silly people—not embodiments of evil not dreadful monsters' (Mullen, in Montgomery, 1996).

So, is this real evil or is it not? Does anything count as evil if these crimes do not? What is more, the fact that the victims are people who can show fear, realize the horror that has them in its grip, and experience pain is important to the perpetrator. Those are evil features of any situation, and if they are part of the motivation for the acts concerned, the acts and agents concerned are evil. These are acts done because they are evil by people whose warped view of life takes satisfaction in producing evil against their fellows. We can therefore offer a tentative answer to Plato, Kant, and other philosophers who have argued about the possibility of radical evil (Copjec, 1996). It is possible for an individual to do evil, not just *despite* the fact that he knows it is evil but *because* he knows it is evil; sufficient individuals of this type stalk among us to come to our attention in newspapers all over the world. Perhaps, we should pity them because their plight is so desperate but we should also fear them and renounce them for the lack of humanity that allows them to foster and execute such black and misguided actions.

Mullen (2007) offers a characteristically reflective and humane comment:

> Psychopaths . . . are not things nor yet sufferers from brain disorder. The label is attached to humans who have often grown up in environments that failed to encourage the habits of virtue but taught that other people were capricious and only delivered care and attention when it suited them, or they were forced. Psychopaths do not have a developmental disorder, but they have usually had disordered development. There is a multiplicity of routes to becoming an anomic adult, suspicious of others, and self-absorbed. Temperament (which is largely genetic), intellectual ability or the lack of it (again in part genetic), and chance all play their role . . . The central problem is how social and criminal justice policies play out at the expense of the wretched and demonized of the earth. (pp. 145–146)

Mullen reminds us that all behaviour has a causal history, of course, that is inscribed in brain function and may even be detectable in certain neuroimaging studies, but what is more needed when such a defect results in ASPD is a humane response to these abject individuals rather than the response of a narcissistic and self-congratulatory society that despises people who do not play the game its way (and in that sense, mirrors the egoistic psyche of the psychopath himself).

9.12 **Further forensic and philosophical problems**

Several philosophical questions are posed by the behaviour of psychopaths and serial killers.

When is bad behaviour proper to be regarded as due to a psychiatric disorder?

(1) A plea based on mental incapacity involves *either* loss of knowledge such that the offender does not understand the nature of his act or that it is wrong *or* an inability to act in accordance with one's own will (irresistible impulse).

(2) A psychopath understands that his act is wrong.

(4) A psychopath carries out a willed intention.

(5) Therefore, a psychopath does not count as insane under either heading.

The psychopath is a hard case for the insanity rules or any other formulation of diminished responsibility and his behaviour may have interpersonal and biological foundations over which he has no control (Elliot, 1992; Raine, 2002). Some psychopaths both understand their cruelty and take steps to enhance it. They are also impulsive in the way that their thoughts and desires give rise to action. Their actions fail to be shaped by the intersubjective perceptions that would inform a normal person's structure of emotion and motivation and, in consequence, they neglect to take account of long-term and socially significant features of what they are doing. They are deficient in their 'other-regarding moral beliefs' (Fields, 1996), and they do act hurtfully towards others and fail to appreciate the gravity of the harm they have caused. This does not excuse their actions, but it may imply that we have a duty of care, as a society in which their malformation has been produced, to mitigate its effects.

There may be biological and psychological causes for the disordered and violent tendencies of ASPD, but the resulting actions are executed in a conscious and malign manner with aggressive and hostile intent. Therefore, the individual is responsible, in as much as anybody ever is, for his actions and should be treated with the dignity that befits a human being (even where he or she is damaged in a profound way). The *mens rea* and the anti-social deed enacting it engage the individual in a moral and interpersonal world that is not a world of production and respecification of faulty machines; at its best (and as far as we can make it so), it should also be a caring world.

This implies that the focus of our corrective interventions must be to reconfigure the second nature of a damaged human creature by drawing the psychopath into the world of real people so as to deepen and enrich his being-with-others. In this way, we have some hope of teaching the (necessarily) painful lesson that otherwise time and human suffering will teach—that we live in a human, intersubjective life-world where the being of each affects the being of all.

What is the will and how can it be pathological in its operation?

A defect of will (or volition) might be caused by an uncontrollable urge (such as in kleptomania), but in psychopathy, we have something apart from mere impulsivity. There is a lack of the moral incentive, a motivational force based solely in the recognition of one's being-with-others. Moral belief has two components, one cognitive and the other emotive or conative (Fields, 1996). These form part of the 'identity structure' (Vallacher & Wegner, 1987) of an interpersonal action and moderate one's dispositions to act for self-serving ends by informing the action in the light of the reality of one's being-with-others.

Elliot (1991) discusses the two forces that must be balanced in a theory of volition where the strength of the impulse and the resistance to impulsive action are weighed against each other in trying to understand practical reasoning. Fishcer and Revizza (1998) relate moral responsibility to reason-responsiveness and, following Kant, we could include in one's reasons a realistic appraisal of one's being a member of the kingdom of rational ends with its pervasive imperatives for mutual regard and respect. The countervailing moral incentives to the impulsive act would then include one's responsiveness to that knowledge and would distinguish psychopathy from disorders such as kleptomania and exhibitionism.

In relation to these disorders, Elliot (1991) speaks in terms of a choice between two compelling but aversive dispositions where the agent feels so much pressure to act in a way that is disruptive to his or her psyche that we can apply the concept of duress where

(i) The individual suffers psychological distress; and

(ii) The agent has only alternatives which are aversive. (p. 55)

Psychopaths do not fulfill these criteria because they are relatively unaffected by the fact that they have acted as they did and, having no particular aversion to doing the morally reprehensible and destructive acts they tend to perform, they seem driven only by self-regarding attitudes.

Thus, the defence of duress will not work for a psychopath in the way that it does for a kleptomaniac or others suffering from impulse disorders. The psychopath has an irresistible impulse only in the sense he does not see reason enough to resist it, nor is the act unreasoned even though it is ill-judged, impulsive, and morally insensitive. If reactive or moral attitudes (and forensic or legal judgements and sentencing) are grounded on action-related ascriptions of praise, blame, and responsibility for the offence, then the psychopath shares many features of ordinary criminality, as has been suggested earlier.

Is there such a thing as freedom of the will?

Arguments against freedom of the will assume that there are causal antecedents of human action undermining claims that those actions are free and responsible in the ways demanded by well-grounded moral judgements and attributions of responsibility to the agent.

(1) A human action is a physical event.

(2) A human action is an event caused by preceding mental or physical (brain) events.

(3) The existence of preceding causes implies that I am caused to do my actions rather than the conscious originator of them.

(4) Therefore, I am not (in any morally relevant way) responsible for my actions.

If (as I have argued) 1 involves a conceptual mistake because human actions are mental or discursive events and there is no sustainable identity theory of mind–brain events, and the physical view of reality is merely one way of describing what goes on, then a human action may be preceded by physical events (and may take place in a human being engaged in brain–environment exchanges), but the (space–time) relations between the physical events and the experiences constituting mental life are not related in the way suggested by 2.

I have argued that a human action is by definition an operation on the world structured by the thoughts of an agent and enacting his or her will to power. Any adequate view of the agent as a being who uses reason to structure actions necessarily implies that the agent is a rule follower who is effective in the world through his or her skills of shaping what happens around him or her and that is what we mean by being free (or to exercising one's will) in the required sense. The assessment of responsibility is therefore a judgement based on experience and interpersonal knowledge of the effectiveness of other human beings in controlling and manipulating events by using their life skills, and it links a person's story to what goes on around them (Gillett, 2001). Thus, 3 involves a mistake (in the type of story being told) and 4 an unsupported assertion.

We must not overestimate the conception of freedom that follows from these arguments. Persons do not have independent and rational control over their actions but are rather constrained by the life skills and the situations in which they find themselves as to what they can do. I have undercut the argument from studies of brain activity associated with human action to the claim that none of us really has any control over our behaviour or that we are all helpless pawns of forces lurking deep within us. We are as free (and as bound) as any chess player or other human agent who has learnt to negotiate a certain domain. The way in which one sees things and therefore the structures available to organize behaviour are highly dependent on the discourses in which one has been formed and the psychic influences that have shaped one's attitudes, but in the end, each of us constructs an autobiography inalienably our own (not always skillfully or willfully). For some of us, that story is deeply conflicted and fraught with all kinds of inadequacies and tensions, but each of us can fairly be reckoned accountable for the use we have made of the personal and intersubjective resources that others have invested in us.

What is morality and what does it mean for an agent to act morally?

I have argued (following Kant and Foucault) that an important part of moral thinking is the moral incentive or a disposition to feel for others and act well towards them (Gillett, 1992). The moral discourse of a psychopath is empty and self-centered so that he lacks moral sense and the ability to be moved by the morally relevant aspects of a situation (to do with how it affects others). Psychopaths instance amoral egoism in that they reveal in their own lives the psychically defective states of mind that arise from an inability to appreciate the force of the moral 'ought'.

Morality turns out on this account to be a set of reactions and habits of action responsive to the needs, vulnerabilities, interests, and so on of others that is refined and developed as one reflects on that complex and articulated set of motivations and considerations.

Can an individual ever act out of an evil motive that he believes to be evil?

The problem of radical evil or evil motivation has taxed a number of philosophers. Kant (1788/1956), in particular, faced a problem of rational and evil action in that he argued as follows:

(1) A rational individual follows the dictates of reason.

(2) When a rational individual obeys the dictates of reason, he acts freely.

(3) One dictate of reason is **the categorical imperative**, the supreme rule of morality.

(4) If you follow the categorical imperative, you act morally.

(5) You cannot act freely, rationally, and immorally.

(6) You can only be blamed for free and rational acts.

(7) You cannot be blamed for your evil acts.

Two possible lines of relieving argument spring to mind:

(1a) What we ordinarily call rational is not Kant's all-in kind of rationality but a reduced, means-end kind of rationality.

(2a) What we ordinarily mean by freedom is acting in the service of your own motivations, a kind of conditioned liberty.

Taking these together, we can generate 5* instead of 5:

(5*) It is possible to act with conditioned liberty, according to means-end rationality, and immorally.

Kant, however, could not take this route as for him premises 1–4 are definitive of freedom, reason, and morality. He could, however, claim that to give in to pathological or self-interested desires and act against the categorical imperative is to slip from the standard of conduct definitive of a properly rational being but you 'are free whether to be free or bow to those interests' (Copjec, 1996, p. xv). On this account, one acts immorally in acting in a way incompatible with the categorical imperative (Kant, 1793/1960, p. 26) just as one might be guilty of other types of irrationality (self-deception, wishful thinking, weakness of the will, and so on). But Kant (1793/1960) made a further claim that there is 'a radical innate evil in human nature' (p. 28). The root of this evil, he claims, is the tendency to put the maxims of self-love above the maxims of the moral law (p. 32), a familiar weakness. But that familiar weakness, evident in the devices and desires of the human heart, does not amount to the radical 'Evil be thou my good.'

I have elsewhere argued that a reading of rational conduct implicating psychic wholeness as intrinsic to right thinking or reason is supportive of a more Aristotelian version of Kant's contentious claim about the irrationality of evil (Gillett, 1993d). On this account, a failure to accommodate one's action to the truth of one's being as a member of the kingdom of ends and so to be (empathically) mindful of the needs, sensibilities, and vulnerabilities of others is a kind of irrationality that allows one to be clever but not virtuous even though the path of reason is inextricably tied to virtue (Aristotle, 1925). For the moment, we are concerned more with those whose maxims seem utterly and cruelly perverse.

Kant contrasted evil with well-being and therefore linked evil to the occurrence of human pain and suffering rather than some supernatural principle. He argued that the occurrence of evil through human acts was a result of an ineffective moral incentive to do the good rather than a positive incentive to do evil but also that bringing about evil for others was causing them harm. Thus, the possibility of radical evil would turn on the question 'Can an individual positively will to do others harm as a primary aim?' Plato and other philosophers who have tried to argue that it is impossible to will evil because it is evil have usually claimed that the individual only acts because he can see some, to him, good reason for acting (perhaps selfish). If this is conjoined with the view that to see evil as being good is to evince a certain kind of insanity, then we are forced to the conclusion that you cannot act sanely and in a radically evil way. But before we accept that conclusion, we might examine a weaker view.

The weaker view in question holds that far more people go along with harmful acts and programmes than have a positive will to do harm. This deflationary view has support from Hannah Arendt (1963) who, having attended Adolf Eichmann's trial in

Jerusalem, argued that evil was often caused by a banal compliance in evil acts by people whose own personality was not striking in any way. The deflationary view of evil still poses three important philosophical questions:

(1) What is the relation between evil and human well-being?

(2) What is the role of a defect or lack in moral sense that allows evil to occur?

(3) Can a human being be motivated by evil?

The first question can be answered in agreement with Kant: evil is that which typically tends to destroy human well-being in those upon whom it is practised and, ultimately, in its perpetrator. This defeats the assumption that there are self-serving and, on balance, egoistically good acts that are also vicious by forging a deep connection between the respectful, healthy, and mutual enjoyment of human relationships and human well-being (as being-with-others). Other-discounting beliefs and actions are bad and other-abusing or exploiting beliefs and actions are very bad (not only for the others concerned but also for oneself).

The defect or lack of moral sense that ushers the possibility of evil into the human psyche is the disengagement of moral discourse from its sympathetic, relational, or personal resonances. The systematic abuse and dehumanization of others occurs when that can be done by naming them as other or conveying to a developing human being that the whole world is other and vicious (uncaring, neglectful, self-serving, and exploitative), whereas it cannot easily occur without that happening. Human beings are often caught in dilemmas requiring a choice between self-serving interests and the implicit demands of others (i.e. of morality when those are justified), but that is no more problematic for a neo-Kantian theory that the common conflicts between urgent desires and either prudence (one's own deferred or all-things-considered best interests) or morality. The psychopath and the badly abused individual have problems forging a truly good life out of the raw materials that experience provides for the construction of an autobiographical narrative. This, in part, is because they have not internalized the moral incentives inherent in everyday life and interpersonal relationships (or what in social and personal life counts as something).

The case of the serial killer demonstrates the mistakenness of the view that it is impossible for a person to adopt an evil maxim believing it to be evil. There is a class of people who do evil to their fellows *because it is evil* and inflict on others payment for the injuries they take themselves to have suffered. Such individuals, in effect, do say 'Evil be thou my good' and their victims suffer as a result. When one looks into the lives of those concerned, it becomes clear that they are marked by a pathetic kind of torment, but even as one recognizes that torment, one is brought short by the despicable expression of it in their actions. It can be no more than a philosopher's trick to somehow recast the evident and striking evil exemplified in the lives of serial violent offenders as any kind of good (even allowing for singular and aberrant interpretations of good). If the person who harms another is not just ignorant but, in fact, uses his moral and personal knowledge to amplify the harm he is causing, then he is evil and what he does is evil and that by any other name is still evil.

Chapter 10

'My name is Legion, for we are many'

The brooding look in her eyes became almost a stare. Eve seemed momentarily dazed. Suddenly, her posture began to change. Her body slowly stiffened until she sat rigidly erect. An alien inexplicable expression then came over her face. This was suddenly erased into utter blankness. The lines of her countenance seemed to shift in a barely visible, slow, rippling transformation . . . Closing her eyes, she winced as she put her hands to her temples, pressed hard, and twisted them as if to combat sudden pain. A slight shudder passed over her entire body.

Then the hands lightly dropped. She relaxed easily into an attitude of comfort the physician had never before seen in this patient. A pair of blue eyes popped open. There was a quick reckless smile. In a bright unfamiliar voice that sparkled, the woman said, 'Hi, there, Doc!'
(*Thigpen & Cleckley*, 1957, p. 26)

This is an account of the transformation of a patient, Eve White, into her alter, Eve Black. It is a truly dramatic (even theatrical) type of report that provokes scepticism in many clinicians who regard Multiple Personality Disorder (MPD) as nothing but theatre. That scepticism, or something worse, is strengthened when one hears of a Wisconsin woman who sued her psychiatrist for convincing her that she had 120 personalities, and charged her insurance company for group therapy in which his hourly rate could be multiplied by a factor of 120 (Akron Beacon 8/4/97). MPD and the related repressed memory syndrome (RMS) have both caused a great deal of controversy in psychiatry and clinical psychology and investigating the controversy takes us deep back into a (neo-analytic) philosophical discussion of the psyche and its layers.

To get a philosophical grip on these closely related problems, one needs to

(1) Outline MPD (or dissociative identity disorder [DID]),

(2) Identify the philosophical problems generated by MPD,

(3) Discuss contemporary philosophical theories of personal identity (also in Appendix H),

(4) Outline the clinical phenomenology of repressed memory,

(5) Discuss philosophical accounts of memory,

(6) Mention some of the theories prevalent in the field, and

(7) Outline an account of personal identity that deals with the issues raised by MPD.

10.1 The clinical phenomenology of MPD

MPD is diagnosed when there is evidence of two or more distinct personalities within the same individual such that the dominant personality at a given time controls the individual's behaviour, and each personality is complex and integrated. Some add a requirement that there be amnesic discontinuities between personalities (a feature of the classical cases). The condition was first described in France and Germany in the 19th century but in its modern form is almost entirely an American production. In 1980, a US survey reported about 100 cases in total and a survey of world literature revealed about 300 cases in 1986. There was a tenfold increase in cases in the two decades 1960–1970 and 1970–1980 (Fahy et al., 1989). Since 1986, there has been a virtual epidemic of alleged cases in the United States and Holland, and at present, such cases number in the thousands (Hacking, 1995; Spanos, 1994). There are at least two possible interpretations of this historical and epidemiological data. The *first* is that there is a real condition, currently called MPD or DID, that is increasingly being recognized as we become aware of its various presentations and that it has certain commonalities with RMS. The second view is that MPD and RMS are both social constructs co-created by therapists and patients in response to diverse maladies of the soul. There are explanatory, socio-cognitive (Spanos, 1994), and hostile iatrogenic variants (Merskey, 1995) of such views, but both believers and unbelievers subscribe to the following dilemma:

> Is multiple personality a real disorder as opposed to a product of social circumstances, a culturally permissible way to express distress or unhappiness?
>
> (Hacking, 1995, p. 12)

This question, as Hacking notes, subscribes to a relatively naive, or at least simplistic, division of psychic disorders into the 'natural' and 'artifactual' and should be modified in the light of an analysis in terms of the enactment of identity and character (Butler, 1989 ; Spanos, 1994). Hacking (1995) himself suggests that we study the 'relationships between multiplicity, memory, discourse, knowledge, and history' (p. 12) to find a way ahead. The guiding orientation of the present work and, in particular, the arguments concerning classification and medicalization suggest that interactions between discourse, subjectivity, interpersonal relationships, and brain mechanisms will illuminate how the experience manifesting itself as MPD arises in a human subject. Indeed, when we examine the concepts (such as identity, divisions in the psyche, memory, and amnesia) surrounding MPD and its clinical phenomenology, interesting answers to a variety of philosophical questions about the mind emerge.

Multiple personality syndrome is described as a disorder in which there is sufficient disunity of the self so that several different foci of mental life are present in the same human individual. Such human beings are said to have 'two or more different personalities each of which is so well defined as to have a relatively coordinated, rich, unified, and stable mental life of its own' (Taylor & Martin, 1944). There are usually striking discontinuities between the personalities each of which has a different name, a distinct set of memories, first-person experiences, and character traits and, in some cases at least, a distinct psychometric and physiological profile. The dramatic differences in personality are evident in the study of Eve and her three alters: Eve White, Eve Black, and Jane (Thigpen & Cleckley, 1957).

> Though Eve Black, when absent or 'in', preserved a considerable degree of indirect awareness of the outer world through Eve White's thoughts and perceptions, she insisted that she was totally immune from any physical pain suffered by the latter and from any other sensations she experienced. The adult Eve White . . . was never able to gain memory of the experiences of Eve Black for which she was punished, though extensive efforts were made, both with hypnosis and without, to bring this material to awareness. After being told in detail what had occurred, she was still unable to establish any shadowy contact with it through memory. It remained extraneous to personal experience. (p. 99)

The marked discontinuities of personal or autobiographical memory evident in this passage are the rule for such patients and it is often the inconveniences that are created by such 'gaps' in the person's life that lead to the diagnosis being made. This is dramatically illustrated when the therapist raises the possibility of making Eve White aware of Eve Black's existence.

> 'She don't know anything about me . . .' She broke off suddenly and a flash of defiance lit her eyes. 'And don't you go and tell her either! When I get out, she don't know a thing about it. I go where I please, and do like I please and it's none of her damned business.'

(Thigpen & Cleckley, 1957, p. 31)

The asymmetrical co-consciousness reported in some cases is very clear in the Eve case.

> While Eve White was conscious and in control, Eve Black, though functionally absent, preserved subliminal awareness . . . Invisibly present at some unmapped post of observation, she remained able when she chose to follow the actions and thoughts of her spiritually antithetical twin. The hoydenish and devil-may-care Eve knew and could report accurately what the other did and thought and could even describe her feelings. These feelings, however, were not Eve Black's. She did not participate in them. The young wife's genuine and natural distress about her failing marriage was regarded by the detached observer as inconsequential and distinctly silly.

(Thigpen & Cleckley, 1957, pp. 87–88)

Recall that what we are hearing is a post-hoc reconstruction of experience (in terms of a distinct identity) by the persona Eve Black; we are not privy to a contemporaneous commentary on a co-conscious entity observing 'at some unmapped post' the goings on in the life of Eve White.

In Eve's case, as in others, the onset of the problems seems to relate to events in childhood when, on occasion, the normally quiet and obedient Eve White would act completely out of character and directly contrary to her parents' orders. Eve Black seemed to retain a memory of these events and of the punishments that followed, but the pain or distress associated with the punishments was not experienced by her in the way that it normally would be. Eve White, we are told, did not remember and found quite distressing the fact that she was punished for these escapades, of which she was unaware and also that she was accused of lying when she reported that she had no memory of them.

Further evidence of the nature of dissociation and character differentiation is found in the case of a young man called Jonah (Ludwig *et al.*, 1972), a 'shy, retiring, sensitive, polite, passive, and highly conventional', 27-year-old, African-American admitted with headaches who was amnesic for what happened during these headaches. It emerged that he had twice attacked his wife with a butcher's knife and beaten her while referring to himself as Usoffah Abdullah. He was found to have four personalities: the two already encountered, *Sammy* who was aware of all the others and saw himself as a memory trace for the group as a whole (he acted as 'lawyer' who talked himself out of difficulties brought on by the more unacceptable behaviours of his co-personalities), and *King-Young* (with some knowledge of the other personalities and a 'ladies' man') who 'enjoys good times, especially with women, is a glib talker, and cannot take "No" for an answer. During interviews, he smiles frequently and radiates a certain warmth and charm, which is accentuated in the presence of women' (p. 300).

Jonah's personalities were distinguishable on psychological, psychophysiological, and neurological testing. The authors' observe, 'we can conceive of no way that these results taken *in toto* could have been produced solely through the mechanisms of deception or intensive role playing or both, even though these mechanisms may have been operative to some degree' (Ludwig *et al.*, 1972, p. 300). Putnam (1991) also reports intriguing psychophysiological findings.

> In another MPD case, one personality exhibited better than average acuity without muscle balance problems, but a second personality had markedly deteriorated acuity with left exotropia . . . which resolved completely when the person switched back to the first personality. (p. 492)

Putnam compares these and other findings to findings in controls tested while simulating different personalities and concludes that patients with multiple personalities are distinct psychophysiologically from normal people and simulators. Thus, MPD is physiologically unlike simulation of multiple personalities, a finding that deserves some explanation in that differential physiologic responsivity has long been clinically noted in MPD patients and often complicates the use of medications, surgery, and other somatic interventions. (Putnam, 1991, p. 493).

Ludwig *et al.*, (1972) offer useful remarks on the development of this syndrome.

> With Jonah . . . certain types of affectual experiences have acquired their own separate historical development and have become relatively walled off from one another. When these affects are elicited, they cannot be expressed as part of the integrated personality except where they are of low intensity or relatively devoid of conflict. With either a single

or multiple personality, however, all affectual expression derives from and is influenced by the inherent abilities or natural endowments of the individual as well as the acquisition of certain basic knowledge and skills. (p. 307)

The authors notice that there is a relation between, on the one hand, the way that affective associations and experiences can become segregated from one another and from the reach of 'basic knowledge and skills' (or the 'discursive knowledge and skills' that enable one to construct an integrated conscious narrative from the stream of brain–world activity) and, on the other, those very skills.

We should, at this point, note a further observation about 'switching' (between personalities).

> From the extensive historical and clinical data (e.g. observation of ward behaviour) gathered on each personality, it is apparent that the experience of a strong sexual, aggressive, or interpersonal conflict within Jonah serves as an 'automatic switch-over mechanism' for the evocation of the appropriate, corresponding personality. It must be noted that Jonah is somewhat adept in dealing with all those situations, provided that they are relatively devoid of conflict or not very intense. It is only when he feels threatened and inadequate that another, more expert, and highly specialized personality emerges and assumes control.
>
> (Ludwig *et al.*, 1972, p. 308)

We meet Jonah as an adult and he and Eve were studied well before current concerns with the condition and its genesis in situations of child abuse were clearly articulated; therefore, it is understandable that accounts of the childhood events at the time of dissociation are less than clear in the case reports.

The development of MPD is now widely thought to be related to childhood sexual abuse and most therapists believe that the individual who suffers MPD can dissociate from the abuse and consequently only have confused (or 'repressed') memories about it.

> Ironically, the extraordinary abuse that is almost invariably at the aetiologic core of the disorder is usually minimized or totally denied by offenders, thus obfuscating the picture. The examiner must, therefore, examine the individual's body, including the buttocks and soles of the feet, to find clues to physical abuse.
>
> (Lewis & Bard, 1991, p. 748)

This moderate view (in which corroborating evidence of abuse is regarded as important) is very different from practices in which the evidence is only 'elicited' after intense, extended, and tendentious interviews with a counsellor but then is regarded as genuinely factual (Freckleton, 1996). The phenomenology of dissociation, and its development into MPD, is described from a first-person perspective in the account of Rene (Confer & Ables, 1983).

> I just knew I could be someone else or cut off one feeling from another.
> I didn't have any friends so I made me some, I would give them whatever I wanted them to have, they grow, get a name; it really becomes a person.
> It would click, switch, like you shut off part of your mind. You know, you feel that you are another person.
> You know you are losing control, but it grows and becomes strong, like an individual, and you sort of trust it more, let it happen.

The description is an MPD stereotype—escape from an unbearable situation—commonly disclosed in a searching history of childhood experience. The condition seems plausibly related to a vivid imagination and a facility for fully entering into make-believe situations.

> Many individuals with MPD have histories of having had very vivid imaginary companions, which continue into late childhood. Many have had intense feelings for particular toys such as dolls, which at times seemed to be real and even to threaten them.
>
> (Lewis & Bard, 1991, p. 748)

The end result of the gradual sequestration of thoughts and attitudes in a child with a vivid mental life is thought by believers to be the full-blown syndrome where a subject lives in different modes of being or identities each of which collects different clusters of memories, attitudes (both direct and self-reflective), ways of thinking, and styles of behaving under different names (Jonah, Usoffah Abdullah, King-Young, etc.) The early writers believed that the individual slips into one or the other identity in order to express aspects of self that have not been able to be avowed or explored as 'self'; 'Was Eve Black a hidden, unconscious, or subconscious side of the whole person, long denied expression by the other side and disowned by its prevailing awareness' (Thigpen & Cleckley, 1957, p. 110).

Most people recognize that a normal human being can selectively attend to various aspects of their personality and selectively express attitudes and beliefs under the influence of everyday shifts in role, motivation, and inclination. The MPD supporters posit that some people, with a dissociative tendency and strong disruptive emotional forces acting on their autobiographical or narrative consciousness, 'lose control' of self-knowledge in a way that a normal person would not. The problem then is to define 'control' and its application to self-knowledge. Here, it seems important to note that in almost all cases there is a personality who is sexually quite promiscuous and that she (it is usually a she) has the most complete knowledge of all the contents of experiences that have been dissociated into different personalities. In fact, one could argue, a priori, that the development of a sexualized *alter* would allow a narrative to be constructed that had any 'shocking' or 'forbidden' content 'screened' out of it. One might also predict that the development of two personalities would not often suffice to accommodate a deeply conflicted personality, in that one personality might be the repressed and inhibited self who presents with the characteristically non-specific maladjusted symptoms and another the uninhibited, slightly psychopathic, sexualized alter, creating the need for a more assured, mature, and 'together' *alter* as an initial attempt at adaptation to the real world of employment, relationships with others, and the conflicting demands we all live with.

In the process of therapy, one usually finds the subject enabled, by some means or another, to explore, in turn, the alternative personalities, or *alters*, in the context of a supportive and reflective relationship with the therapist. Sympathetic observers ('believers') say that therapy allows the patient to begin the painful business of resolving conflicts and overcoming the emotive and motivational pressures sustaining deep divisions in her mental life. Sceptics claim that the therapist encourages the person to think of him- or herself as different *personae* each with their own mind and identity and then brings about a 'reintegration' that should never have been required. A middle road combines the insights from both stances.

These general points are illustrated by the case of Rene, who presented for therapy as a timid 20-year-old female, prone to guilt, depressed, dependent, shy, and retiring (Confer & Ables, 1983). She was at the time in a failing second marriage. She had had a disturbed childhood during which she was beaten by both parents, rejected by her mother, raped by her father, and watched her younger brothers being both physically and psychologically abused. The themes of physical, sexual, and emotional abuse of children are, as noted, often part of the stereotype of MPD. In her younger life, Rene (and her siblings) repeatedly became a convenient scapegoat upon whom the parents vented frustrations arising from their own inadequacies. On her mother's part, there was an irrational envy of her daughter, most marked during Rene's adolescence, and then a perverse resentment because of the sexual abuse of Rene by her father. That abusive relationship in itself casts Rene in two fiercely conflicting roles: on the one hand, she is a vulnerable, trusting, child needing love without exploitation so that she can develop as a separate individual; and on the other, she is a lover or sexual object with all the erotic ambiguities, mutual satisfaction and exploitation, potential violence, physical closeness, and negotiation for power involved in relationships between lovers.

Rene developed five alternative personalities, each with its own distinct personality profile, physiological characteristics, bodily responses, and personal manner.

(1) Jeane—a 19–year-old energetic, expressive, and carefree young woman, both self assured and adventurous

(2) Stella—a sultry, immature, and promiscuous 18 year old who had numerous casual relationships with men and had a tendency to be ingratiating towards others (especially Rene's mother during the time when Rene was still at home)

(3) Sissy-Gail—a 4 year old who withdrew from interpersonal contact and whose bodily responses were dominated by cringing into a thumb-sucking 'fetal' posture

(4) Bobby—a bitter, resentful, and aggressive teenage boy, protective of Rene's younger brothers, and quite prepared to stand up to Rene's parents

(5) Mary—a deeply religious, forgiving, tolerant, and loving individual who enjoyed 'inner peace with God' and prayed for all the family of personalities present in Rene

Each personality had a set of characteristic responses and feelings to express, many of which were not well developed in Rene as she presented for therapy. Each personality, according to the therapists' working hypothesis, was a vehicle for aspects of herself distorted or 'repressed' as a result of her deeply disturbed childhood. Rene, through therapy, eventually integrated all the personalities and 'understood' their development (along typical lines). The working hypothesis is that things happened that Rene could not emotionally cope with or accept as part of her conscious experience or lived subjectivity and that she found that she could dissociate from full personal engagement in a situation. The price she paid for that escape was the ability to deal with the emotions she felt and articulate the ways that others treated her and the messages they gave her. The discursive skills to do this work require a supportive, open, and nurturing context, which she did not have so that the poorly signified and narratively non-integrated

244 | 'MY NAME IS LEGION, FOR WE ARE MANY'

244 | 'MY NAME IS LEGION, FOR WE ARE MANY'

inscriptions upon the young Rene began to split apart and be attributed to others: imaginary friends, named familiars, and so forth.

These part-persons, all of whom, in Rene's words, 'were given whatever I wanted them to have', were not merely or in any ordinary way conscious roles. Rene began to enter fully into each persona; she was Mary or Stella for extended periods of time. For Rene, every reaction in a particular mode of being was sincere and internally consistent within the personality she was at the time. These modes of being therefore became distinct inducing dissociations or discontinuities of consciousness so that some personalities were amnesic about the activities and attitudes of others, a phenomenon also seen in the case of Eve.

Recall that the personality with the most extensive access to mental content is usually the most 'sexualized' personality who is often promiscuous (indeed reminiscent of a psychopath at least in respect to attitudes towards sexuality and relationships). He or she has multiple, casual sexual encounters but forms no lasting attachments. In fact, quite possibly, Thigpen and Cleckley missed something in Eve's history in that her repeated references to dark places were a thread that was not followed in their attempts to resolve the puzzle of her disorder.

Over the course of treatment, often involving hypnosis and extended interactions with the therapist or, perhaps, with a therapy group involving other people, the personalities are 'brought out' and explored by both therapist and patient. There is, however, a problem about who is doing the exploring on the patient's side at any given time in that the autobiographical consciousness (or self) differs from personality to personality and it is unclear how material hidden within a particular stream of memories ever gets to appear in another.

In one of the few reported British cases, the reintegration is described as follows:

> As part of her treatment, our patient was encouraged to acknowledge her feelings as part of her own character and to say 'I' rather than use the name of one of her personalities. She was encouraged to discuss her problems openly, including the experience of sexual abuse.
>
> (Fahey *et al.*, 1989)

The Eve case shows that this process is not always straightforward in that her reintegration begins quite suddenly and dramatically with an episode with a vivid and distressing recall or re-experiencing of events at her grandmother's funeral when her mother instructs her to touch her dead grandmother's face. That 'flashback' provokes a strange reaction.

> 'She isn't there . . . There isn't Eve White anymore . . . She's not there . . . Why, she's gone . . . gone . . . Dead . . .? Yes, she's dead . . . no more . . . They're both gone forever!' As she tried to tell us what she had experienced, her reactions brought to mind other complex and inexpressible subjective events that other men and women have marvelled at and tried by various means to convey . . . After the terror of the moment subsided, however, she seemed to acquire an increasing confidence, to reflect qualities and capacities we had not seen before in any of the three manifestations.
>
> (Thigpen & Cleckley, 1957, pp. 223–227)

Eve or Evelyn reflects on her dissociation and her sense of loss when the alters disappeared.

> Suppose a screen had been put up in front of you. Now for a year you have two sisters. They are behind this screen but you know they are there. You are aware of them working, playing, living, though all the time the screen hides them. You know they go and in a sense you go with them, though you are then behind the screen. All the time I knew they were there. All of a sudden the screen is not there. And they are nowhere. I feel so depressed— something is missing.
>
> (Thigpen & Cleckley, 1957, p. 227)

She describes the last days of her alters in a fascinating way.

> Looking back, I have the feeling that Eve Black may have known she would never see you again. I don't understand how she could have known . . . When she started crying, I began to realize something drastic was happening.
>
> (Thigpen & Cleckley, 1957, p. 228)

The end of the story is as successful an outcome of psychotherapy as anyone could wish.

> Only a few days ago, we had the pleasure of talking again to Mrs. Evelyn Lancaster. It was a delightful and gratifying experience . . .
>
> It was about six months after she was granted a divorce from Ralph White that the manifestations of multiple personality ceased. From that time, she had not been seriously troubled by headaches. There had been no blackout spells. The distressing nightmares that had afflicted Jane never recurred.
>
> (Thigpen & Cleckley, 1957, p. 267)

Therapy seems to enable the MPD subject to explore the alternate selves and their mental lives in the context of an extended and intermittent conversation in which all personalities are recognized and engaged with by the therapist who uses his or her privileged knowledge (spanning the dissociative divisions) to reveal content from one personality to another and thus begins to induce 'spillage' over the partitions in auto-biographical awareness (or narrative consciousness). At first, this is only very partial and gradual, but the pace of breakdown in personality divisions can accelerate so that the reintegration can be quite rapid. At this point, according to the prevailing theory, the patient not only begins to recognize her psychic conflicts but also can embark upon the painful business of resolving conflicts and trying to overcome the emotive and motivational pressures that sustain the divisions in her mind and discontinuities in the narrative of her lived experience (Andorfer, 1985).

As therapy reaches the point where the increasing discursive and narrative skills of the patient seem likely to resolve the disorder, there is often a phase in which each personality 'achieves insight' about the existence of the others and about its own particular place within that 'group'. Treatment is successfully concluded when the disparate elements, until that time represented by distinct personalities, are reintegrated into one lived narrative consciousness (a 'whole' personality). That process may take various forms with various therapists. In Rene's case, an actual acceptance ceremony and a merger of the five personalities was acted out. Jonah (Ludwig *et al.*, 1972) merged as a new individual 'Jusky', regulated by contractual agreements about representation of the four contributing personalities, but his post-therapy assessments indicated that the merged individual was more unstable than any of its constituents.

The mean length of treatment in the United States is approximately three years (Putnam *et al.*, 1986) and the British case report suggests that psychotherapy lasted months not years (Fahy *et al.*, 1989, p. 100). There are no reports of successful treatment with drugs, a fact that can be interpreted in competing ways: either it could confirm suspicions about MPD in many orthodox psychiatric circles (indicating the power of the biological model) or it could point to the fact that 'talk-therapy' is important in understanding the human mind and human identity. We must therefore confront the theoretical and clinical controversies about MPD.

We should note, however, the appeal of a discursive account according to which the individual is trying to master techniques of adapting himself or herself to an interpersonal world in which disturbing things have happened to him or her. 'Alters' as modes of being that explore alternative ways of being human that create their own moral and relational momentum allow us to avoid the real or fictitious dichotomy. A person might find himself or herself in a situation where desperation has led to the construction of an alternative self who is out of control or so appealing that fantasy and reality, as normally construed, blur and, like many, the subject asks 'Who am I?' This view is supported by taking seriously the meconnaissance that is characteristic of the psychic world and the imago that structures it (Lacan).

10.2 **Controversies**

The current psychiatric and psychotherapeutic literature reflects the controversies surrounding MPD. Piper (1994, p. 600) documents five serious concerns with MPD as a valid psychiatric entity:

(a) Vague and poorly elaborated diagnostic criteria

(b) The recent sharp increase in the number of patients alleged to have the disorder

(c) Exposure to malpractice risks

(d) Difficulties with the issue of child abuse

(e) Encouragement of regressive and non-responsible patient behaviour

These concerns are worth discussing before we look to explain or understand the clinical phenomena. Piper, arguing that the diagnostic criteria are vague and poorly elaborated, observes that the presenting symptoms are often ubiquitous indicators of psychiatric illness such as depression, anxiety symptoms, negative features (poor socialization, headaches, or other somatized complaints), and so on. He then turns to the criterial features discernible and distinct personalities identified in the same human individual and focuses on

(i) The issue of interpretation of an ambiguous syndrome in accordance with a strongly held psychopathological theory—linked to 'open versus closed concepts'; and

(ii) The issue of patient denial.

The first is a familiar problem in psychiatry; interpretations of patterns of behaviour pervade the social sciences, and we ought to be suspicious of interpretation biases that can seriously distort the phenomena being studied. But here, MPD is no worse than a number of other clinical syndromes where a strongly held psychopathological thesis can lead to a skewed interpretation of data. Clearly, some statements from MPD believers are risible (except that they seem both irresponsible and potentially dangerous), but that excess is not, in itself, a reason to dismiss the possibility of MPD holus bolus. Piper (1994) summarizes the literature:

> These studies, ranging from case series of 50 patients to surveys of over 350 cases, uniformly find that MPD patients are polysymptomatic with a core cluster of dissociative, affective, post-traumatic, and somatic symptoms. Their polysymptomatic nature often leads to multiple misdiagnoses and apparent treatment failures. (p. 497)

Putnam, a believer, argues for a considerable cross-cultural constancy in the clinical phenomenology of MPD, but his cited sources have similar attitudes to his own so the data, when examined critically, establish no more than the need to be aware of theoretical biases and therefore to exercise caution and well-honed clinical acumen in this area of diagnosis.

The issue of patient denial is a significant cause for concern as yet another manifestation of a pervasive problem in psychotherapy. Examples where the patient's own understanding of their symptoms is discounted by the expert are widespread and can occur when the testimony of any relatively disempowered person is routinely overruled and set aside in the planning of treatment. Kocan (1980), as we have seen, called it 'the snowball' and identified a process whereby behavioural deviations or even normal actions can be woven into a pattern of interpretation that 'shows' that there is something deeply wrong with a person and justifies serious interventions, quite apart from controversies about MPD.

The dramatic recent increase in patient numbers is especially worrying when one considers that in a recent study 'just three psychiatrists—less than 0.5% of the total surveyed—contributed 128 of the 228 MPD cases' (Piper, 1994, p. 604). The obvious implication is that there is a huge interobserver discrepancy in diagnosing the disorder (therefore warning bells for clinical epidemiology), a fact that, in and of itself, requires explanation. The protean clinical manifestations, the difficulty of eliciting clear-cut evidence for the diagnosis, and the elusive nature of many reported alters is not a sufficient explanation in that differences in clinical acumen so profound as to produce such a discrepancy are not often found in clinical life and usually reveal significant differences in theoretical stance towards the disorder in question.

Piper also targets malpractice risks posed by a failure to diagnose MPD in a patient later diagnosed with the disorder and the threat of medical negligence claims. He argues that the diagnostic difficulties should induce caution about findings of fact regarding sound clinical practice in the area and mentions the famous Kenneth Bianchi case in which a rapist and murderer claimed to have MPD but was later considered to be malingering in an attempt to avoid a guilty verdict (Coons, 1991, p. 759). A decision as to the facts of the case was not at all easy and demonstrated the considerable uncertainty surrounding clinical presentation and diagnosis in areas where recognized experts differ profoundly in attitude (Freckleton, 1996). On this basis alone, any malpractice charge should be difficult if not impossible to substantiate; indeed, Putnam freely concedes that the diagnosis may be difficult and that a sympathetic stance towards the construct validity of the disorder may well be important in the clinical setting.

Piper's complaint about the risk of malpractice is therefore probably best dealt with on evidentiary grounds, a robust reasonable practice stance, and thresholds required to establish negligent failure to diagnose or treat where there is considerable clinical uncertainty.

A further forensic complication is raised by the alleged association between MPD and child abuse, particularly sexual abuse. Court proceedings require evidence of actual events constituting the facts for a successful conviction. Thus, there is pressure to be concrete and definite about poorly remembered and sometimes ambiguous incidents from the past in a way that is quite different from the therapeutic attitude (where one believes one's client). What is more, the demanding jurisprudential considerations are compounded by claims that the public validation of memories of abuse is an important facet of 'working through' the material by the adult patient who has suffered in this way. These avowed reasons to pursue a legal hearing for the complaints of abuse magnify the pressure on families and patients when the child-abuse counselling machinery goes to work on an alleged case of MPD. I shall return to this topic when considering repressed memory (see Section 10.4).

Piper worries that the believers in MPD encourage the development and manifestation of immature and irresponsible behaviour as part of the disclosure and working through of the internal conflicts producing the alter personalities. Wholesale licence to indulge one's psychic eccentricities and fantasies is, he believes, detrimental to the development of a responsible and realistic attitude to one's own personal failings. The therapist condoning such behaviour is therefore intensifying rather than resolving the maladjustments of the patient. However, whereas one might concede that a no-nonsense approach to psychiatry is to be commended, one might also want to allow clinical freedom in techniques for dealing with unresolved psychic conflicts. A certain amount of 'acting out', in itself not to be encouraged as a long-term character trait, might be useful in psychotherapy and should not, at least on a priori grounds, be dismissed without good reason.

The criticisms by Piper and others pose philosophical questions as to whether there can be such a being as *Legion* and problems with psychiatric classification should warn us that any simple resolution of the MPD problem is unlikely even though some questions stand out.

Can the mathematics be so extreme?

Does role playing or anything similar to it ever develop into being a disorder in itself?

The first of these questions is inspired by, among other things, the bizarre report (noted earlier) of the Wisconsin woman who sued her psychiatrist for convincing her that she had 120 personalities (and billed her insurance company for group therapy). There are now documented cases in which more than 200 alters have been reported, statistics that cast doubt on the credibility of the whole phenomenon. In fact, it strains credibility that any one of 200 psychic entities competing to take control of the waking hours of a single lifetime could develop 'its own relatively enduring pattern of perceiving, relating to, and thinking about the environment and self' (DSM IV; APA, 1994a, p. 487) given that each would have only about 7 minutes a day in existence (assuming equal democratic representation—$24 \times 60 / 200 = 7.2$).

The second question is interesting for several reasons. Firstly, it indicates the possibility that dissociation is a normal phenomenon in most of us but becomes exaggerated to the point of disorder in MPD: that is, 'dissociation exists along a continuum and contributes to the psychopathology of many disorders' (Putnam, 1991, p. 498). On that view, MPD becomes a limiting (or beyond-the-limits) case of a normal response to a disturbing or traumatizing series of events. It also implies that a role play could develop into something more, indeed into something quite 'alien' (as in Rene's case). Thirdly, it implies that research into phenomena such as state-dependent learning and selective memory may cast light on the clinical phenomenology and genesis of MPD. Each of these strands may help synthesize the divergent analyses.

If we assume that there is such a phenomenon as MPD and that it has some connection with a history of child abuse, it does not follow that there are as many cases as its advocates claim nor that RMS is a genuine phenomenon, nor that MPD is reliably distinguishable (in the raw) from other types of dissociation. An examination of the metaphysics of MPD might then suggest a link between the extreme phenomenology of MPD and psychic mechanisms that are a part of everyday adjustment (and maladjustment). A philosophical examination of the controversies surrounding MPD may also suggest that the theory of iatrogenic production (held by the 'sceptics') and the theory that MPD is a real condition such as rheumatoid arthritis or subarachnoid haemorrhage (held by believers) are both mistaken and that a more nuanced view of psychic reality is the way ahead.

Out-and-out believers tend to treat MPD as being an instance of several persons with distinct identities inhabiting one body, a view that generates thorny philosophical and forensic questions touching on personal identity, consciousness, memory, and responsibility.

10.3 Philosophical tangles

Two philosophical questions are raised in discussions of personal identity. The first concerns numerical identity and is a question about that which individuates me or makes me objectively unique as a countable object of a certain type. The second concerns subjective identity and what it is that makes me the person that I (reflectively) and others relate to as (familiar, lovable) me. The second can be called a characterization question (Schechtman, 1996) and is best thought of as whatever it is that comes to mind or is signified when my name is used. The questions are not totally separable, especially if one holds that my body is the medium that others inscribe by their discourse and that those inscriptions inform my subjectivity. On this view, I am the unique object who I am as a positioned subjectivity even though that unique subjectivity is inseparable from a given body (so that the soul is to the body as sight is to the eye [Aristotle]).

Ask yourself the question 'If my name was not my name who would I be?' The profundity of the question does not strike you until you reflect on what it would be like if, say, as an adopted child you were to find that the name you were given at birth was different from that which you now have. The disconcerting 'who am I really?' thought that results shows us how naming is central in identity even though standard philosophical discussions seem to skirt naming as an institution in the (intersubjective and radically relational) human life-world where identities are forged and take on (forensic, relational, and interpersonal) significance.

Two centuries ago, Locke argued, I think successfully, that we mean to indicate something more than bodily continuity when we mention the identity of a person. He suggested that the mental life of the person was the crucial indicator of identity and argued that this mental aspect was not properly thought of as any kind of substance whether physical or spiritual. He argues that a (psychic) substance is only important because of the functions it subserves and the way that those functions make each of us the individual he or she is. He concludes

> For it being the same consciousness that makes a Man be himself to himself, *personal identity* depends on that only … For it is by the consciousness it has of its present thoughts and actions that it is *self* to it*self* now.

(Locke, 1689/1975, p. 336)

This close identification of personal identity and autobiographical consciousness is a theme common to both Locke and Hume and, if developed, it can lead to scepticism about whether there is a psyche apart from a set of psychological connections and contiguities (Parfit, 1986). Others argue that the psyche is no more than the natural or typical accompaniment of bodily identity so that personal identity is best understood as an open-ended set of functional characteristics that are part of animal identity (Snowdon, 1990; Wiggins, 1987).

However, even if the longitudinal identity of a person is composed of combinations of and interactions between different moments of mental life, there must be a locus (or actual situated nexus) in which the activity is going on so that the discursive view that a person is a named embodied individual inscribed by discourse and using the skills intrinsic to that discourse to structure and make sense of himself or herself yields a unitary embodied subject as the basis of personal identity (numerical and characteristic). The new and interesting reality that emerges out of this quasi-stable subjective being warrants the belief that personal identity is real and more than a mere cluster of psychological states because intentional or psychic states result from the meaning-making activity of a named being formatively related to others (and using shared modes of articulation to structure himself or herself). This author or centre of subjectivity is real in the sense that he or she has an explanatory (and integrative) role in forging a (good-enough) autobiographical narrative unity as the foundation of personal identity.

Schechtman (1996) has argued that the condensation and summarization characteristic of autobiographical memory implies that the rememberer is, in fact, very much an editor, so that personal identity is only misleadingly reduced to a bundle of loosely connected self-contained moments of conscious experience. Memory is quite unlike a video recording in which a record of historical events is inscribed upon a contingent vehicle (the same videotape) that holds them all together such that each memory moment is merely an imprint of the world at a particular time linked to other causally connected imprints but only in a non-intentional or causal (or contingent) sense of 'linked' (as is implicit in Parfit's Q-memory thesis).

> Summarized event memories do not even seem to provide a simple connection between two well-defined moments of consciousness, and so, they present one of the clearest difficulties for views with the structure of psychological continuity theories.
>
> (Schechtman, 1994, p. 9)

Shechtman (1994) emphasizes the authorial or editorial function of the subject so that the longitudinal integration characteristic of memory reflects the way particular experiences are rendered or apprehended by the subject as having a contentful form and autobiographical continuity rather than an impersonal or (austerely causal) relation of de-facto connectedness and continuity.

> If our autobiographical memories are the way we tell ourselves and others the story of our lives, a consideration of the way these memories really work suggests that we are rather subtle authors. We do not need to resort to crude, literal reproduction of our physical and psychological histories but pick and choose the important elements, use sophisticated representational devices, and shape a story that can express what we take to be the basic and essential information about our lives. (p. 12)

The emphasis on the cognitive, emotive, and narrative work that goes into the construction of an autobiography assumes central importance in understanding MPD and personality in general; 'It is exactly this sort of work, which we have seen to be done in autobiographical memory. It is not merely collecting facts about oneself but turning these facts into the story of a life which makes one a person, and underlies the continuation of a single life' (Schechtman, 1994, p. 16). The discursive view locates the author or editor as a subject among others, being mirrored by them, and informing himself or herself through the very personal (and relational) work that makes one into a being who is 'somebody around here' (Gillett, 2008). The more dramatic problems, however, depend on the dramatic metaphysical stands taken about the disorder.

Moral and forensic puzzles

An *out-and-out believers view* of MPD creates moral and forensic puzzles that spark vigorous debates about it (Allison, 1982–83; Braude, 1996; Coons, 1991; Lewis & Bard, 1991).

Who is responsible for an act committed by an alter: The Responsibility Problem?

On the out-and-out believers view, all that matters for personal identity is present in each alter so that the separate names really do indicate distinctness of identities. Thus, if a murder, rape, act of soliciting, or burglary is committed by one alter, say Bela, then it seems just mistaken to hold another alter, say the primary personality Dmitri, responsible for it and charge Dmitri for a crime he did not commit and of which he has no memory. Braude (1996) urges us to ask ourselves an important moral question in such cases: 'Clinicians treating multiples must decide whether it is appropriate—or even just therapeutically beneficial—to hold their patients (or specific alters) responsible for behaviours which they seem unable to control or remember' (p. 37). This worry is provoked by cases in which MPD is claimed to mitigate guilt for crimes.

> Over the past 15 years, a sizable number of homicide defendants have chosen the not-guilty-by-reason-of-insanity . . . defence by alleging that they had MPD at the time of the murder and, therefore, were not responsible for their crime. They usually claimed that another 'personality' killed the victim and that they should not be held responsible.
>
> (Coons, 1991, p. 757)

Is reintegrative therapy the destruction of identifiable persons: The Therapeutic Murder Problem?

This problem arises when we accept that alters are in fact persons because then we must ask what happens to the people who go out of existence if therapy is successful. In fact, we caught a glimpse of this dilemma in the Eve case as Eve thought about the alters she was going to lose. The neo-Lockean view seems to imply that each of the alters instantiates the essence of a person so that any act of causing one of them to cease to exist is morally equivalent to murder. This conclusion, in and of itself, may indicate that something is seriously wrong with the out-and-out believers view, but it does not tell us where we are led astray.

Is there a way of understanding MPD and the discontinuities in consciousness that seem to arise in one human body (and brain): The Explanatory Problem?

On the neo-Aristotelian view, the mind is an emergent and irreducible function of the brain based on shared language and mental ascriptions. Thus, MPD must be explained in terms of a person's being-in-the-world-with-others as it is realized neurocognitively so as to allow the clinical phenomenology of MPD to be seen as a set of adjustments and maladjustments to the human life-world by a situated subject.

A good philosophical theory of Personal Identity (PI)

A neo-Aristotelian approach to the psyche or soul implies it is an aspect (to do with intentional functions) of the form of a human being rather than a separate entity inhabiting a human body. The attempt to reduce the psyche to underlying neuro-physiological functions is, however, a mistake in that it loses sight of the realm of meaning and intentional activity as reflecting the culturally informed interactions between a person and the human life-world.

The discursive view grounds three properties of mind: *intentionality* (in the phenomenological sense), *naturalistic analysis*, and *cultural embeddedness*. Consider, for instance, the mind of a theoretical physicist, the contents and functioning of which can only be understood by looking in part at the discipline of theoretical physics. To engage with the world on the basis of natural human capacities suggests that, even for a discipline such as theoretical physics, we need to be able to trace a coherent story that relates him or her to the world with which he or she interacts (so his or her thought is directed upon what happens there [intentionality] and does justice to his or her nature as a biological organism—hence a kind of naturalism). The third feature, sometimes overlooked in philosophy of mind, is the cultural shape of the psyche and therefore the processing networks of the brain. The physicist has both explicit and procedural knowledge based on his or her learning experiences in theoretical physics (a product of culture). For any Aristotelian, that learning has affected the (microprocessing) structure of the brain. Thus, the physicist's psyche and even his or her brain function are significantly shaped by a cultural artifact—theoretical physics.

That conclusion has implications for the study of disorders such as MPD in that both the psyche and brain have to be understood not only by recourse to biology but also as real products of interpersonal and cultural forces. What is more, the kind of story a person tells about himself or herself is a joint production of the sum of what we might call 'informational transactions' between the person's brain and environment and the cultural milieu in which signifiers are available to structure those transactions and the resulting lived autobiography.

There is, however, a more radical attack on philosophical accounts of personal identity arising from postmodern theory according to which the unitary subject of experience is a fiction so that a person is a series of isolated moments of subjectivity embedded in and inseparable from the various discourses in which they have taken form. But certain questions should be posed.

> How are we constituted as subjects of our own knowledge? How are we constituted as subjects who exercise or submit to power relations? How are we constituted as moral subjects of our own actions?
>
> (Foucault, 1984, p. 49)

If 'the body is the inscribed surface of events (traced by language and dissolved by ideas)' (Foucault, 1984, p. 83), then life events and the way they are signified have an effect on us according to the interplay between signifiers and the particular discursive context in which the subject is located. That (interactive) actuality etches a pattern on the body made up of habitual ways of reacting and responding, psychomotor attitudes, discursive skills, and so on, ways of responding through which the body, as it were, recapitulates what impinges on it to reflect the cumulative effects of the things done and said to the individual concerned. These are, to varying extents, subject to *meconnaissance*, so that the imago and the human psyche are a subjective product of technologies, methods of punishment, supervision, instruction, and constraints on what are considered legitimate ways of being (around here).

> Rather than seeing this soul as the reactivated remnants of an ideology, one would see it as the present correlative of a certain technology of power over the body . . . This real, non-corporeal soul is not a substance; it is the element in which are articulated the effects of a certain type of power and the reference of a certain type of knowledge, the machinery by which the power relations give rise to a possible corpus of knowledge, and knowledge extends and reinforces the effects of this power.
>
> (Foucault, 1984, pp. 176–177)

Foucault identifies the body as the medium in which the soul is formed as a living acting human being embodies the results of various encounters at different times and places. The soul, as mode of interacting with others and as a topic of study, is a construction put on the longitudinally continuous doings of a named and discursively engaged human body that is entangled in temporally extended discourses, a view that undercuts any simple 'identity' based either on the body or on the conscious life of the individual at a given moment.

Foucault's thought therefore implies that the philosophical dichotomy (created by simple body identity views and neo-Humean views of personal identity) needs to be got over so as to recognize that there is in fact a process of creation of the soul whereby a human subjectivity becomes articulated through being exposed to multiple discourses and nexuses of signification. There must be a situated body to allow the interactions between different subjectivities (and thereby between different discourses) to create the complex and elusive 'I think' that denotes the formal principle of convergence required for identity to be enacted (Butler, 1989).

The fact that an individual may co-instance several named and discursively located subjectivities that are not merely passive but (actually or potentially) creative or productive yields a 'thicker' view of personal identity. Jung regarded psychic integration as an active project (based on his clinical encounters), implying that the integration of psychic reality to form a unique identity is aimed at a positive and productive harmony between (possibly) competing forces shaping an individual, as is evident in a contemporary intercultural example.

The Maori explicitly locate the individual within a system of kinship, genealogy, and myths, each directly relevant to a Maori conception of Personal Identity (PI) although any individual may or may not involve himself or herself in the traditional network of ties and symbolisms. For instance, when an individual sees himself as the canoe of his ancestors, he sees himself as having a place to stand, a validated relationship of belonging, and yet also as having (*tino*) *rangitiratanga* or relative autonomy and sovereignty over his own life. But, in post-colonial society, this personal sovereignty is often exercised within a *pakeha* (foreign) context and not that of Maori identity.

> [Y]oung folk can live with a greater amount of assurance if they know who they are. Then, they can move into the Pakeha world full of self-confidence because they have no difficulty about the question of identity. They recognize themselves fully because they know their history.

> (Rangihau, 1992, p. 185)

In the Western European world view, the importance of history and shared myths is often overlooked and Jung forcefully drew our attention back to it. In fact, we find evidence of the importance of such things in the increasingly popular tracing of genealogies, the search for origins by adopted children, the existence of numerous societies dedicated to faithful recreation of experiences of the past, and so on. In contemporary Maori thought, the appreciation of the importance of myth and history is both conscious and explicit.

> Although possessing supranormal powers in an age of miracles, the heroes of myths and traditions behave basically in human ways. They love, hate, fight, and die just as their living counterparts do. Embedded in the stories are themes and myth-messages that provide precedents, models, and social prescriptions for human behaviour. In some cases, the myth-messages are so close to existing reality that it is difficult to resolve whether myth is the prototype or mirror image of reality.

> (Walker, 1992)

The images and significations that inform an individual psyche have to be brought together in some livable-with way in order to give rise to an adequately functioning narrative subjectivity for that human being. That involves narrative and integrative work (a focus of the discursive view of mental reality) and the locus of that work is the body—the inscribed medium producing the soul. A personal identity is therefore an individual production formed on the basis of discursive skills deployed by a subjective body who is 'somebody' around here.

We might compare this view with Clark's (1996a) discussion of the Cartesian light that illuminates the contents of the psyche in all their glorious and often poorly integrated profusion. He recognizes the complexity of personality as I have done but remains skeptical about both the out-and-out believers view and no-self views (such as the strong bundle theory), remarking that the existence of 'many distinguishable thought-lines, moods, and memories need not lead us to believe that there are many different selves nor that there are none' (p. 25).

> We tell ourselves the story of our lives, complete with our commitments and professions. What counts as Me will vary with my context, and with what I can bear to acknowledge. Was it Me that had that dreadful thought just now? That did that dreadful thing some years ago that surfaces in the dull hours of the night?
>
> (Clark, 1996a, p. 25)

Clark reinforces the view that Kant's Trancendental Unity of Apperception as a basis for PI is better thought of as a centre of narrative unity (as in the present account) and concurs that it is an achievement built on discursive skills (as in Harre & Gillett, 1994).

An aspect of the discursive approach often overlooked by analytic philosophers is the role of early interpersonal exchanges in laying the psychic foundations for personality (see Chapter 8). But I have noted that the idea that the child develops as a cognitive agent in a solipsistic (I am the only mind there is) world is more appropriate in understanding autism than ordinary psychological development in that the primary locus for the development of personality and a sense of self is an embodied individual interacting with others (as Freud and Vygotsky noted in psychology and the phenomenologists in the philosophy of mind). Hinshelwood (1995), following Melanie Klein, remarks that 'our experiences of people with whom we develop close relationships can become assimilated into the self' (p. 186). In fact, concepts such as splitting, projection, and introjection are all 'grist to the mill' for a discursive theory of MPD. Hishelwood (1995) notes, 'any theory of personal identity must accommodate the fact that it is a process (rather than a fixed state) that is ongoing throughout life, one that is essentially interpersonal in nature' (p. 202). Thus, there is an inherent multiplicity within the psyche of each of us and a unitary and integrated self should not be taken as a given fact of psychic nature.

> Suppose that the narrative self (or selves) is fiction. So, fractured memories, discordant motives, concealed causes are not anomalies: they are the ordinary human condition, and only the saint, hero, or philosopher has tamed and transformed the squalling horde of impulses so far as to 'know herself' as single.
>
> (Clark, 1996a, p. 25)

Certain observations from cognitive neuroscience confirm this view (as Parfit and others note). Experimenters investigating patients who have had their corpus callosum divided (split brain patients) use tachistoscopic projection to selectively deliver information to either the left or right hemisphere (Glass & Holyoake, 1986; Parkin, 1996). Such experiments show radical discontinuities in the information used to organize behaviour so that some stimuli can be used to guide the right hand and self-report responses but not the left hand (and for other stimuli, the pattern is reversed) depending on which hemisphere the information was delivered to. These disruptions cause response conflicts as in the case of a subject trying to identify a pipe on the basis of selectively delivered information (he had to choose with his right hand, but the information was flashed to his right hemisphere—controlling the left hand). Although these conflicts are not usually apparent in everyday life and are overcome by patients in time (Weiskrantz, 1987), the existence of differential information access creates a problem about the nature of human consciousness and autobiographical awareness.

> [S]ometimes, the disconnected hemispheres interfere with one another, and . . . there is . . . a latent competition, depending on whether the given function falls principally into the domain of the left hemisphere or that of the right. Yet, the two hemispheres can also cue one another; split-brain patients become increasingly skilled at telling when the other hemisphere has been stimulated, by noting, for example, an eye movement or a shift in bodily orientation.
>
> (Gardner, 1974, p. 366)

The conscious self-narrative plausibly comprises information salient in those parts of the brain controlling the techniques used in constructing an autobiography, and in the attempt to make this information as complete as it can be, split-brain patients use various tricks to try and overcome the informational discontinuities they discern within themselves.

This account of split-brain data is pleasingly convergent with the current account of the unconscious according to which the information flow between the environment and my brain is selectively summarized and presented to others and to my discursive self as a 'good-enough reflection' of what has actually happened in the light of what usually happens around here.

The informational capabilities of the narrative centre of consciousness are also important in discussing memory and its role in PI. Schechtman emphasized the fact that the inscription of memory on the body is similar to a reconstructed narrative in which my continuing subjectivity produces for itself a 'non-gappy' life story (as Freud suspected). We are left with a view of personal identity based on the inscribed body and the narrative perspective of the situated individual that takes into account the many and various constraints arising within the individual, affecting his or her access to the totality of brain–world interactions. These features of the psyche are highly relevant not only to MPD but also to RMS.

10.4 Repressed memory and the memory wars

The adult presentation of MPD is often linked to a history of childhood abuse, usually sexual (Putnam, 1991), but the evidence for that abuse may include memories that have been repressed, a concept that is deeply contested. The prima facie evidence for the abuse is often emotional disturbance in the adult when certain topics arise during psychotherapy. The therapist infers that it is caused by unformed or hidden subconscious associations or remembered experiences provoking conflict within the psyche. A naive reading of Freud suggests that these are always episodic memories of actual childhood events excluded from autobiographical consciousness (by the 'censor'). Three assumptions are required to move from these and similar observations to the doctrine of repressed memory:

(a) There is material from the past with definite content to be remembered.

(b) It has the status of episodic memory of actual events.

(c) The memories are stored in a potentially recoverable form.

RMS has divided the therapeutic and forensic community because, if true, the implications are significant for cases in which adults have claimed that they were abused by parents or relatives who deny any knowledge of the alleged events. But do we have on our hands individuals who are living with wounds which have blighted their lives, or are a number of innocent people having their lives disrupted and their names slurred as a result of misinformation, therapeutic misconceptions, and false accusations?

The residues of child abuse are unpleasant and damaging to long-term mental health (Mullen *et al.*, 1994) and include 'fears, post-traumatic stress disorder, behaviour problems, sexualized behaviours, and poor self-esteem' (Kendall-Tackett *et al.*, 1993). People who have been abused find it hard to form close and rewarding relationships, tend to commit violent and abusive crimes themselves, and are denied justice in relation to the actions of their abusers, all issues that should be addressed and, as far as possible, corrected. The tragedy is that some of the worst effects cannot be corrected and society must deal with the resulting ills (ranging from poor parenting through depression, eating disorders, to serial rape and murder, as in Chapter 9). Mullen *et al.* (1994) observe, in relation to the effects of child sexual abuse (CSA)

> In most cases, the fundamental damage inflicted by CSA is to the child's developing capacities for trust, intimacy, sexuality, and self-esteem and that much of the associated mental health problems of adult life are second-order effects. (p. 45)

In the course of therapy, many therapists dealing with MPD observe that their clients report childhood sexual abuse and the use of dissociation as a strategy to cope with the awfulness of what happened to them (Coons, 1984; Loewenstein, 1991; Putnam, 1991; Wibur 1984). In some cases, the patients had no clear recollections of the traumatic childhood events and the claim that these could only emerge during therapy rests on the thought that dissociation, in and of itself, disrupts continuous autobiographical memory in those affected by it.

There has been a steady growth in the discovery of memories of childhood (usually sexual) abuse in a wider and wider group of patients presenting with psychic distress. It has gradually emerged that the memories of alleged abuse are not always forthcoming and may require careful and sensitive questioning to be recovered.

> Of 19 women for whom there was evidence of serious sexual abuse, 14 remembered events corresponding to the original records. Two remembered that abuse had taken place but could recall no details. Three did not report abuse when specifically asked whether they

had been abused as children. Of these three, two described long blank periods for their memory of childhood corresponding to the age when abuse had taken place.

(Brewin, 1996, p. 132)

Similar findings have been observed in other studies (Williams, 1994) and a neural mechanism has been proposed to explain them on the basis of neuropeptides released during stress and their effects on the formation of stable long-term memories (Bremner et al., 1996). That account is independent of Freudian theories about repression and the Ucs and based on work suggesting that the release of stress-related hormones during and after traumatic events interferes with what they call 'the laying down of the memory trace' (Bremner et al., 1996, p. 73; Nemiah, 1989). The data on memory traces and their relation to contexts and affective frameworks imply that the recovery of accurate memories of events experienced in stressful conditions is significantly impaired or disordered (as found in recent work on beta-blockers and post-traumatic stress disorder [PTSD; Cahill et al., 2002]).

Any inherent difficulties in evaluating claims of recovered memories of childhood emotional and sexual abuse (because of physiological interference going on in the formation of stable episodic memories for such incidents) are compounded by the fact that the individuals involved are often disadvantaged in the discursive skills required to form life narratives. The association between child abuse, socio-economic status (SES) status, and 'disturbed and disrupted backgrounds' (Mullen et al., 1994) implies that the very children at risk of abuse are also subject to inconsistent parenting, intra-familial conflict and discord, poor definition of personal, moral, and social boundaries, and regression or immaturity in their behaviour and general psychological development (Kendall-Tackett et al., 1993). All of these would exacerbate any tendency towards a poor articulation of self and autobiographical memory . What is more, there is the issue of knowledge and legitimation to be overcome in the area of memories of infantile abuse: 'Language games about memories are connected to issues of power and ideology as much as they are to empirical evidence and facts about the world' (Potter, 1996, p. 244).

Potter (1996) notes that 'standards of credibility are differentially applied depending on such attributes as race, class, and gender' and that these factors may tell against those who suffer from abuse and produce reports that deeply threaten cherished social stereotypes (for instance, that of the loving supportive nuclear family).

> Many people who recognize the ways in which standards of credibility have reinforced dominant structures while discrediting and silencing oppressed and marginalized groups have argued for the importance of taking a stand on believing reports of abuse and harms that come from members of non-dominant groups because the reports come from members of those groups. (p. 246)

She concludes that even a self-consciously 'socially democratic' approach to epistemology contains hidden biases that may disadvantage the already disadvantaged and that prominent among this group may be the type of people who become victims of abuse. 'When women seek health care, then, they run the risk that their experiences, their reports, and their concerns will be pathologized' (Potter, 1996, p. 247). Her argument is a timely reminder of the evil of neglecting genuine discoveries about child abuse in general and of the potentially damaging effects of that neglect. She highlights the particular injustice of discounting individual reports in an individual who has already suffered as a result of disempowerment and betrayal of trust.

Drawing the battle lines

Public awareness of child abuse and its effects has been raised by media campaigns and highly visible exposes of abuses in schools and institutions.

> Childhood sexual abuse is increasingly invoked as the causative agent for a broad spectrum of disorders, especially in women, ranging from depression through eating disorders to such complex personality configurations as the borderline conditions and multiple personality disorder. More and more troubled people are 'remembering' sexual violations, often under the supportive, encouraging, even coercive influence of therapists who are certain that the vocation and abreaction of such memories is the *sine qua non* of therapeutic success.

> (Esman, 1994)

The calls for public and legal understanding of the suffering of victims of abuse have prompted legislative changes (for instance, to the statutes of limitations) to accommodate the kinds of evidence arising from recovered memories and resulted in cases where individuals have been sued for large sums of money or convicted of crimes that nobody ever knew had happened or remembered happening until the alleged victim entered therapy. One commentator remarks:

> This process has brought psychiatry into contact with a widespread and unexpected social phenomenon. In this case, adults, mostly in the third and fourth decades of life, have begun to accuse their fathers, and sometimes other relatives including their mothers, of sexual abuse in childhood, which was never revealed, and which indeed they themselves had forgotten until the 'memory' was restored to them.

> (Merskey, 1995)

Loftus (1993), in a review of the subject, reports several cases, among them the following:

> One case involved a 27-year-old San Diego woman (K.L.) who began to have recollections of molestation by her father (D.L.) that were repressed but then were later brought out through 'counselling and therapeutic intervention' . . . The daughter claimed that her father had routinely and continuously molested and sexually abused her, performing 'lewd and lascivious acts, including but not limited to touching and fondling the genital areas, fornication, and oral copulation'. Her earliest memories were of her father fondling her in the master bedroom when she was three years old. Most of her memories appeared to date back to between the ages of three and eight. She sued her father for damages for emotional and physical distress, medical expenses, and lost earnings. She claimed that because of the trauma of the experience, she had no recollection or knowledge of the sexual abuse until her repression was lifted, shortly before she filed suit. (p. 520)

Cases such as this have provoked a fierce reaction from both the profession and the general public despite the allegations being relatively modest and plausible.

> Other cases involve richly detailed allegations of a more bizarre, ritualistic type . . . The
> plaintiff, Bonnie, in her late 40s at the time of trial, accused her parents of physically,
> sexually, and emotionally abusing her from birth to approximately age 25. A sister, Patti,
> in her mid-30s at the time of trial, said she was abused from infancy to age 15. The allegations
> involved torture by drugs, electric shock, rape, sodomy, forced oral sex, and ritualistic killing
> of babies born to or aborted by the daughters. The events were first recalled when the
> plaintiffs went into therapy in the late 1980s.
>
> (Loftus, 1993, p. 523)

Even more lurid and implausible memories of, for instance, satanic ritual abuse and alien abduction cast doubts on the whole recovered memories phenomenon so that a *False Memory Syndrome Foundation* has rapidly gathered members throughout Britain and North America. It comprises not only families and sympathizers with those accused but also psychiatrists and psychotherapists who are deeply sceptical. Adults who self-diagnose on the basis of popular psychology and self-help books about memories of abuse are suggestible enough to inflate the problem and further polarize the therapeutic community (Wyatt, 1994)[1].

The criticisms of repressed memory theory and praxis have conceptual, scientific, clinical, and forensic aspects and are both philosophical and psychological in tenor.

Scientific objections

Most scientific objections attack the idea that there can be buried or repressed memories that are sufficiently accurate to be recovered and reported in a way that provides factual evidence about the original events; they focus on the *amnesia characteristic of the early years of childhood*, the *reconstructive and malleable nature of memory*, and the *vulnerability of memory to post event information*.

The amnesia characteristic of early childhood years has led one critical commentator to be sceptical of the whole phenomenon of recovered memory: 'There is little, if any, reason to believe in the validity of recovered memories, especially when a significant proportion are reported from the age of three years or less' (Merskey, 1995, p. 283). This 'infantile amnesia' is best thought of as a function of the gradual development of the skills required to articulate autobiographical memories and is obviously relevant to recalled episodes of abuse. Episodic memory develops from a phase in which the child is composing scripts for types of events and, with that foundation, begins to acquire declarative memories of unique events (Nelson, 1988, p. 252); 'memories of young children are more closely attuned to one class of objectively existing *memoria* (repeated sequences) than to another (unique episodes)' (Neisser, 1988, p. 359). Neisser notes with disapproval that 'most theorists still think of personal memory as if it were just a set of remembered concrete experiences' (p. 356) and argues that childhood memory is designed to equip the child with a set of adaptive expectations and strategies for dealing with the challenges of adult life. Such event-memories are highly influenced by the social and interpersonal milieu in which they are reported so that 'most children between the ages of 3 and 8 years can provide detailed accounts

---

[1] Wyatt, M. (1994) Repressed memory therapy: a critique [Unpublished dissertation]. Otago, NZ: Education Department, Otago University.

of events such as visits to McDonalds and birthday parties—indeed, these children even design their account of an event to suit their audience' (Conway, 1990, p. 147). This latter feature is especially important in discussions of childhood testimony about alleged abuse, as is the observation that 'the two best indicators of clarity of memory were emotional intensity at the time of experience and perceived life impact at the time of experience' (Conway, 1990, p. 91).

One might therefore expect that if children form relatively clear memories of emotionally loaded events recognized as such at the time and form well-organized memories where the events are not unique, then repeated disturbing episodes of child abuse might be expected to be the clearest memories that children form. However, the memories in question in RMS are adult memories of childhood events and not those of children reporting their own experiences. What is more, the evidence for such memories and the thesis that they could be repressed and not accessible to ready recall in adult life is materially conceived and validated in the clinical setting and therefore provokes further questions about its credibility.

> Over-reporting, under-reporting, retrospective distortion, tendentious recollection, responses to overt or implied suggestion—all may play a part in skewing the data, requiring a substantial measure of reserve in their interpretation. This is all the more true in the present climate, in which the information and entertainment media are replete with stories, often lurid, of the prevalence and the dire consequences of abuse.
>
> (Esman, 1994, p. 1102)

The reconstructive and malleable nature of memory is increasingly evident: 'Autobiographical memory is typically inaccurate and . . . memories are reconstructed in terms of schemata so that any plausible event description which does not violate a schema expectancy might be erroneously judged to have been experienced,' and yet 'events which are emotional and personally significant appear to be represented in memory in some detail and may be less subject to construction' (Conway, 1990, pp. 98, 100). Despite the relative robustness of some emotionally charged memories, there is a growing consensus that memory is not like a library or record in which texts or traces encoded by events in the world are stored for later retrieval. 'The underlying processes that account for memory may well be similar to those involved in problem solving. We probably use information from a variety of sources, even some unrelated to the original perceptual experience, to help reconstruct it' (Fisher & Cuervo, 1983).

Loftus (1993) produces many examples of memories induced or changed by experimental devices:

> Since the mid-1970s at least, investigations have been done into the creation of false memories through exposure to misinformation. Now, nearly two decades later, there are hundreds of studies to support a high degree of memory distortion. (p. 530)

The phenomena include not only the creation of pseudo-memories, alteration of the details of remembered events and scenes by post-event information, but also the creation of an entire set of memories of abuse in a suggestible subject. This particular finding was not, of course, an experiment (that would have been completely unethical) but a series of events that happened as a result of the arrest of a person called Paul Ingram (Ofshe, 1989).

The vulnerability of memory to post-event information is well attested and has been studied by several researchers: '[A]n eyewitness's memory is susceptible to the influence of information that is presented after an event is witnessed' (Bowers & Bekerian, 1984). Post-event interference is particularly marked when the original cues and context are not reproduced during recall (Bekerian & Bowers, 1983), as is shown in a number of diverse experiments and in a wide variety of incident types.

> These examples provide further insights into the malleable nature of memory. They suggest that memories for personally experienced traumatic events can be altered by new experiences. Moreover, they reveal that entire events that never happened can be injected into memory. The false memories range from the relatively trivial (e.g. remembering voting) to the bizarre (e.g. remembering forcing one's daughter and son to have sex).
>
> (Loftus, 1993, p. 533)

Clinical objections

These objections concern the clinical practices that generate accounts of childhood abuse by therapists committed to the repressed memory hypothesis. Loftus (1993) tellingly compares them with a number of the experiments that induced false memories.

> The false memories in the examples above were accomplished with techniques that are not all that different from what some therapists regularly do—suggesting that the client was probably abused because of some vague symptoms, labelling a client's ambiguous recollections as evidence of abuse, and encouraging mental exercises that involve fantasy merging with reality. (p. 533)

Merskey (1995) contends that much of the evidence produced for false memories is manufactured.

> In the hands of therapists who believe in immediately searching for repressed memories of childhood abuse, the patient is quickly encouraged to produce evidence of such events from childhood. If memories do not come quickly, more pressure is exerted. (p. 282)

Loftus (1993) reports similar problems, remarking that 'evidence exists that some therapists do not take no for an answer' (p. 526); she outlines the process leading to suspect claims: 'The therapist convinces the patient with no memories that abuse is likely, and the patient obligingly uses reconstructive strategies to generate memories that would support that conviction' (p. 528). The memories produced by such techniques then provoke another set of objections in relation to the forensic use of such reports.

Forensic objections

There are two different concerns: (i) the different attitudes of counsellor and courtroom and (ii) the effects of subjectively 'true' but possibly false testimony.

The first worry is that the clinic setting depends on a supportive, sympathetic, and credulous attitude to testimony about events and experiences that seem real to the patient, but that stance should not be carried into the courtroom. In therapy, the patient's perceptions and psychic reality needs to be taken as revealing a kind of truth—about the patient. Therefore, the therapist, who may be agnostic about the events concerned, has to take them seriously as revealing important features of the patient's subjectivity. But in the courtroom, the facts must be established because they bear on the lives of more than one person, and therefore a high degree of critical judgement and a jurisprudential caution must be exercised.

The second worry concerns the injustices that can result from accounts of child abuse based on repressed memories in that courtroom evidence affects the fate of the defendant as well as to the psychic health of the client or patient in therapy. Loftus (1993) remarks, 'uncritical acceptance of uncorroborated trauma memories by therapists, social agencies, and law enforcement [personnel] has been used to promote public accusations by alleged abuse survivors' (p. 534). Merskey (1995) also notes the damaging effects of reports of repressed memory.

> Once a memory is produced, the patient is told to stay away from members of the family until they acknowledge their wickedness and guilt, and lawsuits may be commenced to pay for the damage done and for further therapy. Families are torn apart on uncorroborated evidence, based upon the solicited recall by individuals who have had no conscious knowledge of the matter in the 10, 20, 30, or even 40 years since the events which are said to have taken place. (p. 282)

What is more, there is no evidence to support the view that the psychic effects of a criminal conviction are beneficial or more beneficial than less adversarial ways of proceeding. Even worse, there is a complete lack of any evidence that the disruption of families is less harmful than an unresolved legal case (this is especially worrying when zealous caseworkers break up the families of children because they believe that the child has been abused.)

The forensic implications of repressed memories make the 'memory wars' both bitter and bloody. Merskey (1995) notes that such conflict 'disrupts families, wipes out the life savings of parents, abolishes their contact with children and grandchildren, and embroils some in painful legal battles' (p. 283). Therefore, a careful look at the philosophical arguments and psychological evidence that bear on MPD and RMS becomes pressing.

10.5 The philosophy and psychology of memory

Traditional philosophical views picture memories as internal traces accessible to the person who has them and able to be recalled as a kind of revisitation of past events (like re-running a video recording taken at the time the remembered events happened). Most hold that 'remembering is the final stage of a causal process and that memory is some sort of causal device or mechanism' (Benjamin, 1967, p. 184). This view implies that we have a store of memories corresponding to past events retrievable with more or less difficulty at later times in our life and more or less accurate in their details. Thus a genuine event memory 'must correspond to a past cognitive and sensory state of the remember' (Shoemaker, 1984, p. 40). Philosophers concede that there might be degeneration in the memory traces, so that the vivid detail that was there at the time of the original experience may not persist into the memory record, but hold firm to a correspondence between present mental state and the past, causally mediated as a recording-like effect of the past event, referring to the relation as *being causally connected in the right kind of way* (Martin & Deutscher, 1966; Parfit, 1984).

Some philosophers have also argued that one person could have 'quasi-memories' of another person's past experiences on the basis of the right kind of causal relationship between the memory and the remembered moment of past experience (Parfit, 1984 ; Shoemaker, 1963).

The causally-linked-sequence-of-episodes theory has remained more or less the account embraced by Hume (1739/1969): memory is the summoning to consciousness of past impressions and their attendant complex ideas. He considers a conversation in which one person is trying to help another recollect a shared experience and supposes that the one 'hits on some lucky circumstance that revives the whole "concluding" as soon as the circumstance is mentioned, that touches the memory, the very same ideas now appear in a new light' (p. 133). This is 'the mental datum theory: to remember is to have a certain sort of mental datum . . . and to tell others what one remembers is to inform them of the details of the datum' (Benjamin, 1967). Benjamin argues that such a theory is linked to a strong Cartesian belief in incorrigibility or transparency of mental contents and therefore faces us with a stark choice between declaring the memory veridical or declaring that the person making the memory claim is a liar. In fact, we recognize that people make honestly mistaken memory claims. He notes that the primary discursive role of memory talk is to mark the logical status of a certain event as being in the speaker's past and a secondary role is to refer to the (hypothesized) mental capacity used in the mastery of memory skills. The analysis parallels that of knowledge talk (remarks preceded by 'I know') where the role of discursive warrants (or giving a guarantee of veracity) is crucial to the 'language game' (Wittgenstein, 1969). We must therefore look at the function of memory talk in everyday life and the natural history on which those linguistic practices are built.

When a person says 'I remember visiting the Taj Mahal when I was six years old,' we normally take ourselves to be hearing a fact about that person's life, and if it were later shown that the person had never visited India, that claim entitles us to demand that she change her statement to something such as 'I have the most vivid impression of having seen the Taj Mahal when I was six years old.' Even if her impression of visiting the Taj Mahal is as strong as any other impression from her childhood, faced with the discrepancy between the normal reliability of memory and the fact that this 'memory' is clearly mistaken, we turn our attention to the second sense of the term 'memory' (to denote the process of remembering) because we infer that the person's memory (mechanism) is faulty in some way. Having detected an apparent memory that is not a real memory—first-person testimony notwithstanding—we want to know how that might have come about. Here, we find help in psychology and neuroscience ('the natural history of memory', to adapt Wittgenstein's phrase).

From psychology, we confirm some things already widely known: people sometimes forget things; people invalidate and mnemonically obscure observations that are disturbing or objectionable; people mix things up or confuse different things when they try to remember an episode; and people tend to get relevant points right and spin a story around them. We also learn some new things, for instance, about the detailed structure and vulnerabilities of memory. Mixed into these latter things is a good dollop of theory and we devise the idea of a memory store holding mental copies of actual events, captured by the term 'memory trace'. But we now find that this (traditional folk) theory is being displaced by the cognitive reconstruction view of episodic and autobiographical memory.

It emerges that memory is not just a self-contained cognitive realm but that 'central knowledge structures relating to the self have been employed in representing the memory' (Conway, 1990, p. 92) so that it has individual, idiosyncratic, and dynamic features (linked to the *imago*). Looking at childhood memories through such a lens reveals that the child's growing sense of self and conception of how he or she fits into various relationships is an important factor in the way that events are remembered, a fact that is explained when we realize that the main cognitive task of early childhood is to develop strategies and expectations relating to the life events that have to be dealt with in adulthood; 'Thus, memories of specific events are used to build knowledge structures representing routine activities and in the process the initial memories of specific events are lost—hence, childhood amnesia' (Conway, 1990, p. 147).

Over and above the general poverty of specific memories for early childhood events, some childhood memories are so disturbing that they are especially subject to disruption. Freud held that such events occasioned the formation of 'screen memories' to register but not depict the actual content of the disturbing memories. 'It is not clear from Freud's writings whether he considered screen memories to be complete fabrications or whether he thought of them as fragments of memories of real episodes which defence mechanisms of the psyche have, as it were, sanitized for remembering' (Conway, 1990, p. 145).

The option central to the memory wars is that traumatic episodes might be stored in some subconscious partition in the mind for later accurate and factual recall in some detail is suggested by the fact that 'the emotional intensity and personal significance of an event give rise to autobiographical memories which are detailed, highly available for recall, and comparatively resistant to forgetting' (Conway, 1990, p. 104). But, it is not clear how this meshes with claims about dissociation or repression from 'damaging' events in childhood.

Many philosophical and psychological conceptions of memory embed a mistaken view that should be revised in the light of discursive and experimental data about the phenomenology of memory. The mistake affecting many philosophical accounts is that our folk belief (and indeed discursive norm) that a memory report is or should be factual is transformed into a philosophical doctrine that there is a string of episodes that are accurately stored in the mind as representations making up autobiographical memory. This view, supplemented by psychological doctrines about memory traces and compartments in the mind called 'short-term memory', 'long-term memory', and so on (depending on precisely which theory is being outlined), underpins the memory wars and the forensic status of memories. But a closer and more extended investigation of the actual phenomena characteristic of memory suggests that memory, far from being a series of recordings of autobiographical episodes, is a skill using (extraconscious) strategic clues and generic scripts that enable one to create a good-enough facsimile of a given autobiographical episode. According to that view, these cognitive skills, hierarchically nested in psychic structures that capture a person's sense of self and subjective history, form the materials for a more or less accurate reconstruction of the past affected by the recency of the remembered events and their meaning to the person (or autobiographical salience).

Therefore, memory exhibits a pervasive feature of psychic life: the contents involved are intentional and involve seeing-as or understanding-as, skills subject to discursive influences. Imagine, for instance, the memories formed during a conference by those who participate in it.

'A visitor from some exotic culture who knew nothing of conferences—if there still are any such cultures—would describe what is happening here in ways that might surprise us. That possibility does not affect the reality status of the events as I have chosen to describe them' (Neisser, 1988, p. 363). Neisser is much clearer than many philosophical or scientific commentators who confuse the fact that intentionality is a feature of mental contents with the idea that they are fictitious or that the things they relate to exist only in the mind.

Armed with a considered view of the philosophy and psychology of memory, we can now attempt to come to some balanced assessment of what is happening in the memory wars.

Idealogical neutrality in the memory wars

Scientific realism has much to answer for in this vexed area of psychiatric controversy. 'The natural science model can assimilate all contradictions to error and thus discount the nuances—indeed the inherent contradictoriness—of many complex psychic phenomena' (Code, 1996, p. 258). Scepticism (based on a rigid empiricist version of scientific realism) is particularly threatening (as Potter has noted) where the people in question are people who are traditionally marginalized, whose testimony is systematically discounted, and whose rights are often abused by 'the establishment'.

> The almost inevitable 'gappiness' of memory that testifiers about such emotionally charged events commonly betray prompts the already incredulous, whose incredulity is reinforced by the dispassionate purity of empiricism, to seek the very loopholes that the dominant social imag[ery] makes available in its construction of women as hysterical, Jews as devious, Blacks as sexually out of control, and children as spinners of fanciful yarns. Empiricist epistemologies have no available apparatus for counting such 'gappy' and emotion-laden testimony as the basis of bona fide knowledge.
>
> (Code, 1996, p. 257)

An emphasis on clear, coherent, and well-evidenced beliefs in our assessments of testimony is bound to tell against the sufferers of abuse, but the traditional positivist approach to knowledge also misses the nuances and shades between truth and falsehood that are bound to arise when subjectivity with all its internal contradictions and psychic complexity is our focus.

Freud was probably at his canny and clinically astute best when he equivocated about the status of 'screen memories' and what they were screening. He was aware that the emotionally charged (intensely cathectic) material involved was a complex mixture of fantasy, symbolic appreciation of the nuances of interpersonal relationships, actual event-memories, life episode meanings, and autobiographical constructions, and that this morass seethed and bubbled according to the dynamics of the primary process. In all of this material are event-memories-as-experienced-by-the-individual concerned who, at a young age, is busy sorting out the techniques and 'nesting structures'

(Neisser, 1988) that will allow her (or him) to compose an integrated and 'good enough' autobiography. In the name of therapy and psychic resolution, we insist that the material (from Ucs, posited as leading to psychopathology) be recovered to consciousness as would ('genuine') episodic memories. But then, we sometimes go further and, in the name of validation and public recognition as an important part of therapy, try to cast the resulting material in the simplistic binary mould of positivistic truth and falsity that is the 'bread and butter' of litigation-related evidence. All this can take psychic distress and turn it into a monster destroying lives. But how are we to avoid the monstrous cascade?

The epistemic claims in relation to RMS are as problematic as other claims about the unconscious. First, they are produced to explain certain adult psychic problems. Second, they derive from testimony by people whose accounts are often discounted and whose views are often marginalized. Third, they represent areas of autobiography about which a person may feel sensitive, guilty, and confused. Fourth, they arise from a time in life when a person has not mastered the techniques of producing good-enough autobiograhical testimony. Crucial questions, therefore, must be asked.

Is there an explanatory gap to be filled between the life events disclosed in therapy and the severity of the adult disorder? This is one of Freud's crucial arguments for the existence of unconscious psychic material, and if there is such a gap, then one might be prompted to look for it in events that have not emerged in the spontaneous recall of the subject.

Is there evidence in transcripts or other accounts of the therapeutic sessions (where 'the memories' were recovered) that suggests coercion by the therapist rather than just permission to produce potentially shocking and highly charged material? When we consider the social norms and the emotional costs of confronting material about child abuse, there might have to be genuine acceptance and permission given to the victim to talk about taboo subjects, but that permission differs (in both its content and conduct) from attempts to coerce the subject into producing reports of abuse that are not otherwise forthcoming.

Are the supposed event-memories independently plausible? Here, we are alert for aspects of the alleged episodic memories so incredible or bizarre as to be inherently implausible. Prima facie indicators of fabrication are such things as stories of alien abduction, satanic rituals involving human sacrifice (where there is no surrounding evidence of homicide or possible victims whose disappearance has caused concern), or episodes which, if true, would almost certainly have led to discovery quite apart from the testimony in question.

Is there any corroborating evidence from siblings or peers or other witnesses that might support the allegations? Whereas this might be problematic because of the marginalization of victims, such evidence affects the balance of probabilities in ascertaining the facts.

These questions are not supposed to undermine the subjective distress or saliencies of the victims. That psychic reality, as Freud seems to have been aware, may be our only indication of significant personal intrapsychic conflict and the need for fantasy affecting recall as to matters of fact and needs to be dealt with on its own (deeply emotive) terms (often in a transference-affected relationship).

We ought also to note the justification for the legal recognition of accounts of abuse in terms of the benefits of public validation of a victim's story to the victim concerned—that is, 'therapeutic jurisprudence' (Wexler, 1996). That has led to at least one finding against a therapist for failure to take due care in therapy resulting in direct harm to a target of abuse allegations. If empirical evidence of this benefit could be weighed in the balance against the relatively incontrovertible damage that can result from an overzealous pursuit of redress for alleged abuse, a more balanced view would result, but no such evidence currently exists. It is therefore significant that the legal system has begun to strive for a balance between justice to accused parties and what is owed to the supposed victims of alleged abuse (Appelbaum & Zoltek-Jick, 1996).

Loftus (1993) has some practical recommendations for therapists in this area (and these, for a pragmatist and realist, are as significant as any other argument):

> Psychotherapists, counsellors, social service agencies, and law enforcement personnel would be wise to be careful how they probe for horrors on the other side of some presumed amnesic barrier . . . Techniques that are less potentially dangerous would involve clarification, compassion, and gentle confrontation along with a demonstration of empathy for the painful struggles these patients must endure as they come to terms with their personal truths. (p. 534)

The 'memory wars' are fiercely fought and involve extensive damage to lives and souls. Both sides have their ardour fuelled by keenly felt injustices. However, even if scientific realists are wrong about value-free facts, they are right about the sometimes adverse effect of passion where wisdom and considered judgement are called for. The debates about repressed memory fall in that category and should make one wary of taking an extreme view on either side.

10.6 Diverse theories of MPD

The writers about MPD and RMS include believers (of different stripes), unbelievers, sceptics, and agnostics. Out-and-out believers accept that MPD occurs when more than one personality or mind inhabits a single human body, whereas unbelievers claim that cases of MPD are complex psychological artifacts produced by the joint efforts of therapists and suggestible patients, a quasi-therapeutic *folie à deux*. Both unbelievers and believers share a commitment to psychic realism—the idea that there is a definite way things are inside the mind. This shared assumption is, however, problematic[2]. Allied to this view is the essentialism that sometimes forces classifications of psychological disorders into the model of disease entities or natural kinds such as endocarditis or systemic lupus erythematosus[3]. In contrast to both realism and disease essentialism (shared by both opponents and proponents of MPD), Hacking, a philosopher of science, is an *agnostic* in that he thinks that both dogmas are problematic from the standpoint of 'realistic' realism.

---

[2] As noted in Chapters 1 and 4, and Appendix A

[3] As discussed in Appendix B

Braude and the realist view

Braude (1991) is a believer of a relatively sophisticated kind, offering an account full of clinical detail and close philosophical analysis of the phenomena of multiplicity and personality. He acknowledges the role of therapists and also of an MPD-believing culture in the genesis of the current 'epidemic' of MPD and has arguments for a 'realistic' (moderate) realism about MPD.

(1) MPD is often found in patients who have not had hypnosis or therapy (Braude, 1991, p. 62).

This point does not quite turn the trick against what we might call 'the social production view' according to which the popular mythology of an MPD-believing culture may encourage people to take on certain culturally validated roles and ways of being unwell (the 'looping effect' of Hacking) and MPD is one of the roles available to be occupied by a disturbed person.

(2) Even if some cases of MPD are cases in which role playing can be demonstrated or, at the extreme, cases in which there is malingering, it does not follow that all cases of MPD are of this type (Braude, 1991, p. 62).

This is a logical truth highlighting a problem with difficult and ambiguous categories of illness. The core cases of any such disorder may be clear-cut but, awareness in the profession having been awakened (perhaps at first among a series of interested and enthusiastic professionals), the previous oversight then may become a public issue or at least an issue in the popular health media. By the time the disorder has moved beyond its original clinical setting and reached the point where it has penetrated public consciousness, it may have gathered to its ranks a penumbra of cases whose status is much more questionable than that of the originals. At this point, critical attention reveals flaws in the diagnosis because a 'mixed bag' has resulted from the influx in the 'penumbra' of false or more dubious cases. This 'mixed bag' then confounds systematic study by diluting the genuine examples and obscuring any striking or salient features they genuinely share.

(3) Genuine cases show subtle and sustained effects that are difficult to mimic (Braude, 1991, pp. 63–64).

One psychiatrist refers to 'the smell of the clinic' invoking the sometimes inchoate or poorly articulated perceptions of the experienced clinician who takes note, perhaps, of elusive and subliminal features of the case before him in assessing its genuineness. The problem with MPD is that the experienced clinicians often include a disproportionate number of enthusiasts who tend to diagnose MPD (or RMS) on relatively slight evidence. Vesting too much authority in these experts and deferring to their opinion can be a cloak for sloppy or dogmatic thinking that is problematic when one takes a critical look at any disorder in that such thinking is usually also imperceptive and unreflective about the subtleties required in clinical assessment and the many relevant supplementary observations properly considered by a careful clinician. In the case of MPD, it may be that certain subtle and sustained effects tend to confirm the presence of the disorder and it is relevant to note minor physiological effects (muscle balance, acuity, exotropia) that evince a change in mode of psychic being sufficiently profound to alter many of the things we would normally think are unconsciously controlled.

This last observation brings us to Braude's discussion of the presumed underlying mechanism giving rise to MPD. He identifies a tendency to dissociation in patients whose psychic states are not well integrated into their autobiographical or 'indexical' self-understanding in the way that psychic states and resulting actions normally would be. This indexical understanding of self is the 'owning' of the psychic contents in question or their being 'assigned' to one's own autobiography (ownership, authorship, and alienation are also relevant in psychotic disorders of the mind affecting thought form and content [Stephens & Graham, 2000]).

Braude argues that certain kinds of psychological events associated with dissociative states may be accessible to the consciousness of the subject from whom they are dissociated but not in the same way as the states he or she autobiographically 'owns', so that dissociation involves 'effaced' co-consciousness. The phenomenon is well illustrated, for instance, in automatic writing where 'the automatist who observes his handwriting is obviously aware of his or her automatic behaviour,' but the writing is not accessible or thought of in the normal indexical way as being an activity in which he or she is engaged. Normal indexical thinking of an aspect of self involves the immediacy of a lived first-person experience apt for autobiographical treatment (Braude, 1991, p. 122) so that the experiences and actions can then be 'owned' morally as something for which the individual is responsible. Braude invokes 'apperceptive centres' with an autobiographical role in integrating indexical states into a single conscious first-person narrative and, in treating them as loci or points of application of cognitive (discursive) skills in a way that converges with the present account.

Braude (1991) recommends a set of attitudes towards multiples accommodating considerable ontological ambiguity: 'One feels concern for the well-being and integration of the multiple while at the same time feeling the naturalness and importance of acknowledging the alters' distinctness and maintaining different relationships with different alters' (p. 209). This realistic, pragmatic, or circumspect (based on dealings with) rather than metaphysical resolution of the philosophical problems posed by MPD has the rationality of good practice to recommend it and that may be the warmest recommendation of all. However, it leaves us with a philosophical task in relation to the metaphysics of identity and the forensic status of MPD.

We must ask why our common discourse about mind and personality forces us to think of multiples in ways that embody apparent contradictions. For instance, distinct apperceptive centres have commensurable sets of learnt discursive skills and yet we argue that they alternate in occupying the discursive sphere in which those skills have been learnt; indeed, the least frequently appearing alters may have the widest range of such skills. What is more, when we try and explain what goes on in therapy or in the recovery of repressed psychic contents, we invoke an account based on the unity of mental life normally shown by a human being. This implies that the belief in a single mental entity is fundamental and the idea of multiple entities is, at best, an 'as-if' belief. There are also the moral and forensic difficulties that arise from even a moderate realist view. Braude (1996), for instance, notices the more dramatic contradictions in our attitudes toward violence or 'considerations of sexual consent with the alleged date rape of a multiple but also in the context of marriage to a multiple' (p. 38). These questions of morality, sexuality, and responsibility cry out for resolution.

Can we justify the pragmatic need to treat multiples as multiple for some purposes and not for others? Clark (1996a) Mental life is essentially unified and in its place outlined a view that, to some extent follows Hacking in pursuing an account of MPD and RMS that is somewhat more sympathetic to discursive analyses.

Hacking's account

Hacking introduces his lengthy analysis of MPD, RMS, and other dissociative states by commenting on the work of Hippolyte Taine, a French positivist and an early champion of the naturalistic approach to dissociative phenomena such as the doubling of consciousness, automatic writing, and what was then called spirit possession. He specially notes the agenda behind Taine's conceptualization of dissociative phenomena such as hysteria and the French cases of double consciousness. For Taine, these phenomena were metaphysically important in that they were evidence against the view that there was a single non-natural soul residing in each one of us—the bearer of moral and spiritual properties. Positivists, such as Taine, looked at the odd phenomena associated with inner 'spiritual' forces disrupting consciousness and argued that they were natural manifestations that could and should be studied by experimental and comparative psychology. Thus, phenomena, at the time, surrounded by mystery and mystical conjecture were placed within the ambit of naturalist science and thereby secularized and legitimated. That move leads Hacking (1996) to remark, 'one of the roots of multiple personality is republican positivism' (p. 163), and motivates a discussion of discourses, the political agendas influencing them, and the social production of truth according to a discursive conception of the scientific method.

Hacking locates certain productive forces influencing scientific theories within sociopolitical contexts and undertakes an analysis of MPD that some interpret as embracing a kind of social constructionism. That interpretation is too simplistic when taken to imply that fashions of belief manufacture such phenomena as MPD and RMS in that Hacking argues that social and discursive configurations influence the *ways of being* adopted by individuals as they attempt to negotiate the task of constructing an acceptable or validated narrative of the transactions between themselves and their environment. The mirror-world, the world of reflection and meaning, is a shared world of significations arising in the human group around here and it provides ways of being human (based on real-life trajectories) to those under its canopy (Berger, 1967).

Hacking traces the historical and cultural roots of MPD and other states in which knowledge of the subject of experience, whether in the first or third person, is conflicted or ambiguous, noting the holistic connections between ways of characterizing what people experience and the significant movements in intellectual and political circles at a given time in history. He remarks, for instance, how the idea of parallel conscious narratives, a key constitutive element in the validation of MPD, became displaced by the growing science of memory and the multilevel conceptions of mind prevalent in the Freudian school. It is therefore ironic that the modern revival of a naive view of Freudian theory has forged the link between MPD and its explanation in terms of repressed memories of abuse. Hacking (1996) also develops a key idea undercutting spurious distinctions between realism and social constructionism in the human sciences—*the looping effect of human kinds.*

People classified in a certain way tend to conform to or to grow into the ways they are described, but they also evolve in their own ways so that the classifications and descriptions have to be constantly revised. (p. 21)

Every self-conception has a formative (not merely a representational) relation to the human being using that conception. Thus, if I think of myself as being a nuclear physicist, then I am not only reporting what I am but also making a commitment to what I intend to be and what I am currently making of myself. The thought that I am a nuclear physicist shapes, according to various models, the way I conduct myself, the experiences I cultivate, the ideas invoked when I describe myself, my actions, aspirations, and so on (the thought can only have those effects if it actually changes the way in which my brain works at a microprocessing level.)

Thus, the creation of ways of being human that a person may aspire to—nuclear physicist, basketball player, scholar, entrepreneur, thief, homosexual, doctor, and so on—provides a repertoire of narratives for a life that can be constructed. In a (sometimes straightforward and sometimes subtle) way, such narratives shape my experiences, their signification, and therefore my memories. Even more subtly, the characters articulated in a narrative type provide each of us with a number of ways, myriad, complex, and dynamic, of following his or her chosen (or stumbled upon) narrative path. One can imagine a complex process of adjustment and interaction between a narrative and a lived life such that the product is historically and numerically but also discursively distinct for each person, even if, to some extent, the resulting narratives gave rise to generalizations, about personality traits, attitudes, and so on, allowing us to discern common features between one person and others (Harre & Gillett, 1994). The commonalities might be of different kinds—biological, psychological, familial, mythological, typological, cultural, historical, or symbolic. They also function in diverse ways to affect both the external and internal story of a life.

By calling this personal production a narrative, we must not buy into an overly self-deterministic or existential reading of the complex process of self-formation. To do so would be to valorize and romanticize it to the point of mythology. Narrative twists and turns are not all conscious choices; a human being is, to some extent, shaped by the images, myths, and discourses in which he or she is embedded and they give content to the patterns that inform the complex tapestry of a lived life, a fact that should influence our understanding both of MPD and of the formation of memories.

We could think of MPD as a syndrome based on a psychological or even psychobiological tendency to dissociation or split consciousness such that, in combination with events of a certain type, extreme psychic strains, for instance, might manifest as a dissociative state. This is a naturalistic reading and therefore scientifically respectable and not dependent on spiritual, moral, or religious beliefs. Historically, the varieties of psychic phenomena preceding the explicit recognition of MPD involved both dissociation and split consciousness, originally described as 'doubling' (Hacking, 1996, p. 159ff). These psychic conditions were controversial, but ways were found to bring the phenomena into the fold of the naturalistic psychology of post-enlightenment thought (by figures such as Taine, Charcot, and Freud).

A second approach is more sceptical and regards MPD as an artifact co-created by credulous, and somewhat histrionic, patients and enthusiastic therapists. The current epidemic is seen as something similar to the outbreak of 'the vapours' fashionable among young women of delicate constitution in the late eighteenth and early nineteenth centuries. Once a condition is welcomed into the universe of natural science, then as in all accounts of natural and therefore law-governed phenomena, questions must be asked about causation (as in the work of Freud, Janet, and others). They focused on neural function and structure, but the science of cognition was in its infancy and cognitive neuroscientific accounts were completely speculative. Freud, however, tied psychic events to brain events in a way that took account of personal psychological history and his claim that adult psychiatry must pay attention to childhood narratives to find the causal origins of psychic disorder set the stage for scientific studies of dissociation. He himself favoured the concept of repression and the sequestration of thoughts in a realm beneath consciousness and, in that respect, did the MPD movement no favours by marginalizing dissociation as a mechanism of psychic disruption.

A number of the therapeutic narratives arising in the treatment of MPD, looked at through the lens of causal theory, suggest that child abuse is an important feature of the development of the disorder. And, as is usual in science, the production of a cause–effect thesis confirms and is supported by the original naturalistic commitment bringing MPD closer to the model of a natural kind, or psychiatric entity with genuine nosological validity, albeit controversial, and giving it scientific recognition as a phenomenon to be researched rather than a curiosity.

Hacking notes that the concept of child abuse makes it possible to think that childhood can be disordered and instances categories of disorder evident in certain patterns of events which we can then be alert for. The idea that child abuse leads to abnormalities in the adult psyche, combined with Freudian beliefs about the unconscious contents of the mind, then paves the way for crucial theoretical developments in the area of aetiology and psychic trauma that culminate in the concept of RMS as part of the pattern.

As the knowledge of MPD spreads in clinical circles and among the public (who provide psychiatry with its clients), we increasingly encounter cases that do not quite fit the classic story. This is bound to happen with any complex social phenomenon, but in this case the theoretical understanding of memory as a store and the concept of the unconscious mind allow us to posit psychic states and events (with their origins in childhood experience and currently psychologically active) that are not readily reportable by the conscious adult subject who has presented for therapy. Thus, repressed memory becomes a valid subject of enquiry and RMS an affliction to which one might legitimately be subject. Increasingly, such memories are 'discovered' and, for those inclined to belief, that confirms the reality of the scientific story (and the natural kinds involved). *MPD on the basis of child abuse* becomes established and reinforces the idea of a cause–effect link that is the hallmark of kosher scientific phenomena. Once the accepted aetiology adds its considerable weight to the legitimacy of MPD, the complex phenomenon encompassing MPD and RMS is 'discovered'.

We now need to step back from the dispute and see if there is a justification for the kind of recommendations that seem to be emerging from our study of RMS and MPD. Unfortunately, the relatively ho-hum remarks to follow will excite no one except those so committed to belief or scepticism that they will not tolerate divergence from their own views.

10.7 **A synthesizing account**

The current analysis of MPD assimilates it to more familiar or everyday kinds of disso-ciative phenomena such as daydreaming, intense role play, the adoption of specialized personae for different life contexts, and self-deception, and likens RMS to intentional and emotionally motivated forgetting without entering the lists on the side of any particular view of repression. To formulate an account based on the reality of clinical experience and the critical concerns one ought to have about both MPD and RMS, one needs to consider the nature of subjectivity and narrative, a narrative theory of PI, and the Explanatory Problem of accounting for MPD within an Aristotelian view of mind and brain.

According to the discursive view of psychology, I have the sense of self-identity that I have because of a process of adaptation to being-in-the-world-with-others. My subjectivity has become articulate as my body has been inscribed, in its reactions, responses, and habitus, by the discursive milieu in which I have developed. The pro-cess of inscription is not existentially ratiocinative (as a free choice) in the way that humanists such as Jean Paul Sartre seem to suggest; rather, I attribute to myself certain attitudes, actions, intentions, and feelings because others have trained me to do so and reacted to me in various ways.

Imagine, for instance, I feel disturbed at my father and his intolerance of my opin-ion on some issue and somebody asks 'What has made you so angry?' Through this exchange and others like it, I learn that I, Grant, am in the state that people call *anger* and this new learning sets up certain connections not only in my conscious mind but also in what, following Jaspers (1923/1997), I would call the 'extraconscious mecha-nisms' and resulting psychic structures that organize my mind. I learn to attach a certain signifier to the state I am in at the moment of learning that I am angry and also gain a certain facility in immediately recognizing and reflecting upon my state of mind as being attributable in part to my system of emotions. This anger is then known to be an emotion (not just a physiological reaction) and to be mine, to belong to the named individual who is me. Thus, when someone asks 'How do you feel?' states that have become articulate in this way are called to my conscious mind and reported as emo-tional states of self. Notice that the physiological reaction (a 'hot' relatively passive state) and a self-signification (a social technique) combine to yield the emotion as experienced and understood. These states serve a distinctive role in social or discursive situations (Griffiths, 1997, p. 245) and they lend feeling tone to the narrative moments that are my subjective life.

What is more, as a result of the discourse (in which I and my states are mirrored), an emotional state is located in my mental economy with connections to a variety of other modes of being such as hostility, resentment, being wounded or hurt subjec-tively, and so on. In a normal situation, there is a coherence to this complex cumulative construction and it allows comprehensible tensions (to do with, for instance, my con-flicts with my father). The attributions of others are coherent with my self-attributions in terms of both their content—for example, <anger>—and their referent—me, Grant. They confirm and strengthen my understanding of the situation—my father pro-voked me—they signify my own reaction—I felt angry—and they contribute to my growing identity—this incident is an experience in which I am somebody provoked to anger and it *should* be recorded with me occupying that particular discursive position. All these aspects of my subjectivity may or may not form parts of a coherent whole and allow me to deal creatively with the tensions that arise between others and myself. (And here we should recall, with Lacan, that the signified or describable elements in my experience fall short of my embodied immersion in the situation, other aspects of which might also, in a variety of ways, influence the extraconscious realization of this conscious experience.)

I stress that we must not overintellectualize this process. My subjectivity, the presented and self-presentational result of myriad social interactions, is that I experience anger and other emotions, not as deliberate responses and not as freely negotiable aspects of my mental life but as self-referred reactions. My subjectivity is also, in an important sense, *me* (as far as I am accessible to myself), an accumulation of narrative moments and themes appearing as constitutive aspects of my subjectivity and the psyche I exhibit or inhabit.

All these considerations are important when we reflect on *discourse*, *subjectivity*, and *narrative* in psychiatric phenomenology. I self-constitute through a narrative integration of subjective experiences signified and connected according to various templates or scripts made available to me by my culture. I take on a discursive or articulate shape in the mirror of discourse that reflects and conveys to me the contours of being in the human life-world

In theorizing about MPD, there may be a fundamental biological propensity in some people allowing certain experiences to completely dissociate from the primary conscious stream of an individual but, given that small concession to *facticity* (Sartre) or nature, the discursive view then treats each stream of consciousness as a narratively integrated subjectivity with its own referent or named subject (e.g. *Grant Gillett* or *Eve White*) both incorporating and rejecting certain experiences as signified parts of itself. The question 'Does that experience, E1, belong to me?' is not necessarily answerable solely on the basis that it actually happened to the body normally referred to by using my name. There is far more in the discursive acceptance of an event as part of my subjectivity than the awareness (at some level) that it happened to the particular specimen of middle-sized dry goods that is a locus for my subjectivity, although autobiographical acceptance on that basis is normally legitimated in our society. The fact that it is normally legitimated (even required) implies that self-attribution on this basis is a habit or disposition regarded as a building block of self. I, Grant, become the being constituted through legitimate habits of self-attribution.

The body, says Foucault, is the inscribed surface of events. We could think of the body as the (partially prefigured) waxed surface on which the stylus of experience writes (Freud's *wunderbloc* depicts the multiple inscriptions or grooves that all leave their trace although the visible conscious surface is constantly being renewed). Foucault speaks of words being etched into the body by the ideas that give them their significance so that the formation of self and autobiography is through the words addressed to us and applied to us as defined in their meaning by the discursive context against which they are pronounced (this is the reality of the living mirror-world rather than that which is written down.)

The brain, we might say, captures any event or situation in terms of the things that happen, their effect on the body, the signifiers applied to those things and their effects, and the bodily and interpersonal milieu in which they happen. Say, for instance, that I am threatened with being cut by a knife when 'playing' with some sadistic playmates in a dark smelly corner under my house. I am young, but nevertheless the experience affects me. The effects and the memory for the details of the experience are linked to the identities of the playmates involved, the under-house kind of darkness, the smell, the time of day when it occurred, the imagined instrument, and maybe other incidental things not explicitly attended to at the time. The memory of this experience, disturbing as it was, fades over time (it is quite stressful to live in the presence of such unpleasant experiences); but, even if my explicit autobiographical narrative has moved on, my body retains an inscription of this event, waiting to be reconstructed should conditions potentiate reconstruction. In this sense, I carry 'memory traces' 'encoding' traumatic events. But is there any evidence to support the idea that such events are not readily accessible to conscious autobiography? Bremner et al. (1996) suggest that the memories associated with emotional stress might be different from normal memories and adduce a number of strands of evidence to support such a claim:

(1) When an animal is conditioned to develop fear to an innocuous stimulus, it might only be evident under certain conditions. They extrapolate to the idea that human memories of stressful events may reside in 'implicit memory' rather than straightforwardly available for explicit conscious recall.

(2) They examine some of the findings in PTSD and conclude that 'dissociative amnesia' is characteristic of patients with PTSD (p. 74).

(3) They note that the hippocampal functions required to reassemble memories of stressful events may be state-dependent—tied to certain affective states or other configurations of stimuli reflecting the stimulus conditions at the time of the events in question.

We might add that the events involved in abuse and dissociation may occur at ages when children have discursively engendered expectations of parental and other relationships and that when those 'protoscripts' or burgeoning cognitive structures are disrupted or violated, the resulting bewilderment makes the memories vulnerable to being masked, suppressed, or moulded by contextual influences at the time of recall. These plausible suggestions lead to the key ideas found in prevailing theories of dissociation and RMS.

Andorfer (1985) suggests a model of MPD involving a complex network of schemata and embedded 'propositions' and 'proposition trees' making up memory structures that combine 'both episodic and semantic organization' (p. 319). He hypothesizes an executive and a set of embedded instructions activating responses based on connections in the psychic system.

> Personality comprises the stereotyped verbal, affective, and cognitive behaviours exhibited by an individual and the interpersonal behaviours that are their derivatives. As such, personality is a product of the specific contents of propositional memory and the specific interrelationships of those contents. (p. 320)

On the basis of this theory, he formulates a plausible story about the genesis of MPD.

(1) 'The childhood environment that predisposes to multiple personality disorder is one in which the caretakers are extremely unpredictable in their behaviour and alternate between nurturance and destructiveness.' (p. 321)

(2) 'Thus, by early childhood, the system's Propositional Memory is already a mass of contradictions.' (p. 321)

(3) 'This is an intolerable state of affairs for the Executive because its purpose is to maximize the predictability of experience.' (p. 321)

(4) Partitions are created, which prevent activation of conflicting tendencies and clusters of information in Propositional Memory. (p. 322)

(5) 'Each propositional subsystem has different ideas about life, different attitudes and values, different memories of the same caretakers, different interpretive themes for evaluating the behaviours and motives of others, and different emotional states.' (p. 322)

(6) 'While a personality subsystem is activated, propositional trees are encoded into its region of memory and not into other regions of memory. As a result, the personality subsystems evolve along separate lines and have unique learning histories. Thus, as time passes, the personalities become more and more distinctive in behaviour and evolve new traits that may not even have existed before the split.' (p. 322)

Andorfer's theory is deeply influenced by computational approaches to the mind, whereas I have favoured a more fluid and phenomenological conception similar to that of Clarke (1996a) and Griffiths (1997, p. 242ff) especially in relation to autobiographical and emotive phenomena.

A discursively based version of this sort of account seems best suited to address the Explanatory Problem. It accounts for the growth of split subjectivities and also for the accessibility of remembered material between personalities. Andorfer neglects the powerful social and naming effects on the development of subjectivity but otherwise provides a possible way in which a single cognitive system (with a primary ecological orientation) could form a configuration such as that seen in MPD. Even if most of the time any strains on the easy acceptance of this or that experience into my subjectivity are psychically negotiable (not, of course, consciously or explicitly), Andorfer shows us how the process might go badly wrong and stray outside those limits in rare cases.

In genuine cases of MPD, the process of autobiography goes seriously wrong and the type of human being who uses dissociation to protect himself or herself from distress might evince a drift in narrative consciousness towards an alternative name (or grammatical principle of synthesis) under which to gather discreet dossiers or clusters of 'cross-grained' experiences inscribed on one's body. Each parallel dossier would have its own internal integrity and could be incompatible with the dominant subjectivity. At times, the person would slip into this alternative mode of being much as one slips into a 'work persona' or a 'party persona'. Those dossiers or experience may then diverge so far from the dominant subjectivity that subsequent reconciliation of the different narratives or subjectivities is impossible; they can no longer come together—their experiences and attitudes are too divergent.

Such a process of growth in autobiographical distinctness and incompatibility seems to be reported by multiples for whom each parallel subjectivity comes to have a fuller and fuller life of its own along with a distinct set of significations and discursive skills. As such, each has its own name and there are increasingly fewer connections at any level between the intuitively self-attributed moments of one consciousness and those of another. At this point, the active nature of the skills involved in self-construction ought to be apparent, as should the coexistence of disruption and distinction and yet deep connection between one psychic stream and another. The disruption and distinctiveness are readily displayed in therapy and popular accounts, but the suffering engendered by the deep connection, although less obvious, may be just as real.

There is a skill in weaving a narrative out of diverse experiences potentially in tension with each other. The skill is normally mastered in childhood along with walking, eating, and excretory continence; but, similar to continence of action or even excretory continence, it requires support and nurture and can be derailed, particularly, one might think, in susceptible individuals. Derailing influences are likely to include the kinds of mystification discussed by Laing, the kinds of fraught and pathological parenting styles evident in many cases of anxiety disorder, the kind of control by others that is encountered (or perceived) in anorexia nervosa, and the kind of unpredictability and abuse that seems to be found in MPD. Absent from the posited abnormal predisposition to dissociation, such influences would probably not manifest themselves as MPD. The claim of discursive psychology is that the combination of the human need for narrative integration and the disruptive effects of the cathectic tendencies in MPD are formative of both conscious and extraconscious structures of split subjectivity.

'Who am I?' has never been an easy question for the philosopher. The more one explores aberrations such as MPD and the schizoid experiences of other mental disorders, the more intricate and ramified it seems to become.

We can now return to the philosophical puzzles posed by MPD.

10.8 Philosophical problems revisited

I have identified a number of problems for philosophers when they turn their attention to MPD; two remain to be addressed:

(A) Who is responsible for an act committed by an alter? (The Responsibility Problem)

(B) Is reintegrative therapy destruction of identifiable persons? (The Therapeutic Murder Problem)

The Responsibility Problem

This is really two problems in one because there is not only a difficulty in determining whether the act of an alter is an act of the human being concerned but there is also a problem of assessing the identifiable, embodied, person's degree of responsibility for the act in question.

Braude (1996) observes that 'it is commonplace and unproblematic to regard two things as the same for certain purposes but not for others' (p. 39). We might, for instance, want to argue that a collective such as a hunt or a club was, in some sense (for instance, in respect of its meeting place, rules, and name), the same over a period of 100 years but concede that, in another sense (for instance, with regard to the individuals making it up), it had completely changed over that same period of time. This does not seem applicable to a multiple. We might, alternatively, want to regard a person as a private citizen for one purpose and as an office holder with a certain public role for another so that as private citizen I might sympathize with my friend who has run a red light but, as an officer on patrol, charge him with an offence (he would probably not make such clear distinctions). This again does not serve in MPD, but it does come somewhat closer in that it credits me with having modes of identity or personae whose reasons for acting might conflict in various situations.

Braude (1996) suggests two conditions (one metaphysical and one cognitive) that should be met in attributions of responsibility. The first involves the possibility of the person controlling the actions that eventuated and the second requires the agent to 'possess certain reflective or rational capacities' (p. 40), namely those required to evaluate and make a reasoned decision about the action being considered (similar to Fisher and Revizza's reason responsiveness condition). He makes a Freudian distinction between 'weak' and 'strong' responsibility, the former where the action arises primarily from Ucs (such as a slip of the tongue or impulsive riposte). He objects to the claim that all actions of a multiple are the responsibility of a 'core personality' as is suggested by some commentators, arguing that 'it is false to say that "the core personality is dominant" . . . an underlying unifying self . . . is certainly not dominant in any interesting sense' (p. 41). Braude finally concludes, 'DID [MPD] is simply one of a large variety of cases in which it is difficult to determine the extent of an individual's ability to control and evaluate his behaviour' (p. 47).

Braude's claim, that multiples might have to be considered responsible in a weak sense but not in a strong sense (for the actions of alters) because 'it may be that the multiple as a whole cannot judge actions in a suitably integrated and comprehensive way' (p. 51), seems eminently reasonable, particularly in the light of Andorfer's analysis and the fragmentation of the discursive self that seems typical of MPD. However, we are left feeling that a pressing moral issue may have been evaded rather than resolved.

Clark (1996b) makes a telling comment when he discusses conditions in which the individuals concerned are discursively recognized as being in states of altered consciousness (and therefore, altered responsibility) such as trances: 'What they say and do reveals their wishes, even ones that they have consciously repressed' (p. 56). We might extend and develop this insight by noting that it is true that the *psyche* initiating the action performed by a multiple is the *psyche* comprised by all the alters however dissociated that may be. It is also true that the named person who carries within their body the personality configurations that appear as this or that alter has within them the capacity to perform an act of the requisite type and has *some* degree of responsibility for his or her behaviour at any given point in time. That leaves us relying on the human judgement involved in an assessment of state of mind to determine the degree of responsibility (but the arguments defending that position have already arisen in relation to psychopaths). Such a judgement may take account of psychic integrity, impulsivity, rational deliberation of the vicious act, and all the other things that are taken into account in forensic assessments of your or my responsibility for an action, and incorporate them into determinations of intent.

The fact that we cannot provide a cut-and-dried procedural rule nor come to an overall stand on the determination of moral responsibility in cases of MPD is typical rather than exceptional in jurisprudence about moral responsibility and indeed is in part the reason for the key role of common law in this area. Common law allows case-by-case judgements sensitive to our understanding of the mind of the agent, something that in 'folk psychology' we do all the time.

The therapeutic murder problem

Must we seriously regard ourselves as destroying a human person or human persons if an MPD patient is successfully treated and achieves a sufficient degree of personal integration to dispense with his or her alters? When we examine the process of therapy, we see that it carries its own reassurances. An example of successful therapy is well described by Andorfer (1985), who treated a patient called Esther with alters named Roxy (borderline, promiscuous, antisocial), Annie (narcissistic, breezy, sophisticated), Marie (inarticulate, tormented, anxious, fearful), and Athena ('inner-self helper', intelligent, rational). A therapeutic alliance is formed and the constellation of personalities is accepted so that rapport with each of them can be established. He notes that '[i]t is important to remember that each personality plays a role in the psychic economy of the overall personality system' (p. 314). On this basis, he recommends that the 'executive' personality be enlisted in the task of reintegrating the alters in terms of their cognitive, affective, and behavioural functions and suggests that this process not be rushed. The gradual opening of the personality and spill between different psychic alters will allow 'repressed or dissociated memories of childhood trauma' to be 'uncovered, abreacted, and assimilated' (p. 314) into the patient's narrative autobiography.

As is obvious from this typical account of the therapeutic process, there is no destruction of psychic material here but rather a process of knitting together of a fragmented subjectivity. Once seen in this light, the Therapeutic Murder Problem begins to look decidedly unproblematic despite the romantic and dramaturgical losses involved.

The overarching philosophical problem of personal identity has been finessed to some extent in the present account by denying that there is a single basis or essence to which personal identity can be reduced. We are each one of us named, dynamic, changing, and responsive individuals inhabiting multiple relationships and incurring responsibility for a lifetime of actions done under varying states of immaturity and maturity and the reality of personal identity is existential. I exist as a being-in-the-world-with-others and therefore can think of myself as me the psychological being I have become.

10.9 Conclusion

It is always reassuring to be able to condemn extremists, if only for aesthetic and moral reasons to do with civilized discussion. It is especially reassuring when sound reasoning and empirical evidence support that condemnation. It seems to me that a moderate attitude, in which there is a judicious admixture of belief and criticism, is the most reasonable attitude to adopt towards both MPD [or DID] and RMS. I have tried to make that moderate attitude plausible in my own treatment of these two fraught topics.

Chapter 11

I eat, therefore I am not

I have rules and plenty. Some things I don't touch.
I'm king of my body now. Who needs a mother—
a food machine, those miles and miles of guts?
Once upon a time, I confess, I was fat—
gross. Gross belly, gross ass, no bones
showing at all. Now I say, 'No, thank you,' a person
in my own right, and no poor loser. I smile
at her plate of brownies. 'Make it disappear,'
she used to say, 'Join the clean plate club.' I disappear
into my room where I have forbidden her to touch
anything. I was a first grade princess once. I smile
to think how those chubby pinks used to please my
mother.
And now that I am, Dear Diary, a sort of magical person,
she can't see. My rules. Even here I don't pour out my
guts. Rules. The writing's slow, but like picking a bone,
satisfying, and it doesn't make you fat.
. . . .
Don't touch
me, Hunger, Mother. . . . Don't you gut my brain.
Bones are sovereign now, I can touch them here and here.
I am a pure person, magic, revealed as I disappear
into my final fat-free smile, where there is no pain.
(From 'To make the Dragon move', in *The Diary of an Anorexic* by Pamela White Hadas)

This chapter attempts to lay bare the ways in which discourse and narrative can transform the desires of the body and, in the extreme case, use those transformed desires (or surrealist collages [Lacan, 1979, p. 169]) to kill the person who holds them, as in the eating disorders. The phenomenology of and current theories about Bulimia and Anorexia—two diseases which are said to be reaching epidemic proportions in our time—reveal the disturbed subjectivity that can lead a young woman to starve herself to death. Subjective autobiographical narratives help us answer questions about the meaning of the disorders to those who live them and evaluate the theories of aetiology and diverse treatments offered by different therapeutic schools.

One of my first experiences with anorexia was the sister of a friend, a girl to whom one was instantly moved to apply stereotypically feminine adjectives—delicate, soft, sensitive, quiet, and helpless. I did not realize then that this stereotype implicitly contained the secret of her disorder which I, like others, found extremely perplexing. One was led in her case, as in so many others, to wonder whatever could lead an attractive young woman, against all reason, to so control her own body and its natural desires that she risks death.

Anorexia therefore poses the question 'What is desire?' just as mania poses the question of well-being, schizophrenia the question of rationality, psychopathy the question of moral action, and multiple personality disorder (MPD) the question of identity. In each case, a particular area of the human psyche, as a discursive production, is thrown into sharp relief. The complex relationship between subjectivity, discourse, and self-worth is limned by examining the inside of anorexia and the anorexic ideal—*lightness of being*. We can then identify conflicts inherent in the social production of a human being, its norms, and its effects on a situated subjectivity rather than conflicts between the 'natural' organism and the 'artificial' culture it lives in (Giordano, 2005).

11.1 **The eating disorders**

The *Diagnostic and Statistical Manual of Mental Disorders IV* (DSM IV; APA, 1994a) describes anorexia in the following terms:

> The essential features of Anorexia Nervosa are that the individual refuses to maintain a minimally normal body weight, is intensely afraid of gaining weight, and exhibits a significant disturbance in the perception of the shape or size of his or her body. In addition, post-menarchal females with this disorder are amenorrhoeic. (p. 539)

Many descriptions note that 'anorexia' is a misnomer in that loss of appetite is a relatively rare feature, females are far more often affected than males, the peak incidence is between the ages of 16–19 years, and sociocultural factors figure in the aetiology.

> Anorexia Nervosa appears to be far more prevalent in industrialized societies, in which there is an abundance of food and in which, especially for females, being considered attractive is linked to being thin.
>
> (DSM IV; APA, 1994a, p. 542)

The other major eating disorders include Bulimia and morbid obesity.

> The essential features of Bulimia Nervosa are binge eating and inappropriate compensatory methods to prevent weight gain. In addition, the self-evaluation of individuals with Bulimia Nervosa is excessively influenced by body shape and weight.
>
> (DSM IV; APA, 1994a, p. 545)

The measures taken to prevent weight gain often involve vomiting induced by fingers in the throat, but laxatives or ipecacuanha may also be used. Regurgitation is usually furtive although the lingering smell of vomit and 'moth-eaten' teeth (due to the effect of gastric acid on the enamel) gives it away. The most serious problems in bulimia (where weight loss is not as extreme as in anorexia) are electrolyte disturbances, gastrointestinal disorders, endocrine changes, and heart changes (Fairburn & Brownell, 2002; Mickley, 1999). Secrecy and obsession with food are important in both disorders and both are marked by desperation and a stubborn refusal to change the abnormal behaviours. Similar to anorexia, 'bulimia tends to start in women in late adolescence or early adulthood,' but there is also a 'high prevalence of depressive symptoms . . . attempted suicide . . . self-mutilating behaviour, alcohol and drug abuse, and low self-esteem' (Freeman et al., 1988). Anorexia is 'clean', self–controlled, and resolute unlike the murkiness and all-too-evident emotional disturbances of bulimia.

> Anorexia was my solution as it is for many females (and to a lesser extent males). By not eating, we attempt to conquer issues affecting our lives. The fact that the denial of food then becomes a physical problem is irrelevant in the drive to find autonomy, assert control, and boost self-esteem.
>
> (McCarthy & Thomson, 1996, p. 17)

Orbach (1993) also mentions denial and control as being a central feature of anorexia (p. 91) so that the patient achieves a negation of her basic appetites: 'It is the achievement, not the thinness that is psychologically important. The anorectic is so used to experiencing herself as unsuccessful that her now obvious ability to wield power over her body is a fantastic achievement' (p. 91). Hilde Bruch (1978) also stresses that the anorexic patient's 'relentless pursuit of thinness' springs from a need for identity and effectiveness through control over the body. 'While others consider her pathetic and in need of help, her own self-image is one she is finally proud of. She feels a strength, for she has become someone with no needs and no appetites' (Orbach, 1993, p. 95).

By contrast, the subjectivity of bulimia is primarily focused elsewhere:

> Although there is no doubt that food and eating is the obsession that drives bulimia, it is the vomiting—the purging—that is the final goal. It is the purging which, as the name suggests, brings with it a transitory feeling of cleanness, purity, and control.
>
> (McCarthy & Thomson, 1996, p. 34)

Both disorders are marked by a subjective preoccupation with food and its preparation despite the fact that the rejection of food and the effect of food on the body is a central motivation. Some writers go so far as to claim that the anorexic betrays an almost obsessive absorption with food and its preparation even though she finds it very difficult to eat the food she may have, painstakingly and quite elaborately, prepared for others. (McCarthey & Thomson, 1996, pp. 102, 122, 133). In anorexia, the fascination with and fixed rejection of food is part of a regime of rigid control over the body and ingestion tied to the positive self-worth accompanying thinness; in bulimia, by contrast, the sufferer feels impelled to eat large quantities of attractive, unhealthy, and fattening food.

Figures on long-term mortality for anorexia vary from 20% to 2% (DSM IV [APA, 1994a]; Eckert et al., 1995; Gelder et al., 1983, p. 368; Treasure et al., 2003). Death can be due to starvation, suicide, or electrolyte imbalance, all risks evident in recent accounts.

In May 1994, Michelle nearly died of anorexia. She arrived at hospital weighing 29 kg (4 st 7 oz). All her vital organs, including her heart, were failing and her blood pressure was dangerously low. It was touch and go for two weeks and she remained in hospital for 12 months.

(McCarthy & Thomson, 1996, p. 167)

There is an association with depression, obsessive symptoms, and suicide, a co-morbidity highlighting the deep unhappiness of the young women concerned, a reality that hides behind an obscuring self-possessed facade in constant danger of breaking down. 'This new apparently needless person she has created out of herself feels precarious. She is in danger of evaporating and making visible her very opposite, the despairing, anguished, needy person buried deep in the anorectic's inner world' (Orbach, 1993, p. 92). The internal conflict within the disorder and the facade of self-possession constitute a paradox for those treating the disorder: on the one hand, the anorectic seems weak and childish, yet on the other hand, she is a crafty, strong, and unyielding opponent (Orbach, 1993, p. 5).

The epidemiology of the disorder is hard to evaluate, despite the widespread perception that its incidence has increased dramatically since the 1940s (Giordano, 2005). A recent review interrogated our detection of anorexia in terms of prevalent social attitudes and expectations: 'The present social context for adolescent girls is very different from that of the late nineteenth century and the motivation, function, and meaning of starvation behaviour may have changed accordingly' (van t'Hof, 1994, p. 38). The author identifies 'detection routes' for 'a case of anorexia' in which prevailing social theories about what a person is doing when she starves or becomes thin, whether behaviour in general is linked to inner or psychic changes, the medicalization of deviations from norms for age, and so on, are all important.

The detection route in any specific period has been defined as the total of four relative probabilities that a girl will be identified as an anorexic patient. First, the relative probability that a girl who is not eating will be noticed by the people in her direct vicinity. Second, the relative probability that such a girl will be seen by physicians. The third relative probability is that the girl will be diagnosed as suffering from psychological starvation. Fourth, the relative probability that her case will be recorded, either in medical records or in publications.

(van t'Hof, 1994, p. 171)

The route from manifestation to becoming an epidemiological statistic reflects our present medicalized environment in which all aberrations of the body are tracked, investigated, and recorded (as cases). Recall, in this regard, categories such as wasting, consumption, neurasthenia, and so on, all of which mark the passing out of sight of thin women, making it hard to be confident about claims of an increased incidence in recent times (Orbach, 1993).

Most authorities agree that amenorrhoea is an important part of the syndrome, and it provokes hypotheses about the hypothalamic axis in anorexia and bulimia. But the bare fact offers little support for the hypothesis because it is clear that '[t]he menstrual cycle is sensitive to the amount of body fat, but also to diet (particularly caloric intake), sex hormone production, and environmental stress' (van t'Hof, 1994, p. 22). Bruch (1978) observes that female survivors of concentration camps resumed their menstrual cycles after release from the pathological environment but before their bodies had regained their normal weight and nutritional status, and others consider the loss of menstruation as part of the denial of bodily processes that is central to the disorder (Orbach, 1993) so that its genesis (but perhaps not its meaning) is unclear.

A further characteristic feature of anorexia is the disorder of bodily perception and self-knowledge leading the sufferer to distort her body image: some anorexics feel grossly overweight although they are normal, and others feel that their body parts are misshapen, or out of proportion, or that selected parts such as abdomen, buttocks, and thighs are 'too fat' (DSM IV; APA, 1994a, p. 540). Self-reports express obsessive disruptions of self-perception and the complex relations between body image and 'the mirror world' of the gazes of others.

> I was six stone when I was at high school. People called me 'little Rita' but I didn't feel particularly little, I felt huge.
>
> (McCarthy & Thomson, 1996, p. 144)

> She was totally hooked into a certain body image—to be as small as possible. Although she was convinced she was looking good, she was haggard, weary, and had begun to grow extra hair on her face, whilst a 'snail trail' was appearing on her stomach.
>
> (McCarthy & Thomson, 1996, p. 57)

The anorectic patient cannot seem to achieve 'clarity' or 'balance' about her own appearance:

> I remember looking in the mirror one day and feeling horrified at how out of proportion my body was. It was because I was starving myself but I didn't see it like that then. I thought it meant I needed to lose more weight, although I had already lost heaps.
>
> (McCarthy & Thomson, 1996, p. 119)

The suffering associated with the disorder can be overlooked, according to sufferers and those who work with them, not least because the sufferer sometimes seems not only untroubled but even euphoric about her puzzling condition (MacLeod, 1972). 'Fifteen years on from my first professional encounters with women with anorexia, I still feel intense pain and outrage at our (the culture's, the individual family's) ability to create the suffering that leads to anorexia as an attempted solution.' (Orbach, 1993, p. xxviii)

One sufferer expresses the pain and hostility of anorexia in a more personal way:

> Our underlying unhappiness ends up hidden behind thinly stretched facial skin, wasting thighs, and lank hair. But no matter how thin we get, we can't diet our unhappiness and anger away. We become thinner and thinner, denying ourselves even the most basic nutrition. It is our cry for help.
>
> (McCarthy & Thomson, 1996, p. 17)

Why does the anorexic want to reject a world that seeks to nourish and accommodate her and why is her self-distancing from that everyday and shared world so resolute and determined? The origins of the psychic conflicts in eating disorders and the transformation of appetite in particular point to something deep within the discursive self that needs understanding. But before we follow a discursive root into the heart of the disorder, we ought to note certain theoretical and explanatory controversies surrounding it.

11.2 **Constructions of anorexia and adolescence**

There are diverse theories about the eating disorders that do not really come to grips with the subjectivity of those concerned. As with any discontent of the mind, a theoretical understanding should embrace both the complex interaction of psyche and soma and the intertwined external, interpersonal, and existential influences that focus on one's being with others as a being of worth. Leading players in the controversies about aetiology, as in any other area of medicine, are those commanding treatments with a degree of success. And here there is considerable diversity of opinion, in that some regard forced feeding and artificial nutrition as exactly the kind of violation that has produced the disorder and others see it as the only recourse in a metabolic and biochemical impasse with mortal risks and a limited time course. Antidepressants may have a significant effect on symptomatology (Walsh, 1991), and some workers infer from that fact the existence of a biological cause similar to that operating in affective disorders (Pope & Hudson, 1988). Medicine in general and psychiatry in particular is, however, on firmest ground where a plausible theory successfully explains the aetiology and phenomenology of a disorder and so it is to theory we must next turn.

Genetics

There are no coherent genetic theories of anorexia nervosa even though some sources cite evidence they take to indicate a genetic or hereditable factor in the disorder (DSM IV [APA, 1994a]; Gelder *et al.*, 1983; Russell, 1995, pp. 87–88; Winchester and Collier, 2003). However, given that family relationship patterns have a role in the disorder, such factors are difficult to evaluate. What is more, certain temperaments (shared by twins) predispose one to cope with the deep distresses of life in characteristic ways and may be genetic in origin. It is therefore unclear whether a genetic predisposition has been, or even could be, shown.

Hormonal disturbances

There are hormonal imbalances evident in anorexia, and it is possible to produce anorexia (or its converse—hypothalamic obesity) by producing diencephalic lesions in animals so that hypothalamic dysfunction is one theoretical construction: 'The hypothalamus is involved in the control of appetite, satiation, sexuality, and emotion, all of which are changed in anorexia nervosa. Drawing all these strands together, it is argued that anorexia nervosa is a primary disease of the neuroendocrine system, notably of the hypothalamus and related areas of the brain' (Russell, 1995, pp. 88–89).

However, we might note the hypothalamus, with substantial connections to cortical and subcortical centres influencing its function, is only part of a much greater whole controlling affect and appetite in human beings (quite apart from the fact that the hormonal disturbances of anorexia are compatible with the effects of starvation and indicate no special 'abnormality of hypothalamic–pituitary function' (Bruch, 1978; Gelder *et al.*, 1983, p. 366).

Sexuality

A popular traditional theory of eating disorder involved dynamic claims about conflicts concerning sexuality. The theory is plausible in that anorexia and bulimia occur about the age when adolescent sexuality and its conflicts are important in a person's life; similar to sexuality, they involve, for a young woman, what will be taken into her body and the relationship between bodily invasion and certain types of pleasure or satisfaction. Anorexics often have serious difficulties forming stable sexual partnerships, and those with eating disorders may not have normal psychosexual interactions compared with others of their age. Although extreme theories involving an association between eating and impregnation may strain credibility (Rohrbaugh, 1981, p. 413), the bodily control and denial of needs prominent in anorexia seems to be linked to a rejection of the young woman's attainment of sexual maturity and therefore of the role of an adult woman.

It is tempting (for a Freudian or psychoanalytic theorist) to invoke an 'Electra complex' whereby the young woman is both craving for and conflicted about attention from 'the father'. A mechanism symmetrical with the Oedipal conflict, it suggests a heady brew of conjecture comprising linked cathexes of competition with the mother, the sexual unavailability of the father, sexual fantasies about attracting and pleasing the father, and a consequent repression of personal gratification in general (and sexual ideation as one aspect of it). Some of the self-reports of anorexics are taken to support this view and Bruch (1978) notes a 'peculiar kind of incest which involves a psychic relationship' as important to some theorists (p. 36).

> The typical bulimarexic woman adored her father and tried to please him by doing well at school and being physically perfect. She consciously despised her mother, however; and . . . the bizarre eating patterns might have been one of the few ways such a daughter could rebel against a suffocating mother.
>
> (Rohrbaugh, 1981, p. 414)

The rejection of sexuality could be seen more austerely as an instance of the rejection of the body as needful (as in other theoretical constructions), and the idea of an 'Electra complex' then looks to be an extravagant overtheorization despite the appeal of invoking, in the dynamics of anorexic patients, varieties of resistance and obsession that are reminiscent of the primary process and its submerged psychic conflicts.

The posited psychic conflicts also fit with the view that anorexics seek to escape the bodily transformation that signals womanhood, with all its demands and inequities, leading, apparently without exception, to the sexualized female role. It is worth noting that a number of anorexics spontaneously report that they were 'tomboys' and competed with their male peers in their pre-adolescent years. Perhaps, a contributing feature in the generation of the disorder may be the fact that the girl has prided herself on being equal to males but finds that she is increasingly required 'to be like (to identify with) . . . mother', which 'means to be male-oriented just as *she* is' and thus to derive 'a sense of identity and self-worth only from pleasing men' (Rohrbaugh, 1981, p. 415). One patient writes, 'I was one of the boys, not a female to be eyed up in that way' (McCarthy & Thomson, 1996, p. 19); and another, 'I was quite a tomboy. Most of my female friends were 'up-the-tree sort of girls' and I had lots of male friends' (*Jo*; McCarthy & Thomson, 1996, p. 53). Both women refer to a 'be-one-of-the-boys' mentality in their pre-adolescent and early adolescent days, and both resented the way they became sexual objects in the gaze of the boys they considered their 'mates'; 'I had huge problems with seeing myself as female when I reached adolescence. Even today, I'm still not comfortable with the beauty image, with males looking at me as someone sexual' (*Jo*; McCarthy & Thomson, 1996, p. 53).

Orbach (1993) remarks on the 'general cultural attitudes towards women's bodies' (p. 5) and goes on to identify two contradictory imperatives in women's relationship with food:

(1) The imperative to be 'an object of pleasure for men'; and

(2) The imperative to be the provider of food. (p. 10)

These imperatives require a woman to 'feed others but restrain her own desires for that very same food' (p. 10) and explain the perceived need for self-control and effective, unsupplantable authority over her own body whereby its demands (the demands inscribed upon it by a set of discursively mediated expectations) are nullified by subjugating the body to the will.

> A dominant motif for all the anorectic women I have worked with is thinness as ultrafeminine and, at the same time, thinness is a rejection of femininity.
>
> She is oddly desexualized and degendered. She demands to be related to originally. Reflexive responses—for instance, flirtatious or patronizing ones from men, or the 'once over' from another woman who needs to position herself vis-à-vis this woman—are confounded. She defies easy, comfortable definition.
>
> (Orbach, 1993, pp. 66, 68)

The 'original relation' and defiance of stereotypy inextricably interweaves sexuality and gender politics with the moral discourses in which a young woman is enmeshed (Giordano, 2005).

Object relations theory

Orbach explores the idea of the definition of self in object relations theory, whereby the caregiver and nurturer is initially seen as a pole of the (infant–mother) dyadic unity that must be psychically separated so as to form a genuine dyadic relationship (Winnicott, 1964). Through this process, the infant begins to appreciate *self* and *other*, developing a sense of separation or difference from the other and an inner world of objects and relationships so that the self and its needs are distinguished from others (who themselves gradually become seen as having their own needs and actions). Part of normal development is to recognize the mismatch or potential mismatch between the needs of self and the responses of others to those needs perhaps leading to anger at the other for not meeting one's needs but also to self-directed inner hostility because of the fact that one's needs make demands of others. The theory posits that anorexia and other self-harming behaviour can arise from the development of an inner 'false self' in response to such self-directed hostility. This 'false self', unlike the real self, has no body (and therefore no needs) and is not dependent on others so that the bodily demands of the real self are identified by the subject as a cause of disharmony, the body is seen as a bad object, and the false self constructs a schism in relation to the subjective body.

> The real self has needs, and the mother's early failure to meet those needs are the proof of their 'illegitimacy' and 'the badness inside'. The needs are what send people away and the needs are the reason the person is not adequately related to. But since she does indeed live in her body, the bad object encroaches insistently; she cannot be released from it.

> (Orbach, 1993, p. 71)

This schism is, similar to any primary process phenomenon, unconscious and therefore cathectically in-formed in a way that is not transparent to reason and not amenable to rational revision. The body becomes the enemy and must be subdued; its enmity to the (real) self is deep, existential, almost primeval, and not open to conscious negotiation.

The theory explains the conflicts and irrationality of the drive to thinness operating as a fundamental attitude, but it does not adequately explain the seemingly close relationship between anorexia and bulimia, and the evident conflicts of early adolescence. If anorexia, on some occasions, is triggered by or sensitive to adolescent and peer-group evaluations and the realization of imminent sexuality with all its confusing demands, we are confronted by another potent source of inchoate influences on the self—the discursive and political position of a young woman as subject—participant in familial, sociocultural, and political relationships.

Dysfunctional families

Laing and Esterson linked schizophrenia to the internal conflicts of the discursive context within a family, focusing on the situated subjectivity of the sufferer. The same perspective illuminates the psyche of the anorexic in terms of family (dys)function and the internal conflicts produced in a young woman. Minuchin, with wide clinical experience in this area, observes that the families of anorexics exhibit 'enmeshment, overprotectiveness, rigidity, and lack of conflict resolution' (Minuchin et al., 1978) such that the individual with anorexia may be a subject in whom family conflicts are focused and acted out. In some of the families, the mother seems to have effaced herself in response to abuse and exploitation, or just in legitimated deference to her husband. One young woman remarks, 'He controlled my mother who in turn controlled us to keep him happy' (Rita; McCarthy & Thomson, 1996, p. 142). Another reports a father changed dramatically by significant head injuries and yet another, 'He had an unpredictable temper and you never knew what kind of mood he'd be in when he got home' (McCarthy & Thomson, 1996, p. 39). In each case, family conflicts and tensions are immediate and formative.

In many families, food is 'an issue' even for (female) children when quite young.

> I was in standard three [about 7 yr] when Mum stopped me having a slice of bread with my dinner, although my brothers were allowed it. Then she stopped giving me school lunch, so I'd look for money on the ground . . . It was at intermediate that I started to worry about food and being very fat. I was 11. When I look at photos now I realize I was just average, but I remember always feeling fat and hungry and I began comparing my body to other girls.
>
> (*Rita*; In McCarthy & Thomson, 1996, p. 143)

Some families of anorexics can be dysfunctional in diverse ways and many clinicians use family therapy as a therapeutic tool. One woman mentions the pain of her parents' divorce: 'I felt good about hurting her because of being so unhappy at home with her and my stepfather. My father had left when I was three and when things got bad I'd sometimes fantasize about going to live with him. He was the goodie because he wasn't around' (*Kim*; McCarthy & Thomson, 1996, p. 117).

In many cases, there is a history of sexual abuse compounded by feelings of guilt, uncleanness, and worthlessness and deeply ambivalent attitudes to the body that affect the victim's sense of sexuality and ability to be comfortable with intimacy.

One woman mentions, 'The empty space that my mum was supposed to be fulfilling by love' (*Jacqui*; McCarthy & Thomson, 1996, p. 76), encapsulating the dilemma of the woman who has had to give of herself and sacrifice her own life to try and meet a cultural ideal of what a mother should be. In each case, the disturbance in the child's relationship with the home as the environment of nurture and care closely implicates the role of mother as primary caregiver.

The broader meaning of the woman's role within the family falls under the analytic gaze turned towards the typical nuclear family as the setting for the development of anorexia. Orbach (1993) notes an inherent and structural conflict in the meanings of daughter, mother, and food.

> A mother's presence is always implicit in food. It is almost as if food, in its many and varied forms, becomes a representation of the mother. From the child's point of view, the essence of its mother is distilled through food . . . Food personifies the mother and she is rejected or accepted through it. (p. 35)

Ultimately, this intrafamilial process is a discursive incarnation of something wider: 'The process of psychological internalization of the mother's personality . . . central in the construction of the daughter's personality, is always imbued with the impact of the social structure' (Orbach, 1993, p. 39). That social structure both links the young woman to others (as her mother is linked) and inscribes on her body the deep ambivalence she must (is bound to, is condemned to, finds it in herself to) feel towards food: 'A woman comes to know that the food she prepares for others as an act of love and an expression of her caring is somehow dangerous towards herself' (Orbach, 1993, p. 41).

By implication, this reality is also dangerous to her daughters who will also be affected by (or imbibe with their food) the danger or threat contained within it. This deep ambivalence infuses the intrapsychic structure of the young woman in a potentially disastrous way for her growing sense of who she is and how she should feel about her own body and its needs, and confounds her self-knowledge; 'In every case of anorexia that I have come across, the woman does not respond as one might to internal cues of hunger, satisfaction, sexual desire, or fatigue. Nor does the individual really know how big or little she is' (Orbach, 1993, pp. 72–73).

Political theory

Russell (1995), Orbach (1993), Bordo (1985), Szekeley (1988), and others highlight the inherently conflictful subjectivity of women situated in the discourse of male-oriented society. 'The key question then becomes: What in the sociocultural context of women's lives has created the possibility and the necessity for women to engage in the relentless pursuit of thinness' (Russell, 1995, p. 94). Orbach (1993) examines the significations in play: 'Anorexia exemplifies through the language of the body the woman's attempt to enter and at the same time disappear from a culture that derogates and deifies her' (p. xxii). The 'derogation' is the subsumption of the woman under categories and evaluations arising directly from the shape of her body. The deification is the worship of the female body and of the woman as its 'owner'. In both attitudes, relationships to the woman are conditioned and contextualized by the presentation of the body. Consequently, the message shaping the lived experience of the woman is that her being and worth is inescapably tied to the way that she can shape her body: 'The receptivity that women show (across class, ethnicity, and through the generations) to the idea that their bodies are like gardens—arenas for constant improvement and resculpting—is rooted in the recognition of their bodies as commodities' (Orbach, 1993, p. 17).

We could see anorexia as an embodiment of the imposed role of manipulator-of-the-body to fulfil the agendas of others so that the anorectic body is a 'crystallization of culture' (Bordo, 1985). The unconscious of the woman becomes the medium allowing culture to be inscribed upon the female body.

> Psychological symptoms and the meanings sought in them by analysts and analysands render alive the unconscious world of the individual in her time. Decoded, these symptoms allow us to enter, in the most detailed way, women's everyday experience. As windows into generalizable experience, they call attention to deeply painful but salient aspects of women's existence which are so often obscured.
>
> (Bordo, 1985, p. 4)

This passage recalls Lacan's claim that the unconscious is the network of signifiers loaded with evaluative meaning such that the woman's psyche becomes the battleground of the internal paradoxes and contradictions of cultural attitudes towards women in general. In sources attending closely to women's voices, an increasingly persuasive view is that 'maintaining empathic rapport and bounded connectedness with the patient promotes a therapeutic alliance that, over time, allows the patient the psychological space to get to know herself and to recapture a sense of her own body and mind' (Zerbe, 1996, p. 818).

The lived nature and cathectic content of those paradoxes must, of course, bracket my (male) attempts at analysis, framed and constructed from a position of distance and otherness so that it requires phenomenological validation by those of the appropriate gender.

Any good theoretical analysis should take adequate account of the critical nature of adolescence in human development. We might, in fact, usefully distinguish the *persona* from the *subjectivity*. The persona is literally 'what is sounded through', named after the Greek mask through which the actor's voice was presented to the public. The subjectivity is the experienced and narrated life of an individual, subject to discourse and the effects of power. Embodied human subjectivity speaks through and from the body of which it is an aspect so that we are all personae and subjectivities. As personae, we deploy skills of self-presentation by drawing on the discursive contexts around us and latching on to discursive techniques, and weaving them together, more or less purposively, to form an identifiable personality—the psychic essence of the named individual who is me. A named being-among-us experiences in herself the discursive impact of the world and, depending on her discursive skills and techniques, incorporates the values and connections embedded and intertwined in that discourse. Thus, if people around me are saying that it is cool to smoke or to have sex and that these things show that I have got it all together or really know where it is at—positive attributions—then these attributions have a good chance of being built into my story and becoming part both of my subjectivity and of the persona I present to others. But there may be a gap between the two.

It may be that I know that my presented persona and my subjectivity are incongruent, or they do not match: one is not the obverse of another but in fact a distortion of self that I can hardly admit to myself let *al*one present to others. In that case, I have a problem: I am living a lie and living with the anxiety that my lie will be uncovered. Many adolescents experience this anxiety. It provokes defensive hostility in situations that reveal the mismatch and force me to confront it. The risk of disclosure threatens me with an adolescent tragedy—exclusion from among those whose discourse helps to hold my life together. For this reason, adolescence is a tightrope walk between anonymity and anomaly. I do not want to be anonymous, but I also do not want to be so anomalous that I am *alien* or *outre* and attract descriptors that marginalize—'geek', 'loser', 'try-hard', 'uncool', 'heinous', and so on (they change from generation to generation). What allows me to walk the tightrope is my mastery of the skills of discourse and my ability to deal with the way my body is reacted to within that discourse, but a young woman obsessed with thinness has a precarious and perhaps fatally flawed set of life skills in that area.

These theoretical constructions need to confront the phenomena of a situated, lived, and narrated experience of eating disorders. Autobiographical accounts convey the reality of a situated subjectivity and the significations to which it is prone and, taken together with other testimony and the shreds of scientific evidence we do have, enlighten us about anorexia and can therefore serve to synthesize an understanding of the paradox of eating disorders.

11.3 **The thin lady speaks**

Sheila MacLeod (1972) in her autobiographical account identifies the key to the anorexia as follows:

> In becoming anorexic, I did the only thing I could. I adopted the only strategy open to me in order to preserve any sort of identity, however precarious, and in order to believe in myself as an individual being, separate from both the family and the school. Anorexia nervosa is fundamentally about an identity crisis. (p. 54)

MacLeod's account is so compelling and rings so true to other autobiographical accounts and the clinical puzzles of dealing with anorexics that it offers an understanding that is unique. Comments from other anorexics lend both support and credibility to her claims and converge with recent critical analyses (Giordano, 2005) in a way that illuminates the complex negotiation of meaning and being in human psychology (Harre & Gillett, 1994; Winch, 1958).

MacLeod grew in a home where emotions and the needs of the body were not often discussed or openly shared in any healthy or honest way. She was not abused and she explored her childhood sexuality much as other children do. In her family, she was the older sister and thought to be clever, so she was under some pressure to achieve. At a certain point in her life, when about 13 years old, she overheard her aunt make the following remark to her mother:

> 'She's going to be stout—just like Dolly' (Dolly was my mother). At once, all the light and colour seemed to be drained from my surroundings. I was blazingly angry with her and wanted to shout, 'No, I'm not! Why the hell should I be? And who are you to say so?' But of course I said nothing.
>
> (Macleod, 1972, p. 15)

She goes on to dissociate the single, ill-considered remark from the onset of her disease, and as her narrative unfolds, it becomes clear that the desire to be beautiful and to be herself are twin themes important in her developing anorexia. Similar observations are made by others.

> Around the same period, I had started dieting after being called 'Kauri trunks' by a fellow male basketball player. The term had affronted and disturbed me . . . How dare a mate, a male equal, criticize my body—especially that part of my body! I knew my bodily faults full well and my thighs were the absolute worst part of my 16-year-old body.
>
> (McCarthy & Thomson, 1996, p. 19)

The same feature, a casual insulting remark about body weight or appearance, appears in many histories and has the same radical effect on the psyche of the young woman concerned.

> I did have a boyfriend in my fifth form year. When we were on the bed one day, I asked him for a pillow and he said, 'Pull up some of your back.' That must have had a huge effect on me. I've never forgotten it.
>
> (McCarthy & Thomson, 1996, p. 41)

From an early age, some of the conflicts of the mother's role became part of Sheila's life as she assumed the mantle of the dutiful older daughter. Even though she would often bully her sisters by pinching them and pulling their hair, 'outwardly I was all sweetness and patient understanding, continually being congratulated in the role of "little mother"' (Macleod, 1972, p. 25).

That discontinuity between subjectivity and self-presentation is only one of several. Because Sheila was destined to be the clever one, she was expected to work hard academically and this became the focus of resentment directed at both her father and her mother. Her successful entry into boarding school began a life of secrecy designed to conceal the relative poverty of her home and the humbleness of her origins rather than anything to do with her sexuality.

> I'm also sorry to disappoint all those writers on anorexia nervosa who insist that the disease stems from a longstanding aversion to sexuality and childbirth. To me, it all seemed quite natural and even rather exciting—if a bit strange, but then no stranger than any other activities or preoccupations belonging to the adult world.
>
> (Macleod, 1972, p. 38)

However, Sheila found the onset of menstruation quite disturbing and began to experience 'a split in self-perception' (p. 39), recalling the thesis that the body is disowned and a bodiless self is conjured into psychic being. This did have implications for her sexuality: 'I think it was at this stage that I made the unconscious decision, later to manifest itself in physiological terms, to postpone sexuality until I found myself ready to cope with it' (Macleod, 1972, p. 47).

She identifies two prime needs of adolescence: the need for privacy and the need to belong. She felt compromised in the first because of the boarding school dormitory context and the second (her sense of belonging) in that she was in boarding school but not a social peer with her school friends. Privacy is related to self-containment, dignity, and self-ownership; she remarks, 'The anorexic has sufficient sense of identity to know that identity is something to be fought for . . . If anorexia is about identity in general, it is also specifically and most importantly about autonomy' (Macleod, 1972, p. 55). Against this driving desire to assert identity, the body becomes enlisted as an inalienable weapon in the anorexic's struggle. MacLeod (1972) uses her body to assert herself against all those that would control her: 'I felt my battle to be with authority, whether in the form of teachers, matrons, parents, or even nature itself' (p. 65). She summarizes the anorexic response to the conflicts of adolescent identity in the following way:

> It seems to me that anorexia nervosa acts as a metaphor for all the problems of adolescence. But instead of meeting each problem separately and assessing it for what it is, the anorexic thinks she has a master plan, designed to solve them all at one stroke. She is convinced that it works; it can't fail. It is like a dream come true. It is euphoria.
>
> (Macleod, 1972, p. 65)

She speaks of the euphoria of anorexic control in powerful terms.

> My diary, in my pre-anorexic days, often refers to a 'weight of depression', which I felt myself to be carrying around. Once I became anorexic, that weight vanished with my

flesh. My step lightened, I was full of energetic high spirits, and during the summer term I even became keen on playing tennis . . . At night, I would often get up and go for long walks in the school grounds, especially when the moon was full and I felt particularly restless, enjoying the silence and solitude of the woods.

(Macleod, 1972, p. 66)

Her control over nature is a significant achievement.

I didn't want my periods to start again. That I had managed to stop them was a major achievement on my part. Instead of growing up, I had, as it were, grown down, and thus reversed a natural biological process. I was no longer a woman. I was what I wanted to be—a girl.

(Macleod, 1972, p. 67)

She graphically expresses the plight of the sexualized woman who becomes the target of the desires of others that objectify her, constructing her as a provider for their demands so that a distorted body-image is portrayed as a phenomenological response to the control and denaturalization of a female body that has transcended its fleshly constraints.

To see my starved self as beautiful was to dissipate a large part of this confusion: I was literally and metaphorically in perfect shape.

The distortion of perception extended itself to areas other than my body. Having disposed alike of unwanted flesh and unwanted menstruation, I had become pure and clean, and therefore superior to those around me.

(Macleod, 1972, p. 70)

The identity of the anorexic was one to which she clung for all she was worth; 'Perhaps, this may explain the determination of the anorexic to go on starving herself: without anorexia, I should have been nothing. I know that I had no intention of stopping the procedure, whatever anyone said or did to influence me, I was determined never to give in' (Macleod, 1972, p. 73). A young woman's immersion in anorexia conditions attitudes and self-conceptions affecting every other facet of her lived experience. MacLeod speaks of her depression and the way she romanticized images of death to accommodate them in her unrealistic self-image and denial of reality. Her starvation assumes a dramatic and symbolic significance for her linked to Sylvia Plath's Lady Lazarus and the 'art of dying'. 'I, too, thought I was doing something unique and practicing an art exceptionally well. And the irony entailed in starving myself in order to survive was not altogether lost on me' (Macleod, 1972, p. 77). Her attitude of denial and paradoxical control of the possibility of her own death is evident: 'death, like sexuality, is a biological fact, but anorexia nervosa entails the denial of biology, and in particular, the notion of biology as destiny' (Macleod, 1972, p. 79).

One would think that physical reality would make evident what the anorexic patient is doing to her (real) embodied self, but a discursive move transforms the evidence and its implications: 'My self wasn't my body. And cold was a property of my body— some tiresome thing which was nevertheless now completely under my control—and not of my self' (Macleod, 1972, p. 86). She projects on to others her own evaluations of the body and its physicality: 'What really disgusted me was the sight of other people eating. It seemed to me shocking that they should engage in such a crude, almost obscene activity in public' (Macleod, 1972, p. 90).

Faced with her self-construction and the network of meanings driving her anorexia, the choices facing an anorexic woman are tightly constrained. 'The anorexic who has achieved her emaciated state is faced with two choices: she can relax her control and surrender her will, thus admitting defeat, or she can allow herself to die of starvation' (Macleod, 1972, p. 99). This dilemma focuses on the control of self that MacLeod sees as the pivotal feature of her anorexia even though serendipity and the vagaries of the psyche may combine to open other paths undreamt of in the stark (moral) logic of anorexia (Giordano, 2005). MacLeod's life actually begins to turn around not under the influence of therapy but when she realizes just how distorted her perceptions of herself really are.

The change occurs when she is home from school and has no access to scales so that she cannot monitor her weight. Prior to the crucial moment, she has already come to the realization that she feels herself unaccepted both at school and at home and begins to explore the possibility that there is some deep cause within her for the alienation between herself and her contexts. She began to feel that she did not deserve the guilt and wrongness she unconsciously attributed to herself at a level far beneath her superficial superiority and romantic unworldliness. She visits a railway station, four and a half miles from her village, to verify her conviction that she has put on a great deal of weight. To her shock, she found that she had lost 7 pounds. She was bewildered and realized that her body was following its own laws and 'it was my first intimation that all was not right, that there was something abnormal going on in the workings of my mind' (Macleod, 1972, p. 106). Here be alienation!

The same interrupted 'contact with shared or public reality' has equally striking effects for other anorexic patients. 'I'll never forget the day I arrived. All my friends came running down the corridor to meet me, but when they saw me some of them started crying. To this day, I still hear how awful they thought I looked. Of course, I thought I looked normal' (McCarthy & Thomson, 1996, p. 88).

MacLeod's mother played an important part in her recovery; a process that was triggered by her mother reciting a poem which, for the first time, suggested to her that her mother recognized and had sympathy for her condition. The role of her mother in her recovery emphasizes the important part played in the developmental history of most girls by an ambivalent attitude towards identification with the mother. MacLeod (1972) remarks, 'What I do feel sure of now is that my recognition of myself as others saw me had to come from her, from her first and so, perhaps, from her alone' (p. 109).

Macleod's account is impressive because it starkly reveals the investment of the young woman in her starvation and also the way in which food represents far more than the self-denial that is its most obvious feature. The symbolic link between food, womanhood, sexual and physical maturity, and the development of identity provide an explanatory nexus that makes comprehensible the paradoxical phenomenology of eating disorders.

11.4 **Lightness of being—the narrative quest**

Casual but hurtful remarks aimed at the body and the language of beauty have been closely implicated in triggering the transformation of self in anorexia.

> People would say you look great, you look fantastic, and I felt great and I felt fantastic. I felt that I looked wonderful. And the thinner I became—this wasn't so apparent to me then, but in later years I saw it clearly—the more popular I became. So my whole sense of self-esteem became bound up with what I looked like, with my weight.
>
> (*Susan*; McCarthy & Thomson, 1996, p. 42)

We see here, as with Sheila MacLeod, a quest initiated and then maintained by discourse—to achieve lightness of being and resist the 'cloying nature' threatening to transform one into a lump of stuff. Through lightness, the anorexic rises above the world of mundane and massive objects and pursues a distinctive path. The false self is mythical and fantastic, noumenal, spiritual, or superior, in the way that the human is distinct from the brute animal or physical side of our nature (Giordano, 2005, p. 115), and anorexia itself an heroic and lonely protest against a world that threatens to absorb the individual into its potentially deadly embrace (note the sliding of the signifiers). It is easy to valorize the disorder rather than seeing that it thrives on a romantic denial of the real self as embodied, sensitive, and needy in relation to the regard and evaluations of others. The purity of the delusory quest to be as light as a feather, a being of spirit rather than flesh, is characteristic of anorexia but effaced in bulimia.

In bulimia, the central paradox seems to arise from a desire for food out of proportion to bodily needs and then the guilt and equal desire to eliminate the food so that it will not have its natural nourishing role. Again, the meaning of the food is important and a mind focused on food is a central feature, but ingestion is conceptualized as an evil to be expunged and the pattern of alternately bingeing and purging has the telltale form of repetition, the indicator of deeply paradoxical cathexes attached to food and operating at the interface between signifiers and the world. On the one hand, we encounter the loving and nurturing qualities expected in womankind, but on the other, the ever-present threat to beautiful femaleness. In dieting also, a self-imposed disruption of one's relation to food becomes explicit. 'Bulimia is linked very strongly with dieting. Bingeing frequently begins during or after an episode of dieting, when food becomes an obsession in the woman's mind, and the obsession grows until she can think of nothing else. It is an imperative which must be obeyed' (McCarthy & Thomson, 1996, p. 33).

The anorexic opts for total control so that the unconscious conflict and self-hatred is hidden underneath a calm and assured (false) self-narrative, which the bulimic does/will/can not create. 'After every binge and throwing up, and the terror of being caught, I would be asking myself "Why do I do it?" It was so out of control, but I so much wanted to stop' (*Yvonne*; McCarthy & Thomson, 1996, p. 100). The apparent contrast to the pure and fleshless narrative of the anorexic hides what, at a deeper level, the two eating disorders have in common.

The network of signifiers is similar in each case with one set of significations operating in relation to food and ingestion and quite a different set operating in the subjectivity of starvation, self-denial, lightness, and purification. On the one side, we have terms such as *fat, big girl, heavy, losing control, weight, solid, earthy, bodily, fleshy, disgusting*, and on the other, *control, overcoming, thin, light, transparent, slim, perfect*, and *the denial of biology*. One set of images ties the young woman to incarnation and the insistent body with its messy engagement in the world; the other is on a different ontological plane, taking her out of herself and yet into a self that is more truly hers than any other mode of being because she writes her own rules and does not obey laws put upon her by nature or any other more fallible controls.

The connections in the network of signifiers render the self-images and evaluations even more vividly. Swollen, polluted, dirty, consuming, well nourished, and puppy fat, all lock the self into a world of natural processes changing the self in ways that have nothing to do with the spirit. But signifiers such as cleanness, purity, control, rising above, invisibility, and superiority lift one out of the cloying nexus. Signifiers also surround acts of purging. In both cases, the solidity of ingested and digested food and its threat to the value of the woman lurk in the connections between the signifiers and capture the underlying dual attitude to the body and its needs and those contexts in which the relevant signifiers are the discursive currency.

> The feeding relationship resonates far more deeply than simply at the level of physical satisfaction. The process of feeding sets up a whole tableau of feelings that affect not just our relationship with food but our experience of closeness and intimacy.
>
> (Orbach, 1993, p. 33)

This close relationship between love or intimacy and food becomes important in trying to understand the problems of relationships characteristic of eating disorders. All eating disorders share signifiers such as *secretive, furtive, possessive, private*, and *control* expressing the need to distance the self of the sufferer from others, suggesting that the self is protecting itself from an expected encroachment. It remains to delineate the intrusion and thereby to situate anorexia and bulimia as two different narrative responses to an unliveable subjectivity.

11.5 Images of food and womanhood

Orbach notes that a life of nurture, support, and self-effacement are built into the attainment of womanhood and the images clustering around it so that there is a continuity between the self-control of the anorexic and the experience of many women who 'unthinkingly envy the anorectic her willpower and ability to withstand the temptation of food' (Orbach, 1993, p. 78). But the untramelled and light surface being of the anorectic hides deep pain and need.

Orbach links that pain to the conflicts generated by demands to defer to others, to meet the needs of others, and to achieve self-definition and refers to the encoding of this conflicted social role of women in the complex that is fundamental to the anorexic–bulimic mode of being as a situated (and gendered) subjectivity. The needy, normal, and natural self is, at some level, hated and rejected because, if acknowledged and realized, it will usher in the anonymity of the role of food-bearer and support person for the lives of others. The woman who craves recognition in and for herself cannot allow herself to be absorbed and made anonymous in that way. Through the physical negation of her needy self, she is protesting against the symbolic negation of herself as an independent identity and also protesting, albeit in an inchoate way, the lack of recognition for her self-sacrifice in adopting a role as the source of nourishment for others. This 'unconscious world of the individual in her time' is palpably continuous with the 'normal' experience of the homemaker who may pour herself into the danger-fraught realm of food and its preparation and yet have her sacrificial love scorned or treated with negligent disdain by a family who, through their attitude towards her food and herself, seems uncaring and heedless of her presence and identity. 'A lot of creative energy goes into planning meals, and you badly need them to be appreciated. It hurts when they're disregarded. They are, indeed, a kind of offering' (*Penny*; McCarthy & Thomson, 1996, p. 186).

Orbach (1993) comments that the woman with anorexia has 'uncannily strong opinions' and has not accepted 'the strictures and constraints of her role'. She is often a person who has been a 'good girl' and 'reasonably contented but chaotic inside' because her needs for self-expression and self-worth 'plague and disturb her'. They have to be managed and denied and their control 'requires a tremendous and ever-increasing vigilance' (pp. 122–123). Food refusal is the visible symbol that she is defeating her internal wants and needs (in the required way but also, paradoxically, as an expression of her own power). The tenuous internal warfare is therefore won or lost depending on how successfully she refuses food (with its associated images and life trajectories). The strain is too much for some and they binge but then rescue themselves by restoring control through purging (nullifying the lapse).

Food and the woman, both problematized by discourses comprising inherently conflictful signifiers, fill 'the unconscious' with transactions between self (as body) and world that are chaotic and threaten the integrated subjectivity of the young woman. The chaos engenders the self-hate and bodily self-negation of anorexic and bulimic patients. But how can the depths of the self be reconfigured so they are no longer the seat of such a psychic aporia (impasse, immolation)?

11.6 **Retransforming the self**

The embodied self transforms either into the anorexic self (through a heroic act of self-denial) or into the bulimic self (through a deep-seated acceptance of guilt about the needs and nature of the body). In each case, the natural dispositions of the body enact a combination of signifiers that disturbs life-maintaining physiological functions. But the control is false and the distorted subjectivity threatens to obliterate itself, so the difficult existential path allowing a young woman to relinquish rigid control of herself and yet preserve her autonomy must be found. Orbach (1993), attentive to this balance, lists the objectives of treatment as follows:

(1) The creation of an understanding of food refusal.

(2) Focusing on the body.

(3) Restarting the development of self. (p. 110)

The treatment of eating disorders is widely acknowledged to be extremely difficult. The basic problem centres around a young woman not being allowed to compose and retain control of a life narrative that she can regard as worthwhile in its own right.

Orbach identifies the key points of a therapy that respects the woman and enables her to construct a coherent narrative (and moral and political) position apt for a real (embodied) being-in-the-world-with-others.

> By helping the patient come to reckon with the depth of her being, the truths of her past, and the efforts to extinguish her despair by turning to her eating disorder, the therapist, working within a feminist psychodynamic framework, entreats the patient to embark on a journey where her singular personhood is paramount. In the process, the patient learns to exist again—sometimes to know herself for the first time.
>
> (Zerbe, 1996)

Therapy creates a discourse in which the refusal of food can be recognized for what it is and the patient can begin to understand her quest for thinness or lightness and its relation to the needs and conflicts producing it. This discursive context allows the young woman to engage with the underlying significations that have shaped her subjectivity and reconfigure her perception of her body. In Sheila MacLeod's case, that was triggered by a problematization of her own perception of herself. Only once the apparently assured but false self-perception had been 'dethroned' could a competing self-perception begin to form. Orbach's last element, the rebuilding or restarting of the development of self on more secure foundations, shows us that the embodied self must be accepted as being OK, nourished appropriately, and also seen as the only realistic basis on which to pursue the project of identity.

Identity and autonomy are mutually defining and sustaining, and the anorexic's strength of will should not be broken but rather delinked from the self-hate and the disdain for womanhood that makes it self-destructive. Zerbe (1996) talks of a young woman's need to regain ownership of her body and mind and Giordano (2005) of her need to regain her sense of right and wrong in an authentic, self-validating way that is able-to-be-lived-with (p. 264).

It is evident that coercive feeding and the imposition of bodily changes from outside the identity of the individual, perhaps required as a life-saving measure, are not in any way addressing the underlying problem to which the anorexia is a solution. 'In trying to get her to eat and to become the "right size", they negate her protest. They unwittingly deny the meaning of her symptom and in so doing contribute to its perpetuation' (Orbach, 1993, p. 9).

Respect for the patient as an individual and for her difficulties with relationships, acceptance, and trust are basic to the treatment of anorexia so that the very idea of intrusive and self-violating treatment or care is an oxymoron as far as the meanings clustered around anorexia are concerned. Apart from the assertions of feminist psychotherapists, other studies note the effectiveness of treatment aimed at self-conceptions and relationships. A study comparing behaviour therapy, cognitive-behaviour therapy, and group therapy led the authors to conclude 'that bulimia nervosa is amenable to treatment by structured once-weekly psychotherapy in either individual or group form . . . Provided that such patients complete the course, roughly three quarters will be symptom-free at the end of 15 weeks' (Freeman et al., 1988). General claims about relative efficacy are hard to justify from good empirical evidence (Kaplan, 2002), but the current analysis suggests that 'interpersonal therapy' particularly focused on issues of identity and self-acceptance might be soundest approaches as the mainstay of treatment (McCarthy & Thomson, 1996; Orbach, 1993). The patient as a moral agent with a life of her own must be taken seriously and allowed to construct her own narrative but encouraged to weave into that her embodiment among others and their reactions to her so that she is able to give herself permission to be in the (natural) world of others rather than withdrawing from it to preserve her being as a being of worth.

11.7 **Silence, resistance, power**

Anorexia is an extreme response to an inherently conflicted set of social demands preying on a young woman's soul. The problem can be posed, in discursive terms, as follows:

> What is the proper mode of being a self, if the self you are trying to be is subject to the shaping of others?

The mother is saying 'Eat, partake of my bounty' but is also conveying and legitimating the message 'Be sylph-like, pure, deny yourself, be light and beautiful.' The conflict reduces the young woman to silence. What can she say when the meanings offered to express her plight are equal in power and carry opposing implications for her worth and identity? Words fail her (indeed threaten her). Her resistance to the process that is moulding her into the mature shape of womanhood can only take the form of action. Her power is limited to her own body; over that alone, she can permit or withhold permission, to comply with the demands of others or refuse to comply with them. That locus of power is inalienable from her.

As an embodied subjectivity, she hates those aspects of herself that are intrinsically demanding and so resists them, making them subject to her will. Thus, 'the pure and cleansing fire' of her will burns away her susceptibility to the demands of the flesh and her nature is overcome. What is more, freedom from the embodiment engaging her with the world of others gives rise to another freedom and point of resistance.

As the young woman progressively releases herself from the demands of her body, she releases herself from the medium through which she is subject to the evaluations of others. Those evaluations convey an ideal of beauty and enviability that is legitimated and powerful. But her inner self—her essential self, by contrast with her outer embodied self—is not open to the public gaze and her inner strategies of control are solely her own. If she is bulimic, she can react to food by eliminating it so that it does not affect her essential self; her loss of control is negated by purgation, her point of triumph. Both bulimic and anorexic patients therefore devise strategies to prevent enslavement by the body becoming doughy and stodgy through the food that will incarnate them or make them carnal if they allow it to.

In the eating disorders, the young woman resists the law-like connection between ingestion, growth, and incarnation (in accordance with the expectations of others), thereby bending nature and the world to fit her narrative. Without nature to aid them, the forces seeking to control her are rendered impotent. The power threatening to shape her in an undesirable way succumbs to her magic (or spirit), a magic of autonomy and the power of veto over what others want her to do and be. With such powerful magic in her armoury, nothing controls her although many try to—she can say, 'I choose who I am and I dictate who I will be, light or heavy, woman or girl.'

This triumph is profound. It is far above the petty manoeuvres of parents, teachers, headmistresses, or even doctors (shocking as that thought might be). It is a triumph, among other things, over nature and time itself—the primal forces of the universe.

> When I am pushed, there is no limit to my control; I can even control my hormones, my sexuality, and therefore my biological nature. I can reverse my growth and become smaller, a girl not a woman. Time, marked inexorably by my periods, has lost its hold on me and if I choose I need not move on into adulthood. 'I am Pan (or is it Tinkerbell); I have transcended nature and time.'

It is not really surprising that a resistance capable of constructing this discourse is able to persist in the face of most coercive assaults upon it. If nature itself cannot control one, then what respect can rationally be sustained for the petty authorities and restrictions that attempt to impinge on one's life through human institutions.

11.8 A postmodern disease and the primary process

> I am a protester on a hunger strike. I am not sick and I insist that my protest be taken seriously. I do not want to be treated. You ask me what I am protesting about; I will tell you. I am protesting about motherhood and apple pie, about friends and boy-not friends, about Mrs. John Doe and her daughter, about bleeding, about being a good girl, about being clean and dirty, about Naomi Campbell and the virgin Mary, about pâté de foie gras, and about the heaviness of being, especially when that means being pressed down upon; I am protesting about fertility and flirtility, and I will be heard whether you read my lips or not, because you will not be able to ignore my body.

Anorexia is the postmodern disease par excellence, literally inscribing the values that are legitimated in a certain discourse on the bodies of its sufferers through their own produced subjectivities. The inherent conflicts in the discourse—the conflict between health and emaciation, between self-expression and submission to the evaluations of others, between woman as nurturing food provider and woman for whom food is her enemy, and between the woman as object of appraisal and woman as autonomous moral being worthy of respect in herself—are all realized in the network of signifiers that shape the discursive and bodily ideal of the anorexic and her moral quest for lightness of being (Giordano, 2005).

The irony of self-control itself obsessively controlled by an ultimately self-destructive end is, from MacLeod's testimony, not lost on anorexic patients. In fact, irony, inherently superior (but not Mother Superior) to the concerns and projects within its gaze, is likely to be an attractive feature of the narrative voice in anorexia. The tragedy of the situation is that the lightness of being and ironic superiority of the narrator is built on a false belief in the narrator's power over nature and over her own narrative. She is in anguish about who she is and her worth in the scheme of things, anguish that infects her every healthy instinct. She is therefore secretive, tormented, and depressed (a significant co-morbidity [Bulik *et al.*, 1995; Walsh, 1991]) and her euphoria is merely another negation forming the complex subjectivity of a false self.

'I don't know how it was that I came to internalize so early those ideas about fat and repulsiveness and self-hate' (*Penny*; McCarthy & Thomson, 1996, p. 185). This puzzlement demonstrates the characteristic intensity—immediacy—of the primary process, driven by cathectic force and with no respect for rationality. The hurts or wounds are deeply felt despite being inchoate so that it is relevant that girl babies are, on average, cut off from breastfeeding and held for less time than boy babies (Orbach, 1993, p. 26). Deeply ingrained dispositions to self-deprivation and denial of one's basic bodily and emotional needs might therefore condition a woman's sub-subjectivity. But that thesis is as problematic as the primal wound.

It is clear that the deprivation is relative to the amount of contact and affection given to infant boys. But an infant girl does not have an intrinsically comparative experience; she has a singular experience statistically comparable with that of boys but without sufficient intrinsic information to allow her to develop a sense of deprivation and denial from within her own subjectivity unless further aspects of her experience rescue Orbach's claim.

The first depends on there being a basic and absolute level of need for breastfeeding and cuddling required for a healthy (psychic) start in life. It then posits that girls tend to fall below this level whereas boys do not. A second posit would be that the mother's ambivalent attitude towards nurturing a girl infant is subliminally communicated and influences the primary process shaping her developing narrative of bodily and emotional self-needs. The (real) self, despite a number of overt and explicit messages about being loved and valued, then has a deep-seated ambivalence about its basic needs, a schizoid process lying at the root of the pain of eating disorders and the self-destructive tendencies characterizing them. The intensity of that conflict, on this account, results from the lack of rational mitigation (in the primary process) and the elemental and subreflective force of the complexes formed. One cannot reflect upon self-love and its wounds if the relevant cathectic realities are inarticulate.

A further plausible posit would be that the signifiers in play in the discourse surrounding a girl infant during the articulation of her psyche carry an implicit message about the worth and validity of her needs. This message is inscribed very deeply in her body and her attitudes towards it. A systematic comparative disregard for girl children (even in so-called egalitarian societies) would plausibly strengthen any already sensed (from the mother's attitudes) ambivalence in relation to the self so that she is devalued with respect to her male peers. Again, this orientation affects but does not appear within the conscious autobiographical narrative so that it is not rationally revisable by 'insight'.

The latter two posits complement one another and, if true, would shape a damaging complex of attitudes to the self within the subjectivity of a young woman. The entwined effects of legitimated signification and unsignified but active cathectic forces—*l'autre or petit a*—are (*ex hypothesi*) difficult to unravel because the primary process is characteristically insistent, immediate, incorrigible, obsessive, and emotionally disturbing. The resulting synthesis is highly congenial to the conceptualization of the unconscious as the cumulative result of inscriptions on the body (including the brain) or the extraconscious configuration of the brain–world exchanges that form the raw material for my autobiographical narrative and that is interpreted according to the discourses forming me. What is more, the post-Lacanian 'take' on those psychic moments that form the primary process relates them to irrational but legitimated and valorized inscriptions on the body locating or positioning the self-as-subject in a value-laden world of being-with-others in which one forms one's self out of the inchoate flux of being-there so that conflicts in the symbolic realm can create multiple aporias.

> Problems that can fade away in a flash of insight do not require solutions as dramatic as anorexia.

> (Orbach, 1993, p. 125)

11.9 **Philosophical puzzles**

The current topic has focused attention on the nature of desire and its relationship to the definition of self and the psyche within a lived human narrative.

A desire or bodily need is normally portrayed as playing a fairly simple part in psychological explanation: it is a biological given with a more or less univalent direction of psychic influence aimed at its satisfaction. Hunger, for instance, seems straightforwardly related to serum glucose levels and the ingestion of food under homeostatic regulation. Such unambiguous vectors in the motivational structure of an individual participate in causing behaviour based on conditioning and experience. However, anorexia problematizes this simple biological model and therefore our 'flat-footed' constructions of human motivational structure in general.

The simple conception appears in the following kind of argument:

(11.9.1) Desires are primitive and univalent elements of human psychology.

(11.9.2) Desires play a straightforward biological role throughout the phylogenetic scale.

(11.9.3) Desires can be modified in their expression but not in their psychic role by conscious mechanisms.

(11.9.4) Desires such as hunger always tend towards their satisfaction. *But,*

(11.9.5) Hunger can destroy an anorexic by acting against her preservation of self.

The paradox comes about because human desire is a surreal montage (Lacan) with signifying and motivational roles based on meaning and value. The anorexic takes her hunger to signify her unworthy and negatively valued biological nature. This is not a conscious decision (although the significations valorizing starvation may be partially conscious). The desire for food is, therefore, not just a mechanism tending to survival; it is a montage with moral and spiritual qualities based in the world of human meaning. The ultimate effect of reassigning a negative valence to hunger is to destroy health (as one might predict from the laws of nature), but the psyche also lives in the world of meaning and value. At that level, the young woman must negate the forces producing her in a certain way so that she can be or find the way she wants to be. The theme of her narrative quest is therefore aptly summarized as

I eat, therefore I am not.

This dictum, inscribed on the body at a subconscious level, indicates the shaping of culture, and the complex relation between intersubjectivity, resistance, and the formation of self that is driving the young woman out of this world for her source of validation. The paradox of her drives cannot be dreamt of in the philosophy of biological naturalism, and the way that she reacts to the inscriptions on her body represents a desperate attempt to harmonize the unharmonizable demons that enliven her as a being-in-the-world-with-others.

Chapter 12

The meaning of hysteria

The young lady, aged 30, carefully dressed in black, who comes into the hall with short, shuffling steps, leaning on the nurse, and sinks into a chair as if exhausted, gives you the impression that she is ill. She is of slender build, her features are pale and rather painfully drawn, and her eyes are cast down. Her small manicured fingers play nervously with a handkerchief. The patient answers the questions addressed to her in a low, tired voice, without looking up, and we find that she is quite clear about time, place, and her surroundings. After a few minutes, her eyes suddenly become convulsively shut, her head sinks forward, and she seems to have fallen into a deep sleep. Her arms have grown quite limp, and fall down as if palsied when you try to lift them. She has ceased to answer, and if you try to raise her eyelids, her eyes suddenly rotate upwards. Needle pricks only produce a slight shudder. But sprinkling with cold water is followed by a deep sigh; the patient starts up, opens her eyes, looks round her with surprise, and gradually comes to herself.

(APA, 1994b, pp. 498–499)

This graphic description, of a classic case of Emile Kraepelin's, raises familiar problems for psychiatrists and neurologists. Contemporary presentations may not be with a 'swoon' but with hemiplegia, a 'convulsion', blindness, or some other striking (quasi-neurological) symptom. We apply various labels to patients who show one of these disorders: hysteria, conversion reaction, somatization, factitious disorder, and malingering. There are significant differences between them and each has its own profile, best explored if we focus on the stream of brain–world interaction and the conscious narrative arising from it in hysteria.

12.1 The sickness that is not

Hysteria is inherently problematic in that, alongside the physical manifestations, injuries, or overt trauma in the patient's history, there is always 'the subjective element' (Havens, 1966, p. 507). First, it is a psychiatric condition more often diagnosed by neurologists than psychiatrists. Second, some clinicians would like to abolish the diagnosis completely, arguing that it produces nothing but clinical confusion by masking real diseases and leading to misdiagnosis (Slater, 1965) given that at certain times as many as one third of the individuals may have had neurological conditions (DSM IV; APA, 1994a, p. 453). Even though the number of misdiagnoses seems to be decreasing (29% in the 1950s, 17% in the 1960s, 4% more recently [Stone et al., 2005]), some argue that to treat hysteria as illness is to buy into a damaging and disabling game (Szasz, 1962/1972). Third, the patient reports physical symptoms without a physical basis and yet, in many cases, is neither pretending nor 'out of touch with reality' in any obvious way. What is more, although hysterical patients seem to lack insight into their disorder and misconstrue the real state of their body, they are often preoccupied with the changes they perceive in their body.

Prima facie, hysteria offers us an interesting perspective on the contemporary tendency to biologize psychiatry because it seeks to explain apparently physical abnormalities in mental or 'functional' terms, thereby implicitly demanding that we clarify the terms 'mental' and 'physical' framing that contrast. Consider the following statements:

(i) There is an inverse relationship between the electrical activity of certain parts of the precentral motor cortex and the activity in the lateral corticospinal system.

(ii) We have observed that human beings react not primarily to the occurrence of an event but to the socially mediated perception of the occurrence of an event.

Both are objective truths about human beings, one framed in terms of brain function and the other mental function; one might conclude that (i) is concerned with physical reality and (ii) is concerned with the mental domain, but the dualism soon breaks down. In explaining human psychology, we are always trying to link the two types of description because facts about human beings and their function are discovered and used in areas such as pain management and understanding behaviour in the light of personality characteristics, as in the following:

(iii) There is an inverse correlation between the tendency of a subject to develop a premotor or 'readiness' cortical potential in the frontal lobe under certain conditions and impulsivity.

This is an objective, mathematical finding about brain activity relating it to a psychometrically defined mental trait—impulsivity (Howard, 1986); the identification of that group of patients showing a significant deviation from the normal pattern of event-related premotor activity depends upon the (psychological) assessment of impulsivity. Thus, not only the significance of the electrophysiological finding but also its very existence as a documentable fact depends on the prior determination of a 'mental fact' (that subjects a, b, c, f, and g are impulsive). And sharpening our analysis only deepens the metaphysical fuzziness.

Statement (i) embeds certain basic mathematical beliefs. Mathematics is a human tool or invention (the universe did not arrive complete with mathematics any more than it came labelled by divinely preordained science or logic) so that physiological characterizations impose human categories and measures on a natural field the 'regularities' and 'order' of which are framed in terms that aim at true beliefs ('mental states'). Thus, try as we might, we cannot rid scientific inquiry in general, and neuropsychology and psychiatry in particular, of core statements philosophically grounded in characteristically human ways of constructing things. Therefore, we should investigate hysteria aided by the framing stance that human beings inhabit a world of meaning as creatures of flesh and blood who are inscribed by (and articulate their lives in terms of) the meanings and values they encounter in a shared (intersubjective) world of discourse.

The key words signalling the need to attend to discursive relations in an account of hysteria prominently include explanation, cause, the unconscious, roles, pretence, power, subjectivity, knowledge, insight, and self-worth, and they combine to configure or produce what we call hysteria, malingering, and conversion reactions. A clear philosophical analysis provides a phenomenological and categorical apparatus adequate to understand these disorders and their meaning to the human beings caught up in them.

12.2 **Hysteria in the clinic**

Hysteria and conversion reactions, as used in the *International Classification of Diseases-9* (ICD 9), 'occur in the absence of physical pathology, they are produced unconsciously, and they are not caused by the overactivity of the Sympathetic Nervous System (SNS)' (Gelder et al., 1983, p. 169). Janet identified the 'stigmata' of hysteria: 'paresis, anaesthesia, amnesia, coma, and loss of function of the special senses' (Meares et al., 1985, p. 257) and a recent review focused on 'motor and sensory symptoms—such as paralysis, seizures, and blindness—that are unexplained by disease . . . and account for 1–9% of the inpatients and outpatients' (Stone et al., 2005). The criteria on which to diagnose a 'conversion disorder' (DSM IV, 300.11 [APA, 1994a]) are as follows:

(A) One or more symptoms or deficits affecting voluntary motor or sensory function that suggest a neurological or other general medical condition.

(B) Psychological factors are judged to be associated with the symptom or deficit.

(C) The symptom or deficit is not intentionally produced or feigned. (p. 457)

In such a condition, meanings influence or cause the *perceived* bodily state of that person (as distinct from a psychosomatic reaction affecting the *actual* body state of the patient—e.g. stress causing a gastric ulcer or an attack of asthma).

Kraepelin's suffering lady lines up beside cases of monoplegia, blindness, paraplegia, or hemisensory loss without any discernible neurological or organic origin. Despite seeming impressive to the uninitiated, such presentations are rarely convincing to an experienced clinician because of the significant anomalies in them. For instance, pseudoseizures look similar to grand mal convulsions but are not accompanied by urinary incontinence, tongue biting, or other serious physical harm (even though a 'savvy' patient may self-harm in a way that approximates genuine epilepsy). Hysterical monoparesis often presents with a history of minor head injury or some other anomalous feature such as a non-anatomical configuration. Hysterical tremor does not have the rhythms or morphologies characteristic of recognized extrapyramidal syndromes. Hysterical dementia and amnesia is often transparently inconsistent to neuropsychological examination as in Ganser syndrome when the patient does so spectacularly badly that if their apparent cognitive problems were real they would be unable to negotiate even the simplest tasks. The characteristic *belle indifference* is just such an anomaly—an almost unbelievable lack of real and deep-seated distress in the face of what, if real, would be extremely distressing (Gelder et al., 1983, p. 171). *La belle indifference* almost transparently signals that the patient knows that nothing serious is actually going on, quite unlike a genuinely affected person.

A careful psychiatric history, illuminating the patient's psychosocial context, usually reveals a secondary gain or gains derived from the illness behaviour. Often, the synthesis of the case requires insight into and understanding of the various people involved in order to make the 'gain' evident. However, along with discerning the gains derived from the 'illness', one often realizes that the protagonists own recognition of what is happening is quite deficient. Some things that the patient and others do seem to show is that they know what is going on but are defensive about it and others suggest a disarming naivety about the interpersonal dynamics of the situation, an ambiguity that makes the clinical problem intriguing, complex, and frustrating.

The interwoven subjective, interpersonal, and self-evaluative features of these disorders demand a philosophical account that

(1) Shows us why certain physical symptoms are produced by a disorder of the psyche;

(2) Explains why a psyche prone to such disorders has other features found in hysteria;

(3) Explains why the psychological symptoms often coexist with or even indicate an underlying physical disease;

(4) Conforms to a good account relating consciousness and neural phenomena;

(5) Helps us appreciate the social and interpersonal role of hysteria; and

(6) Reconciles the secondary gains associated with the disorder and the self-deception involved.

Each of these desiderata invites us to examine the narrative of the hysterical patient and locate it in the discursive context surrounding the patient and shaping his or her conscious and extraconscious reality, as the following case illustrates.

> Robert was a 35-year-old man who had been injured in a truck accident. The accident occurred a few months after he had started his own trucking enterprise. The injury left him confined to a wheelchair with flexor posturing on his left side and a loss of strength for most movements of the left arm. He also experienced a great deal of pain in his left arm and the whole left side of his body. His legs were stiff and difficult to examine and he had minimal well-coordinated movement in his legs when examined clinically. He had an unsettled insurance claim for the loss of his truck and for his disability. No objective neurological abnormalities could be demonstrated by any means including radiological imaging, electromyography (EMG), and nerve conduction tests, or careful and repeated clinical examination.

Phenomena related to hysteria include somatization disorder (DSM IV, 300.81 [APA, 1994a]) and hypochondriasis. This group of disorders is usually distinguished, to some extent, from malingering or factitious disorders in that the latter imply conscious deception and an awareness of the relationship between one's behaviour and certain rewards or gains attached to it. A good account should not only respect these distinctions but also illuminate them.

12.3 Constructions of hysteria

After initial interest at the turn of the century, the topic of hysteria fell into neglect until Szasz revived interest in it. He highlighted a number of features readily observed in the clinic and developed a novel approach based on the work of pioneers in the subject.

Charcot and Freud

Charcot viewed hysteria as a disorder of the mind requiring careful elucidation, thereby giving it the status of a genuine condition from which people could suffer and posing the problem of causation: how could a change in the mind or soul cause such a bodily manifestation? As is typical of the medicalization of life's ills, his synthesis marginalized the role of meaning in human life and endorsed the patient's perception of himself or herself as suffering some malady. Freud's theory of the unconscious causation of psychic states and disorders allowed hysteria to be classified as an affliction that, although psychic rather than neurological, was nonetheless causative in a way that undercut conscious construction by the person involved. Szasz notes that Charcot himself seemed to be well aware that the symptoms of hysteria were psychogenic and that many of his 'demonstrations' of hysteria and hypnosis were not quite as they might appear to be.

> We must conclude that Charcot's orientation to the problem of hysteria was neither organic nor psychological. He recognized and clearly stated that problems in human relationships may be expressed in hysterical symptoms. The point is that he maintained the medical view in public, for official purposes, as it were, and espoused the psychological view only in private, where such opinions were safe.
>
> (Szasz, 1962/1972, p. 47)

No such irony is found in Freud's belief that cathexes, usually erotic, are sublimated in the unconscious and converted into symptoms of bodily dysfunction where the particular symptoms have a symbolic connection with the objects and situations provoking them. Freud (1922) includes conversion hysteria among the transference neuroses: 'these persons have fallen ill owing to some kind of privation which they suffer when reality withholds from them gratification of their sexual wishes' (p. 252). The relevant (sexual) desires and impulses are, according to Freud (1922), repressed and the hysterical symptoms result from 'two opposed tendencies acting on one another; they represent both that which is repressed and that which has effected the repression' (p. 253). He conceded that the connection to sexuality was sometimes far from obvious but, in quasi-hydraulic terms, invoked pent-up libidinal energy and psychic resistance to its normal expression to explain the hysterical conversion reaction. Consider the following (imaginary) case:

> A young woman, Marie, has a hysterical right monoparesis affecting the upper limb. It emerges in psychoanalysis that the image that comes to her mind is of her father's strong right arm around her shoulders. She may know that her father and mother sleep with him always on the right hand side of the bed and she has an inchoate thought that when he fondles her mother during sexual relations it is his right hand that is involved. The symbolic connection of the libidinal energy fuelling her *Electra* complex and the right side of her body is now potentiated in the primary process (where the links do not have any logical structure but are connected more irrationally). Her hysterical conversion reaction involving a right arm monoparesis now becomes explicable.

Freud (1921/1985) confidently asserted that hysteria and the other neuroses 'are psychogenic and depend upon the operation of unconscious (repressed) ideational complexes' (p. 38). The fabricated example (not one of Freud's) illustrates an important thesis detaching hysteria from actual sexual and particularly incestuous events; 'A hysterical symptom is based upon a phantasy instead of upon a repetition of a real experience' (Freud, 1921/1985). Freud argues that phantasies, associated with the traditional libidinal complexes, create material for repetition (or psychic revisitation) in much the same way as disturbing and conflictful memories of actual events (as noted in the discussions of the unconscious and of repressed memories).

An actual case discussed by Freud serves to introduce Szasz's quite different conceptualization:

> Supposing that a little girl (and we will keep to her for the present) develops the same painful symptom as her mother—for instance, the same tormenting cough. This may come about in various ways. The identification might come from the Oedipal complex; in that case, it signifies a hostile desire on the girl's part to take her mother's place, and the symptom expresses her object-love towards her father, and brings about a realization, under the influence of some guilt, of her desire to take her mother's place: 'You wanted to be your mother and now you are—anyhow, so far as your sufferings are concerned.' This is the complete mechanism of the structure of a hysterical symptom.
>
> (Freud, 1921/1985, p. 136)

Freud discusses a young woman who actually imitated her father's cough so that 'identification has appeared instead of object choice', a case that seems made for Szasz's analysis.

Szasz: it's all in the game

Thomas Szasz likens hysteria to a game in which a type of role playing according to well-known rules is a response to an impossible moral and social situation. He thus renders hysteria as a discursive and interpersonal production appearing as a bodily affliction bringing one under the discursive rules (replete with social expectations) normally (and normatively) applied to illness.

'Under the new rules, however, persons disabled by phenomena which only look like illnesses of the body (i.e. hysteria) will also be classified as ill—that is, mentally ill—and they will be treated by the same rules that apply to persons who are bodily ill' (Szasz, 1962/1972, p. 54). To the problems surrounding a decision about how to respond to the person who acts as if ill, Freud added the possibility that the person himself could be caused (by unconscious forces) to react as he did so as not to be regarded justly (or even truly) as responsible for his situation. Szasz acknowledges the moral problem of conversion reactions for caring and compassionate professionals but deconstructs it to look at the discursive moves made by the individuals concerned and the agendas served by them. 'The premise that the behaviour of persons said to be mentally ill is meaningful and goal-directed—provided one is able to understand the patient's behaviour from his particular point of view—underlies all rational psychotherapies' (Szasz, 1962/1972, p. 73).

He examines Freud's treatment of a young woman with hysterical pains in the legs and disability evident in walking, noting the complex psychosocial situation surrounding the presentation, and suggests that the young woman was evincing a desperate psychological response to a difficult life crisis. Szasz (1962/1972) argues that 'the distinctive feature of hysteria is the substitution of a "bodily state" for communications by means of ordinary language concerning personal problems' (p. 102). For Szasz, the body expresses itself in a more basic and less rational way than ordinary language and appropriates the term *protolanguage* (cf. 'protofeminism' of hysterical protest [Showalter, 1987, p. 161]) to refer to signs conveying a message that is ambiguous, cathectic, or emotive (p. 115): 'one may readily express by means of protolanguage that which is not explicitly known or socially acknowledged' (p. 117). But how can a person convey something embedding a purpose or intention (e.g. to elicit help or sympathy for one's state) without knowing what one is doing? The answer, as Charcot, Freud, and Breuer suspected, lies in 'the unconscious'.

Szasz (1962/1972) argues that the patient's suffering is translated into a bodily sign according to an informal game or set of rules governing human exchanges around the issues of suffering or illness; thus, '[t]he principal informative use of a typical hysterical body sign ... is to communicate to the recipient of the message that the sender is disabled' (p. 121). He calls such language *promotive*.

> By communicating through such symptoms as headache, backache, or menstrual pains, a housewife who feels overburdened or dissatisfied with her life may be able to make her husband more attentive and helpful ... This action inducing meaning of iconic body signs may be paraphrased as follows: ('I am sick therefore ...) Take care of me!' ... 'Be good to me!' ... And so forth.
>
> (Szasz, 1962/1972, p. 126)

Szasz (1962/1972) remarks on the fact that whereas verbal or linguistic symbols have an arbitrary connection with the objects and events signified, hysterical conversion symptoms and signs do not: 'Body signs portray—they literally present and represent—in exactly what way the sufferer considers himself sick' (p. 130).

He acknowledges that the connection is usually mediated by a 'symbol system' and that hysterical symptoms have a 'greater impact on the receiver than do communications framed in the idiom of polite conversation' (Szasz, 1962/1972, p. 141). The impact factor is both important and reminiscent of the insistence or immediacy (Kierkegaard) of the primary process (i.e. of the classical Ucs) because hysterical patients have desperate needs that must be disguised even as they are pressed on those who have to meet them: 'The point to remember is that the more injured and vulnerable a person's self-image, the greater will be his need to protect and bolster it' (p. 148).

Szasz's (1962/1972) final conclusion about hysterics seems harsh: 'The hysteric plays at being sick because he is afraid that, if he tried to participate competently in real-life activities, he would fail' (p. 249). But he softens when he acknowledges the ambiguities in hysterical self-knowledge.

> When it is said that the hysteric cannot afford to be aware of what he is doing—for if he were, he could no longer do it—what is asserted in effect is that he cannot afford to tell himself the truth. By the same token, he also cannot afford to know that he is lying. He must lie both to himself and others. (p. 227)

Our psychosomatic unity is nowhere more clearly revealed than when the hysterical patient's dual needs—to maintain self-respect in an impossible life situation and to express disempowerment—produce the bodily signs of illness in ways that bypass reflective self-knowledge.

Showalter: the body speaks when the person cannot

We have encountered the moral protest of anorexia mounted by a young woman with prodigious powers of self-control, but in hysteria we can trace a similar meaning differently incarnated. She remarks that there is a sense in which psychoanalysis is 'the child of the hysterical woman' literally creating out of the union of suffering and unspeakability the doctrine of the unconscious mind and its ideational contents (Showalter, 1987, p. 147). Charcot and his colleagues, she argues could, if so inclined, have heard the messages that his patients were trying to convey; of the famous Augustine, she remarks, 'they might have predicted that she would eventually have run away' (p. 154), but instead Charcot pronounces, with the incontestability of the clinical ringmaster, 'you see how hysterics shout . . . much ado about nothing' (the Shakespeare is apposite). The language that speaks when speech is impossible (as in Dora's 'complete loss of voice' [p. 159]) was, however, not completely ignored by the time psychoanalysis developed the 'talking cure'.

> Freud and Breuer saw the repetitive domestic routines, including needlework, knitting, playing scales, and sickbed nursing, to which bright women were frequently confined as the causes of hysterical sickness.
>
> (Showalter, 1987, p. 158)

Nevertheless, despite the recognition of aspects of the suffering in interpersonal and other woes,

> Freud failed Dora because he was too quick to impose his own language on her mute communications. His insistence on the sexual origins of hysteria blinded him to the social factors contributing to it.
>
> (Showalter, 1987, p. 160)

Was it onanism or oneirism that led Freud to his synthesis, one might ask, and is it the same or a resulting blindness that leads to a medicalization of 'the self-destructive and self-enclosed strategies of hysteria' (p. 161)? Perhaps, we need to pursue 'the germ of a vastly broadened conception of trauma . . . including snatches of conversation, or little scenes of the apparently most innocuous sort but able to light up thoughts and feelings' (Havens, 1966, p. 516).

12.4 Gains

The hysterical patient gains from the conversion symptoms, usually in terms of relaxed expectations and demands on him or her but often also in terms of extraordinary levels of attention and care forthcoming from others. One young woman, for instance, had a mysterious painful paralysis of her legs and, when assessed, her sickroom had become the centre of family life. The entire family focus had shifted from the living rooms into her space and everything happened there, including meals, watching the family television, household tasks such as ironing and folding of the washing, and so on, so that this young woman's need had so transformed the family's universe of discourse that it axially centered on her.

The cost of this gain is considerable because 'the tactic of dominating others by displaying helplessness cannot be maintained unaltered in the face of a high degree of competence in important areas of life' (Szasz, 1962/1972, p. 240). The hysteric is, therefore, always a pathetic figure whose life skills are extremely underdeveloped and not conducive to what normally counts as success in interpersonal, occupational, or social spheres. That puts the hysterical patient at risk and makes him or her vulnerable, not only if unaided but also if, perchance, unmasked. The anxiety, desperation, and conflict hovering around this delicate intersubjective artifice, despite *la belle indifference*, are revealed by autonomic arousal studies of the disorder.

> By and large, such persons impersonate the roles of helplessness, hopelessness, weakness, and often of bodily illness—when, in fact, their actual roles pertain to frustrations, unhappiness, and perplexities due to interpersonal, social, and ethical conflicts.
>
> (Szasz, 1962/1972, p. 233)

How can a person so effectively produce the moves and responses perpetuating the gain without any apparent cognizance of what they are doing? The contrast between hysteria and malingering rests on a convincing answer to this question.

12.5 Meaning and communication: discursive and subdiscursive constructions

The analysis of 'meaningful connections' (Jaspers) between behaviour (or bodily signs) and the psyche is at the centre of an understanding of hysteria and redirects our attention to meaning and the connections between signifiers, signification, and the body.

Words play a central (and validated) role in the ways that human beings confer significance on the events and things around them; they focus and direct our attention to things that happen to us, casting those events into the light of the reality principle that provides a structure framing one's mental life, replete with a certain 'cognitive style', a network of beliefs and dispositions, and a set of memories. Our words inform our thoughts and attitudes and are the currency or, better, the overt currency of most of our relationships. The 'situations in which the use of our language is taught and learnt' (Quinton, 1955, p. 51)—interpersonal situations—are the basis of our intelligible (or legitimated) understanding of self and world so that experience is replete with emotive or cathectic resonance. The intersubjectivity of one's valued relationships therefore pervades perception, knowledge, and beliefs about one's (psychosomatic) being-in-the-world-with-others.

One's reactions to events and situations are both articulate and inarticulate. The inarticulate aspects are not captured by a person's autobiographical narrative because they evade the discursive techniques available to him or her, those techniques that allow people to comprehend and develop conscious strategies to deal with the moral and interpersonal challenges facing them. Such techniques are not merely intellectual but also productive, participating in the development of life skills and reflective strategies for their improvement. Therefore, as Freud suspected on the basis that the line between Ucs and Pcs/Cs is drawn by language, words and their use (or non-use) are a key to unravelling the issues surrounding hysteria, and the articulation of experience characteristic of hysterical patients is an important clue to its peculiar and effaced (indeed marginalized) phenomenology.

12.6 Hysteria as a way of thinking and acting

Hysteria is marked by a distinctive 'cognitive style' that interacts significantly with the social and interpersonal factors increasingly implicated in its genesis. First, hysteria tends to occur in people with wandering minds rather than wandering wombs. Shapiro (1965) observes that the psychological or cognitive characteristics of hysterical patients 'are aspects of a general mode of cognition. The first of these is the hysterical incapacity for persistent or intense intellectual concentration; the second is the distractability or impressionability that follows from it; and the third is the non-factual world in which the hysterical person lives' (p. 113). These features, taken singly or in combination, indicate a lack of certain discursive skills at work when the person characterizes and then responds to things that happen. They are the skills that take meanings and map one's experiences on to them in a way that fits with the anticipations, articulations, and action schemata structuring one's lived narrative.

> When a hysterical person is asked to describe someone else, the response is likely to be something like 'Oh he's so big!' or 'She's wonderful!' or 'I hate him!' . . . When one asks a question of a hysterical person, in other words, one is likely to get for an answer not facts but impressions. These impressions may be interesting and communicative, and they are often very vivid, but they remain impressions—not detailed, not quite sharply defined, and certainly not technical.
>
> (Shapiro, 1965, p. 111)

The hysterical style is *impressionistic* so that 'the hunch or the impression is the final, conscious cognitive product' (Shapiro, 1965, p. 114) and there is an associated *impressionability* about hysterical thought (note Janet's 'suggestibility' [Havens, 1966, p. 513]); 'this style of cognition makes for great susceptibility to that which is vivid, striking, or forcefully presented' (p. 115). As a result of the poor reflective skills and tendency to be impressed without detailed enquiry or examination, 'hysterical people are often remarkably deficient in knowledge' about 'general factual information' (p. 116). Shapiro (1965) argues that these three features imply that the hysterical mind tends towards 'not seeing a highly and uncomfortably charged fact or, more accurately, not bringing into clear, sharp focus of attention that which may be dimly or peripherally experienced as uncomfortable' (p. 117). Already one begins to suspect that negative or painful features of a hysterical person's experience can 'lurk' relatively unexplored and implicit in the twilight of explicit consciousness.

This cognitive deficiency is conjoined to a second feature of hysterical subjectivity, its 'romantic and sentimental' quality, a tendency to think stereotypically : partners or love objects are all things good and wonderful; opponents are bad, frightening, and revolting; and illnesses are always devastating, intense, or desperately serious. This slightly unreal or unbalanced presentation of a hysterical or conversion syndrome, its 'theatrical or play acting quality' (Shapiro, 1965, p. 119), relates to hysterical romanticism, a dramatic quality of conversion reactions that makes crusty and relatively red-necked clinicians 'see red' in that nothing could be calculated to be more irritating to the straight, often judgemental cast of certain medical minds.

These features of hysterical cognition help explain the puzzling ignorance of the patients about their own disorder so that 'as flagrant as the play-acting or dramatic exaggerations of hysterical people may sometimes be, these people do not seem simply insincere' (Shapiro, 1965, p. 120). 'The capacity of hysterical people to become so ungenuine without being aware that they are so is quite striking and it seems to reflect the nature of their relationship to reality and to matters of fact in general' (p. 120). The mismatch between appearance and reality is not easy to accept especially when, transparent as the implausibility of the symptoms might be and try as one might to offer such patients a more realistic characterization of their ills, the (apparently sincere) pathological farce goes on, sometimes obscuring the real pathology underlying it.

The hysteric clearly has a great deal invested in the pathetic presentation (as Szasz notices) and the deficient life skills make it impossible to wean them from the immature coercion of those who care for them. The combination of self-indulgently romantic conceptions of one's emotional life, poorly focused cognitive techniques, impressionistic and impressionable modes of relating to new experience, and self-dramatization are a potent enough set of antecedents to explain the genesis of a conversion reaction out of 'an accident, some external event . . . experienced as a traumatism' (Havens, 1966, p. 507) or 'predicament from which all other avenues [are] blocked' (Leslie, 1988, p. 506) and to distinguish it from deliberate pretence or malingering.

The famous *la belle indifference*, the 'attitude that it doesn't really count' or 'a lack of awareness of the seriousness of things' (Shapiro, 1965, p. 124), is plausibly linked to a deep-seated but inarticulate awareness that 'this is not serious' because it is inarticulate; it is not open to reflexive scrutiny so as to reveal that 'I have brought this about and am getting the following gains from it.' Despite the emotional disconnect between the indifference or even cheerfulness and the paralysis, blindness, or severe neurological deficits affecting the patient, the cognitive fuzziness makes it so unlike a pretence that a doctor is often genuinely puzzled as to how to react.

The puzzlement is reflected in the fact that hysterics are often misdiagnosed as having dread diseases they do not have, or discounted as 'putting it all on' so that real pathological conditions are overlooked. The hysterical style often results in a vague, impressionistic history with overindulgent and often circumstantial digressions that render the actual history and symptomatology so unclear as to make diagnosis a very difficult task. Often, the story is not well articulated and it is only by dint of creative and shrewd 'reading between the lines' of the dramatized, disturbing, and implausible presentation that the genesis of the problem or the real pathology underlying the conversion reaction can be suspected and elucidated.

The stereotype that hysterics are malingering or faking is fuelled by the *secondary gain* produced by the syndrome. It may allow the patient to escape a difficult situation, to deflect or avoid punishment or retribution, to obtain compensation, or defuse stress and conflict. The 'lack of insight' into the real nature of the suffering may also affect the hysterical patient's pickup of the cues and signals from the clinician that 'the game is up'. The mind of the hysteric has a slightly 'flakey', approximate, and inexplicit understanding of human exchanges that do not match the complex self-constructions despite her or his acute sensitivity to the emotional and relational nuances of any move that threatens the intricate and quasi-stable structure.

The neurophilosophy, such as it is, of hysteria helps delineate the contours of this puzzle.

12.7 **Neuroscientific findings**

A neo-Aristostelian account of a disorder of the mind thrives on the combination of philosophical argument and a keen eye for significant findings about brain anomalies in affected patients. Normal subjects show a characteristic orienting response to a novel stimulus. Such responses are detected by averaging electroencephalograph (EEG) recordings (as in any other cerebral evoked activity) and normally habituate or diminish once the stimulus begins to lose its novelty. However, among patients with conversion symptoms, other stigmata of hysterical disorder, or a history of presentations with hysterical conversion reactions, 'the majority showed no tendency to habituate' (Meares et al., 1985, p. 261). What is more, the extraverted personality type most prone to develop hysteria showed an accentuated set of late (attention-related) components in sensory evoked potential studies (Friedman & Meares, 1979), similar to auditory evoked potentials in cases of functional hearing loss (Fukuda et al., 1996), all findings related to the attention systems of the brain.

The attention systems make a stimulus, usually with a strong emotive loading and a low epicritic (or articulated, cognitively elaborated) profile, salient and accessible for interconnections in the cortical networks. There are immediate links between this neurophysiological anomaly and the cognitive anomalies of hysteria in that signals that would normally take a 'normal' or smoothly integrated and elaborated place in cortical activity remain unduly salient in the brain activity of hysteria-prone individuals similar to novel or unfamiliar stimuli the information content of which has yet to be articulated within the processing structures that define its significance for the organism. The hysteric, we could say, cannot relativize and moderate the impact of stimuli in the light of previous learning experience in terms of the balanced processing equilibrium that results from collating current inputs with other cues and connections. This collation or moderation of the effects of an input is part of delineating the significance of events.

The finding of electrophysiological abnormalities of this kind in hysteria is reminiscent of the aberrations of brain function in sociopathic personalities (Howard, 1986) where there are defective premotor or readiness potentials established in the frontal cortex. I argued that this defect is related to the psychopath's inability to fine-tune (or articulate) his responses relative to complex prudential, social, and moral considerations (or positive and negative contingencies of responding). Patients classified as having a sociopathic personality disorder (psychopaths) are, in fact, more prone to present with hysterical conversion reactions, suggesting that in both groups we have immaturity of the discursive techniques by which human beings adapt their behaviour to the human life-world. The relevant techniques depend, at a neurophysiological level, on well-integrated processing pathways (but the anomalies are slightly different in each case and different again in the unselective association of psychosis).

The sociopathic personality type is bad at playing according to the rules that pervade interpersonal situations because he or she does not appreciate the relatively subtle moral, evaluative, or other-regarding resonances of his or her actions (he or she cannot moderate them in the light of their effect on the feelings of others). Psychopaths characteristically have deficient frontolimbic systems, the brain systems that register negative contingencies and affect the action structuring essential in skilled rule-following behaviour attuned to certain (non-obvious) constraints (including long-term, removed, and complex outcomes and the interests and feelings of others). The psychopath therefore acts in ignorance of other-regarding and prudential consider-ations but may be clever in terms of self-centered intellectual strategies (in Aristotle's terms).

The hysteric is different in that, along with a possible insensitivity to the needs of others, they have an intense and overdramatized awareness of the emotive significance of situations for themselves, but it is not clearly and distinctly articulated in terms of the details of a current challenge or situation. *Ex hypothesi*, this is because their general attentional mechanisms are hit and miss and not finely attuned to actuality (according to the reality principle rather than psychic salience or wish fulfilment) so that their interpersonal and social skills are imprecise, impressionistic, and unstable and they are as approximate in their reactions to practical and complex social situations as in their general cognition (and in their self-awareness).

A neuropsychophilosophical synthesis of these strands of thought elucidates hyste-ria and the related conditions of somatization, malingering, and factitious disorder, thereby generating a more sensitive understanding of psychic disorder than that of the disease model.

12.8 A neuropsychophilosophical perspective on hysteria

Janet (1901/1983), following in a tradition of distinguished physician philosophers, sketched a diagnostic account of hysteria focused on the type of personality that pre-disposes to hysteria and the need to explain the 'mental states' involved. He consid-ered that the hysterical person was 'often very humble, incapable of doing anything, discouraged by trifles, and diffident', perhaps a reflection on the sociopolitical status of his patients (p. 213).

He noted the stereotyped symptoms involving loss of neurological function caused by factors in the unconscious precipitated by 'psychic conflict' and based his account on Kant's 'synthesis', a term that denotes the integration of a sensory presentation into a conceptual representation apt to contribute to knowledge (Kant, 1789/1929). Janet noted that the hysteric had feeble powers of cognitive differentiation and integration and was poor at fixing attention and attaining a clear synthesis of events so as to yield veridi-cal experience (Janet, 1901/1983). As an active, intelligent operation of the rational, rule-governed mind, synthesis used logicomathematical laws of construction awakened by experience to structure the experiences of the thinker in terms of ordered mental content providing articulate knowledge of what was happening around him or her. But Kant is often thought to neglect 'the social character of our concepts, the links between thought and speech, speech and communication, communication and social communities' (Strawson, 1966, p. 151), and the current account aims to correct that oversight.

The corrective strand of cognitive and developmental psychology derives from Vygotsky (1962/1929), and is continued by Bruner (1990), Donaldson (1979), and Bower (1977). In neuropsychology, Luria (Vygotsky's pupil) has incorporated the social character of cognition into our understanding of human psychology and its aberrations (Luria, 1973, 1976) by arguing that meanings—the ways in which we classify, refer to, and think about things—structure cognitive processing thereby representing a (shared, cultural) resource used by an individual to make sense of his or her world. The current account of consciousness articulates experience in terms of concepts that enable reflection and evaluation using discursive techniques based on individual capacities that have been conveyed and refined intersubjectively and interpersonally.

In developmental psychology, Vygotsky and his followers have provided strong empirical evidence and Wittgenstein (1953), in philosophy, has argued that natural language orders and structures the cognitive life of a human individual (Karmiloff-Smith, 1986). Lacan relates signification and the signifiers available to the subject to the 'mirror world' in which each of us develops an *imago* (image-ego) that helps us build an awareness of our own mental lives. Hysteria forces us to consider the skills and the style of this productive process and the many potential influences that can disrupt it. A hysterical thinker uses the discursive skills that are made available through language sloppily or impulsively and is markedly affected by emotional associations with information. Thus, even if the social milieu has a shaping (reality-imparting) role in cognition and rules (and techniques of applying them to one's psyche), potentiating self-reflection and self-knowledge as part of that milieu, the hysterical style is not suited to overcome *meconnaissance* and its distortions of the *imago* (Glowinski et al., 2001). The hysterical thinker, similar to any other, signifies the moments of his or her subjectivity through the medium of language and its powers but cannot achieve clear thought about his or her being in the world as an embodied subject. Thus, the aim of signification—to structure the content of experience so that it is fit for adaptive activity—is thwarted.

The child both figuratively and literally *internalizes* language as a tool for inscribing the events of a life on and within the body and psyche. The raw materials of one's encounters with the world are thereby transformed into psychologically informed responses, reactions, and habits of behaving manifest to and comprehensible by others. That process configures brain processing networks away from instinctive and relatively rigid adaptive responses to the environment towards cognitive plasticity and culturally mediated activity. Meaning is inscribed in the body through the brain systems subserving complex recognitional and adaptive activity replete with (acknowledged, validated, valorized) significance. Thus, 'language is to thought what a catalyst is to a chemical reaction: it starts it, speeds it up, facilitates the progression of a process that would go extremely slowly or perhaps not at all without it' (Beadle, 1970, p. 163). As one's language and thought take shape, so the world and its furniture become intelligible and one's behaviour increasingly shows articulated intelligence and purpose

(Luria, 1973, p. 93ff) forged in the fires (warming and searing) of interpersonal relationships (as seen so clearly in relation to autism and epistemic development).

What is more, the many possible translations (narrative transformations) of one's being in the world to one's lived experience are, for a human being, socially mediated and discursively structured in ways that reflect our relations (of dependence and mutual evaluation) with others.

Hysterical thinking structures experience badly so that one cannot deal with emotions and moral conflicts in a mature or constructive way. The patient has failed at key points to moderate his or her hyperreactive, imprecise, impressionistic, and romantic narrative and integrate that story into an adaptive orientation towards the world. Life therefore becomes 'too much' and adaptive techniques are foregone in favour of a relatively primitive and urgent cry for help. This is the meaning of hysteria: 'I am helpless; life is crowding in on me. Rescue me!'

A hysterical person makes moves in the game of life that are immature and dependent and these can often be related to social and personal influences directly affecting his or her reports and evaluations of bodily and psychic events. Deficiencies in self-articulation explain why his or her needs become expressed to others in melodramatic, coercive, or somatic form although the descriptions used are implausible and unbalanced. The patient may neither be consciously insincere nor calculated and manipulative (unlike the malingerer) but rather unable to present to others his or her real needs and worries. The lack of a biological 'punch' or urgency to his or her distress is manifest as *la belle indifférence* and doctors lose sight of the real ills of an hysteric amidst his or her general tendency to make use of inappropriate cues and meanings to express his or her cry for help.

The hysterical psyche may evince poorly developed skills of self-understanding quite possibly related to detectable changes in brain processing, but even in the transient case the person presents as needy or vulnerable by using dramatic and manipulative devices such as resorting to the 'sick role', 'coma', 'amnesia or loss of identity', and so on. Such overblown presentations are not the 'canny' competence of a duplicitous fraud but rather outrageous and patently false so that one notices the secondary gains and feels manipulated. As Janet realized, the person is *impaired* but not in the somatic way depicted and perhaps not in any way that he or she clearly understands.

Those cognitive competencies that transform self (brain)–world transactions into conscious experience are not well organized or articulated in hysteria so that the meanings or significances of what befall one do not potentiate socially adaptive coping strategies and instead provoke desperate measures designed to elicit crude responses from others such as sympathy, protectiveness, and paternalistic indulgence, more appropriate for children than adults. Thus, the hysterical conversion reaction is a product of conferring concrete, immature, and inappropriate meanings on one's situation that are ineptly enacted but vitally related to deficiently articulated and cognized needs affecting the patient's well-being.

12.9 Hysteria and the philosophical puzzles surrounding it

Psychopathology in general is a domain of phenomena where cognitive skills are distorted and the human stance straddling the gap between the world of meaning (the mirror world) and the actual, causal, somatic world is twisted. The distortion may be explained by a biochemical aberration or by a lived experience strained beyond sustainability by forces at work in the meaning-giving milieu shaping the psyche. The brain is a final common path for the genesis and expression of psychic disorder, faithfully reflecting, in its own ramified, plastic, and therefore highly creative way, our engagement in the human life-world. Clinical psychiatry, through diagnosis and intervention, needs to attend to the duality of meaning and cause inherent in the human psyche as was illustrated in the case of Robert.

Robert became severely disabled, presenting in clinic in a wheelchair and capable only of minimal and painful movements of his paralyzed limbs. Every achievement in Robert's life is a minor act of heroism. If he cut the wood with a chainsaw, that was an amazing feat for a man in his condition. If he succeeded at ordinary tasks during physiotherapy, that also was commendable. His disability transformed ordinary living into a noble endeavour against great adversity. Did he know how much he could move his limbs? How much pain did he really get when he tried to move his arm? If you were to hold your arm flexed and your hands clenched for hours at a time, how good would you be at discerning these things? If your posture is abnormal and uncomfortable so that you stiffen up, how good are you at telling the difference between psychically created disability and genuine muscle cramps? These questions pose a significant challenge to self-knowledge and clarity about one's body and the faculties required are exactly those faculties deficient in hysteria. I do not know if Robert had any clarity in his mind about those things and about the very significant gains that arose from his disability; I do not think he did either, but it did all become too much for him and he committed suicide as a result.

The philosophical puzzles are therefore not only intriguing but have a sharp clinical edge.

(12.1) The self-deception puzzle

(12.1.1) A hysterical patient produces his or her conversion symptoms.

(12.1.2) A mental phenomenon produced by a subject is introspectively known to be so.

(12.1.3) A hysteric does not know that he or she has produced his or her symptoms.

This puzzle is resolved by modifying 2 and inserting the following premises:

(12.1.2a) Understanding the genesis of an experience is a reflective skill called self-understanding.

(12.1.2b) A person can be good or bad at such discursive skills.

(12.1.2c) The articulation of bodily states and their genesis depends on well-developed self-understanding.

(12.1.2d) The hysterical patient has poorly developed self-understanding.

(12.1.2e) Hysterical self-knowledge is poor.

A hysterical patient may therefore not know whether his or her symptoms are psychically or physically produced and, because of their general cognitive immaturity, may have little idea how to overcome them and through what physical, or even spiritual, process of healing.

(12.2) The subconscious gain puzzle

(12.2.1) A hysterical patient achieves certain gains through his or her conversion reaction.

(12.2.2) To achieve gains, we must aim at them.

(12.2.3) Aiming at something means adopting means–ends reasoning to achieve it.

(12.2.4) Means–ends reasoning must focus on (have a clear idea of) the gain it aims at.

(12.2.5) The hysterical patient does not seem to be consciously aiming at certain gains.

2 seems false given the fuzzy and ill-focused thinking characteristic of the hysterical style of cognition. Hysterical unclarity about one's psychic life may therefore extend to the connection between certain behaviour and the gains it produces. Thus, hysterical patients may not use means–ends reasoning to achieve the gains they make from their behaviour.

Being human engages us in a world of meanings and values, and a world articulated by discourse and this potentially schizoid existence is normally negotiated by the discursive skills we learn to master in a good-enough upbringing. In fact, we are all prone to the deficiencies in self-understanding writ large in the hysterical psyche, as is quite evident in the psychopathologies of everyday life that are the topic of my penultimate chapter.

Chapter 13

The pathologies of each are the pathologies of all

I am travelling to my grandmother's place and I find as I drive that there is a street, Anders Road, one block away from her place, which I am reluctant to drive into. Even looking at Anders Road makes me feel vaguely uncomfortable as if 'I don't like that street.' But it is a street like any other and I can think of no reason not to enter it. As it happens, it is not essential or even particularly on my route to go into Anders Road and so I carry on.

I am chatting to my grandmother over coffee and mention my discomfort about Anders Road. My grandmother then tells me that when I was a very young child she was walking me along Anders Road. As we walked, a dog rushed out at me barking. It was much larger than me and gave me a real fright, causing me to clutch on to her dress screaming and sobbing. Ever since that time, even when I was a child, I would not let her take me into Anders Road. This was all forty years ago.

I drive back past the street to go home now with the conscious knowledge that the dog is dead and that any fear I might feel is completely irrational. I somewhat naively expect that, the ghost having been laid, I will feel no fear but know perfectly well in my heart of hearts that it is not true. Of course, it is not true. I still do not like that street and still feel reluctant to go down it.

This story provokes thoughts about the many inchoate and ill-understood aversions, attractions, impulsive thoughts, and so on that affect each of us every day. The story also suggests that insight does not overcome the source of disquiet. I knew the dog to be dead, but that did not cure my subconscious fear because personal transformation requires psychological restructuring that may not be rational or conscious at all but rather a deep communication that you are OK no matter what gears are clashing in the psyche.

In this chapter, I will uncover some of the pathologies of reason and action that afflict every one of us at various times in our normal working life, and although they draw extensively on neurosurgery, the examples are not so remote from similar situations in many walks of life encountered by other than neurosurgeons. I will touch on akrasia or weakness of the will, self-deception, losing one's temper, defense mechanisms, feelings of inadequacy, and hostility to the self, and even slips of the tongue.

Throughout this minitour of the psychopathologies of everyday life, the fact that one's psyche is articulated by discourse operating through one's social and interpersonal relations is an underlying theme structuring the whole and uniting 'us normal folks' with the 'poor unfortunates' who suffer 'maladies of the soul'.

13.1 **The heat of the moment**

Philosophers often discuss the overwhelming of reason by passion or of moral decency by a rush of fleshly appetite and explain many of our failings and weaknesses this way. Some elevate this framework into a whole context of life whereby the flesh (or Satan through the flesh) must be opposed and resisted at every turn. A well-known comedy sketch depicts the African-American wife of a fundamentalist pastor coming home from a shopping spree and switching on the 'The devil made me do it' routine.

> I was jus' walkin' down the street mindin' ma own bisness and then that Debbil he grabs me and he sez 'Go inta that shop!'; that ol' Debbil he jus' drags me inta that shop. And I is sayin' ta him, 'Debbil I cain't go in dis shop becos' we cain't afford none o' them dresses.' And he jus' pushes me over to that rack of purty dresses and he sez, 'Go on now, you try on dat dress.' An so I sez ta him, 'Get thee behind me Satan,' jus' like the Good Lord, but he don' do that thing, he jus' makes me try on that dress. An nex' thing I know I's jus' buyin' that dress and thinkin at leas' that Debbil gone way now, but no! I's jus' walkin' pass that shoe shop an' again he jus' grabs me an' I sez 'Don' you make me go in here you Debbil.' But it ain't no use. ... An' so I's goin' pass that hat shop.

Here, a set of impulses subvert what the agent feels, all things considered, to be the best thing for her to do in the long term. (Or, perhaps, she is making a statement about her husband's miserly ways and her value and image as a woman.) What exactly did happen in her mind during her shopping spree? Is her story further evidence for the indeterminacy of subconscious mental content aside from the narrative endorsed by the agent? Do we see a set of 'impulses' (demonic thoughts) that, according to her, overwhelm her reason and cause her to behave thus and so or do we see an aspect of the self, unable to be endorsed by the self of discourse, unsettling her legitimate (Godly) self-control?

This can happen even in clinical life. It happens to surgeons who lose their tempers (other fleshly appetites prevail more commonly in such callings as psychiatry and general practice). It may seem incredible that a surgeon should lose his or her temper, particularly during an operation, and to be fair, I have not yet struck a female surgeon who has. But I have seen male surgeons do just that, even throw instruments on the floor like a child in a tantrum, shout at a scrub nurse until she was so upset she had to leave the operating theatre, and unbelievable as it may seem, treat a registrar in such a way that the registrar has 'downed tools' and left. Without doubt, the surgeon would not, in his perfect mind, choose to act this way or defend such behaviour in another (otherwise, the picture of defence and denial would be complete). But why are we prone to these immoderate moments; are they best thought of as 'the beast within' escaping, as in Freud's picture or is there another synthesis available?

Most surgeons (of a 'choleric' stripe) admit that their behaviour was not ideal in such moments and apologize afterwards even though some may not actively seek the opportunity to do so. Most realize that their behaviour was inexcusable, acknowledge that fact, and try to make amends (even though the right moments are *so* hard to find). But what are the origins of 'the heat of the moment'; are they 'the beast within'?

A professional who 'loses it' is often facing impossible conflicting demands.

> Mr. A has promised his wife to be home at 6 p.m. for his dinner guests at 8 p.m. At 5 p.m., he has one case to do, an anterior cervical discectomy; all being well, he will do it in time even if he has to get the registrar to sew up. That thought prompts an association with his discussion of the case with the registrar the day before when he said the registrar could do the case. He knows that if that happens, the case takes one and a half to two hours instead of about one hour. He feels bad about disappointing his registrar, but he cannot contemplate facing his wife yet again an hour later than when he said he would be home. He knows that a convoluted and inevitably lame-sounding excuse about promising the registrar that she could do the operation will lead to the 'You always put other people before me' bit, which he finds so disturbing (because it has a grain of truth in it). He decides to do the case himself, feeling very guilty. He is now in a no-win situation and feels disgruntled and off his mettle. The anaesthetist takes a little longer than usual (not a problem in other situations, but here critical in finishing at approximately 6 p.m. rather than 6.30).The nurse is not his regular scrub nurse, who has had to go home to her daughter's birthday party at 4 p.m. The dissection goes well, notwithstanding the guilt he feels, apart from one blood vessel inadvertently cut because of haste but not in itself important except for the three minutes it wastes trying to control and deal with it. The registrar is the model of politeness, but one can hear the self-control and disappointment in her voice. The X-rays to check the level of operation take ages—but show that he is at the correct level in the neck. The disc removal goes well except for the fact that he prangs another little vessel postero-lateral to the disc and can't control the bleeding. The sucker is, at this crucial point, allowed to waver from the critical area of work and he erupts at his registrar, 'Can't you hold the bloody sucker in the right place, I can't see anything.'

A peccadillo one might say. Requiring only an apologetic word and an explanation but, in view of the pressure, the word is not spoken as the surgeon leaves the theatre to rush off home. He feels guilty all night and arrives grumpy and aggrieved the next day.

Note the genesis of this problem: a deep commitment by Mr. A to not disappointing his wife yet again; a conflicting value to do the right thing by the registrar in training; no way of resolving the conflicting demands; and lastly, some, in themselves, minor events that disrupt a delicately poised plan of action. Some of these factors concern fundamental commitments and ways that he feels about himself; they all touch on the sources of the self and his engagement in a complex discursive situation. Perhaps, he has been working hard to transform himself from an uncaring, career-driven, and inconsiderate husband to being a caring partner for his wife. At a stroke, a great deal of the good work in this project close to his heart is undone, not by anybody or anything malign. His registrar, who may have a partner of her own, gets the backlash of his conflicted self because she is the nearest available target (and perhaps because women are always targets as the embodiments of many of the demands men construct and experience). But note that 'the beast within', rearing its head in the heat of the moment, is not a force produced by a primitive level of his psyche; it is a product of his highly civilized plans and moral engagements. The beast within may have aggregated cathectic energy, but it is, in a very real sense, a social product of the human (cultural) life-world.

Thus, the first form of action failure—hot akrasia—though beastly in its force and crude in its manifestation, is produced by a conflict only explicable by appealing to some of the most complex significations realized in Mr. A's brain. As is typical of the discontents of the mind, his failure is irreducibly complex and results from a conflicted entanglement of meanings and commitments in his life-world rather than being produced by a simple opposition between the primal and the civilized facets of his being. 'The heat of the moment', despite its primal aspects, shows us that sometimes the skills we acquire through immersion in social and interpersonal reality are insufficient to deal with the forces operating on us within that same milieu.

But akrasia, incontinence, or failure of action also comes in a 'cold' variety with a philosophical history stretching back to Plato and Aristotle. Both puzzled over the fact that an agent could sometimes act in a way that he or she knew he should not, all things considered, and many contemporary discussions broaden the scope to include all types of irrationality, both failures of right action and failures of right belief.

13.2 **Cold akrasia**

Akrasia, weakness of the will, or practical incontinence is what all of us show when, for no apparent reason, we do what we know we should not. Aristotle notes that the incontinent man cannot benefit by reason because even though he knows and sincerely affirms the reasons he should act on, he still does what he knows he should not so that he lacks *phronesis* (or practical wisdom), the ability to act on his best reasons all things considered. Practical wisdom, for Aristotle, arises from training whereby one learns to respond well to a range of situations. In some situations, one mimics the conduct of a wise teacher, and in others, one follows his or her instructions or corrections of one's previous responses. In either case, one develops self-control (or not, as in the failure of volition in psychopaths).

One's development as a moral agent under supervision and shaping of one's attitudes and actions enables one to act according to one's best reasons (all things considered) and also to have sufficient self-control to (most of the time) negotiate the heat of the moment. The *akratic*, however, knows what he ought to do and say, and all the reasons why he ought to do and say that thing, but does not do it. Therefore, further reasoning is of no avail because, as Aristotle so nicely puts it, 'If water makes a man choke, what can you give him to wash it down?' You cannot improve such a person by reasoning because he lacks a skill: his body is not disciplined so as to provide the right patterns of response and action. But does this kind of failure ever happen in clinical life?

Consider three different kinds of situations. The first (already discussed) is the flood of passion—the heat of the moment. The second is when one says, 'Why am I doing this operation?' and the third when one says, 'Why did I do that?' during an operation. The second, the intention I am enacting I cannot now endorse, is evident in everyday life when I realize that I am doing something that there is no good reason to do, such as eating a sticky pudding when I am already not only overweight but also full on that particular occasion and trying to keep my credit card expenditure within reasonable bounds. The third finds me realizing that I have just done something that I knew was foolish at the time but did not stop myself from doing it for long enough for the realization that it was foolish to sink in and get built into the control of my activity. What kind of being am I if I am prone to these failures of intention and action? And here, Davidson's discussion of weakness of the will and self-deception further illuminates the relation between mind or psyche and brain.

Davidson on irrationality and weakness of the will

Davidson's (1982) account has two essential elements: (i) the mind can create partitions between systems of mental states producing potentially conflicting intentions to act such that each system has 'a supporting structure of reasons, of interlocking beliefs, expectations, assumptions, attitudes, and desires' (p. 300); (ii) reason may or may not 'cause what it is a sufficient reason for'. Once we accept that partitions can be produced, then it is a small step to accept that rational connections may hold within each division but not operate between them and the field is open for the production of actions (or intentions) not in accordance with one's all-things-considered-best-judgement (or lacking the best rational warrant). The problem in his account is the lack of explanation for partitions and the fact that it tends to buy into the psychic reification (the 'inner me full of states and events') that is metaphysically suspect. If we cannot explain how partitions occur, then it is unclear whether the partitions themselves have any explanatory force. How does the subject place thoughts and attitudes in different parts of the psyche so as to explain the actions and intentions that are irrationally generated as result or is this just a characterization at the functional level based on an inference to the best explanation of the type that we find in Freud's account and elsewhere? (Mele, 1987, p. 80).

Davidson's solution in terms of intrapsychic partitions distinguishes between prima-facie or conditional evaluative judgements and 'all-out' or unconditional evaluations, the things I have called all-things-considered-best-judgements (hereinafter, 'best judgements').

> Our 'best' judgements . . . could naturally be taken to be those conditioned by all the considerations deemed relevant by the agent; but action is geared to unconditional judgements. Since there is no principle of logic or psychological law that says we must

> trim our unconditional judgements of what is best to our best judgements, someone can judge, and act, contrary to his own best judgement. (1985 p. 201)

Between 'best' judgements and 'unconditional judgements', Davidson (1980) interposes a (second-order) 'principle of continence' to the effect that we should act only on our best judgements, but does not spell out whether this is merely a causal disposition (glossed that way to make the rational story work) or whether it actually has that explicit form.

> There is, I suggest, [a] . . . principle the rational man will accept in applying practical reasoning: perform the action judged best on the basis of all available reasons. It would be appropriate to call this the principle of continence. (p. 41)

The principle of continence implies that the undivided psyche will always act on the all-in best judgement and any divisions in the psyche make room for the posit that the reasons rationally or consciously dominant in the intrapsychic domain are not all the reasons affecting behaviour. Therefore, an apparent (as far as the present reasoning is concerned) best judgement may not be an all-in best judgement and the akratic action can result from that lesser 'best' judgement. But why reify all these explicit psychological states when they can so easily be disconnected from causal or explanatory efficacy? What is more, the phenomenologies of akrasia and self-deception imply that the overlooked reasons produce conflict so that, even if he knows all about his perfectly good reasons for not having the sticky date pudding and yet does it anyway, the agent does not feel good about it. What is more, In the case of self-deception, the agent's (negatively evaluated) belief (she does not love me anymore) often seems to be the very thing that makes him form (and defensively shore up) evidence for what he wants to believe (she is trying not to show that she really does love me but I see through her little game). If so, it must be engaged with the system forming the (self-deceptive) belief that is formed. His response to this phenomenology both illustrates Davidson's attitudes towards mind and brain and reinforces a variety of anti-realism about subconscious mental content.

Davidson (1980) argues that the reasons behind our actions cause those actions so that what we call reasons (or pro-attitudes) are in fact physical or brain states causing behaviour. But the (physical) descriptions that are the key to their causal efficacy and the laws governing them are not part of mental explanations (pp. 161–162) so that our reasons and our evaluations of them may not track the causal efficacy or strength of the states and events they pick out. 'There is no paradox in supposing a person sometimes holds that all that he believes and values supports a certain course of action, when at the same time those same beliefs and values cause him to reject that course of action' (p. 41).

Thus, 'in the case of incontinence, the attempt to read reason into behaviour is necessarily subject to a degree of frustration' (Davidson, 1980, p. 42) because the reasons and their rational persuasion may not be what is doing the work. Therefore, even though a surgeon may have good reasons not to do an operation on some occasion, he is caused to act otherwise by other motivations such as the desperate appeal of a manipulative patient.

Davidson (1986) has a parallel account of self-deception, again in terms of partitions in the mind (as in the case of akrasia, ultimately resting on the causal–rational distinction).

> It is now possible to suggest . . . where in the sequence of steps that end in self-deception there is an irrational step . . . What must be walled off from the rest of the mind is the requirement of total evidence. What causes it to be thus temporarily exiled or isolated is, of course, the desire to avoid accepting what the requirement counsels. But this cannot be a reason for neglecting the requirement. (p. 92)

The desire that p be true is, obviously, never a reason for believing p to be true because rational constraints proscribe the grounding of belief on wishes; to do otherwise is what we call wishful thinking (to which we will come shortly). Davidson again invokes the fact that states and events may cause outcomes which their rational descriptions would not warrant because they are causal states obeying certain causal laws. Thus, the desire that A should love me can *cause* me to develop a belief that reason would not support—<A does love me>—despite the fact that (causally inoperative) beliefs in another division of mind—<all the evidence indicates that A does not love me>—would, if attended to, defeat that project. Within each partition, rationality rules, but the mental states in question are partitioned off from each other. However, recall the phenomenology.

The beliefs and reasons concerned are formed because of their relations to one another: I persuade myself that A loves me and desperately reinterpret the evidence because, at some level, I know that she does not. Davidson must adopt the strategy of claiming that the true beliefs and the conflicting desires operate on belief formation because of their causal force rather than because of their content (which is neither fully operational nor rationally reflected in the trains of reasoning going on).

However, the hook is not slipped so easily. If there is a 'queer kind of sense' to irrationality, it must be found in the relations between the beliefs and desires in terms of their mental contents (as in Freudian analyses). If we disconnect their mental effects from their mental or reason-giving content, we have not explained why they function as they do except to say that somehow, on some level quite apart from that of their intentional nature or their meaningful content, they do and therefore 'we also need to know how it is that reasons can have causal efficacy in virtue of their reasonableness' (Antony 1989). Davidson's reasons cannot be partitioned if they have to be co-present in my psyche to explain what I do and why I try to deceive myself. Davidson (1982) is therefore forced into either denying the phenomenological force of the conflict (and partitioning the reasons *qua* reasons) or arguing (with functionalists) that 'the breakdown of reason relations defines the boundary of a subdivision' (p. 304) while allowing what is thereby divided to interact causally at least (but not in the meaningful way our explanations normally appeal to).

This two-level shuffle with the rational or conscious mind not reflecting what is really going on in the causal machinery preserves the theoretical requirement that action be explained by reasons but sacrifices the claim that reasons derive their force from their meaning to the subject. Davidson (1982) concedes the point—'a thought or impulse can cause another to which it bears no rational relation' (p. 303)—thereby posing an impossibly difficult conundrum. How can we respect the reason-giving content of beliefs and desires, claim that the way they are combined reflects that content, and allow the strength of their connections at another level—the physical or causal—to do all the work in explaining irrationality? Presumably, the principle of continence is a requirement that the causal force tracks the reason-giving force without explaining how that is secured. These inadequacies have motivated attempts to go beyond Davidson's account to explain the phenomenology of failures of reason in a meaningful way.

Sorenson's (1986) analysis of self-deception as a scattered event comes closer to a focus on the experience of the person who demonstrates irrationality of various kinds.

> The deceiver is a person who fosters his victim's belief that p despite the fact that the deceiver does not believe p when he begins the fostering. It is possible for the deceiver to change his mind before the deception is completed. The self-deceiver is a person who fosters his belief that p despite the fact that he does not believe p when he begins the fostering . . . Self-deception is a gradual process.

Sorenson suggests that the irrational belief (in the light of all the evidence) results from a psychic process (involving selective attention to evidence, failure to pursue pointers contrary to the desired belief, enhancement of ambiguous support, and so on). The self-deceiver believes not-p (she does not love me) but wants to believe p (she loves me), so he or she sets in train an accumulation of reasons that end up producing the desired belief (she does love me). As a result, he or she is successfully deceived and succeeds as a deceiver.

This analysis overcomes some of the problems with irrationality, but why should a reason that is part of the subject's economy at t_1 become inoperative (rationally) at t_2 yet play a role in sustaining the accumulation of further (rather shaky) evidence for its contrary. A better account would preserve enduring explanatory roles for inscriptions in the psyche both in rational and irrational cases (allowing for extraconscious factors described by Jaspers: forgetting, dissolution over time, habituation, and so on) but loosen the connection between the explicit moments of the subject's lived experience and what is felt in an inchoate or affecting way on the basis of the individual's being-with-others.

The right kind of account would therefore respect the intuitions that

(i) Akrasia and self-deception make a queer kind of sense; and

(ii) Irrationality works according to familiar principles of mental explanation; and

(iii) We should account for the force of the reasons involved in terms of their meaning in interpersonal or relational terms and not merely their causal efficacy.

The present account sees akrasia as a reflection of our engagement in a world of deeply important relations with and evaluations by others that require an individual to develop the well-articulated skills (adapted to a shared life-world) required to construct a coherent narrative of their trajectory through that world.

Reasoned action

To act with a given intention is to organize one's present and/or envisaged activity under a guiding conception with ramifying and constitutive links to experience through the network of signifiers and associated disciplines and techniques inscribed on the body (Gillett, 2001). An action enacts a focus of reasoning about and coordination of one's activity as part of a self-narrative. 'Normative reasons', articulated as all-in considerations taking account of a wide range of one's attitudes and motivations and structuring one's experience as being coherent over time, add a facet to the account stressing mental integrity (Smith, 1994). Thus, the ability to act well (in accordance with one's all-things-considered-best-judgements) rests on discursive skills that are part of one's identity as an agent who is seen as worthy of recognition and validation.

Lacan notes that our system of signifiers is something intrinsic to but also intrinsically alien to a subject's own psyche and serves as the framework in which one takes shape and forms an *imago*. The complex many-way interaction between my psyche, the language informing it, the relationships delineating my developing soul, and the discursive techniques available to me structures and influences (but does not completely determine) the way I enact my story. In deciding to act in a certain way, I appropriate certain modes of being, adjusting and refining them so that they come to define a self and project an image of self adapted to my situation. If most people around here act so as to respond to a personally directed adverse comment with *anger* rather than, say, *shame*, then that affects me (and 'around here' can be very local, perhaps even intrafamilial). As one masters the skills shaped in the discursive practices around here, so one learns to engage adaptively with one's situation in response to the traces that inscribe one's subjective body.

However, the work of agency is not done once a psyche has been formed because to act in accordance with intention one must be able to guide one's activity through to the point of completion in the requisite way. This is a skill developed through practice and training and it affects every area of one's life. It combines energy and reality so that when children (and young researchers) announce their projects we may need to negotiate with them to inject some realism into the plans. Not only that, we often need to give judicious help and nurture the skills of independent, action-guiding, commitment needed to become an individual who can do what he or she says he or she will (the scaffolding of educationalists).

Disruptions to this commitment are common because human beings respond to novelty and constantly re-evaluate their intentions in the light of new information or shifting weights attached to those evaluations. Thus, an immature thinker finds it hard to keep hold of a steady guiding conception in the hurly-burley of life, whereas maturity tempers flexibility with the resolve that comes with the experience of successfully seeing things through. What is more, certain interactions with the agent might undermine his or her continence: for example, highly critical, aggressive, or aversive modes of relationship may result in hesitancy and fear of failure (a possibility often overlooked in training doctors). But reflection about thought and motivation, bolstered here and there by encouragement and 'cheering on the sidelines', some even-tempered and judicious criticism, and the occasional positive suggestion or handy tip, could support a good intention, just as many ropes can anchor a tent in a storm.

On the present view, inferential and other connections actively maintained by argument (in the broadest sense of the word) articulate one's actions broadly within one's psyche so that personal integrity (or normative reasons, in Smith's terminology) allows one to act coherently in the face of desires, commitments, relationships, and beliefs. A fine sensibility to others and a well-articulated conscious life allows one to bring many diverse considerations to bear on any particular action. Thus, I might think that <*apfelstrudel* would be so nice, I must order it> but my better self, taking due account of my weight, my heart diet, my Visa card balance, my gastric fullness, and so on, enables me to exhibit continence.

The relevant skills draw not only on a sensitive and balanced appreciation of the situation and its features but also translate that assessment into action despite being vulnerable to disruption. Think, for instance, of my delicately poised decision not to eat the *apfelstrudel*; imagine that I still feel a tad hungry, I have just received an unexpected financial windfall, I have chosen all the low-fat alternatives on the previous three days of my visit, and this has been recommended as the best German restaurant in town. Imagine, at the crucial moment, that the waiter walks past with a delicious looking *apfelstrudel*; I am gone.

Such delicately balanced intentions understandably fare badly in conflicts of will because salient influences (such as insistent drives, the need for affection and self-affirmation, or unreflective 'moral' reactions) do not require carefully maintained psychic checks and balances to give them their force. In particular, primitive, forceful, or unsettling motivations tend not only to induce an evaluative loosening of my 'action-structure' (Vallacher & Wegner, 1987) but also of my 'perceptual and imaginative asymmetry' (Peacocke, 1985) that displaces rationally favoured goals in the midst of evaluative disarray. Phronesis is the ability to enact all-things-considered best judgements so that they 'win out' even in a vulnerable moment of deliberation (such as that envisaged with the *apfelstrudel*).

Phronesis is related to a strong will (as in Appendix F) and akrasia applies to immoral as well as moral behaviour. Moral reasons are likely to be vulnerable (as noted in relation to the psychic and neurophysiological characteristics of psychopaths) because they depend on complex interpersonal patterns of sensitivity, reasoning, and reflection, often opposing one's own unmoderated tendencies. But moral judgements may also be salient and urgent and triumph over an 'all-things-considered best judgement' of a less worthy kind.

> A bank robber, having committed a violent robbery in which he shoots both a guard and a bystander who tries to interfere, rushes from the bank and leaps into his car to speed away. As he is about to pull out, he sees a young child, confused and crying, step in front of his car and he stops although there is a clear sense in which he 'ought' and he knows that he 'ought' to escape and that any delay may well lead to his arrest.

The bank robber enacts his intention (to rob the bank) sustained in the face of possible confounding contingencies (the actions of the guard and the bystander) but even though he has killed to achieve his goal and injuring the child would be a lesser evil, he stops rather than injure the child, despite the fact that his 'better' judgement tells him that he ought not. What is more, his akratic action makes 'a queer kind of sense' (we don't need a fanciful inferred mechanism) because we intuitively recognize the salience of the moral appeal of the vulnerable child. Whereas the robber may have reckoned with having to injure adults, he had not reckoned on a child entering the picture and his commitment to a premeditated structure of motivation and readiness to respond is discombobulated by the child's pathetic intrusion. As a result, he stops although he knows he should not all-things-considered (of course, we regard him as a better man for that). Recall the 'perceptual or imaginative asymmetries' (Peacocke): the robber formed an intention—a coordinating and guiding conception—suitably bolstered in his psyche against disruptions that he had anticipated as, in imagination, he 'walked the path' of his robbery. But the particular disruption that unhinged him had not been foreseen; the child's presence had not been integrated into his guiding conception, he had not rehearsed an adequate mental response to it, and so he was vulnerable to a sudden re-evaluation of his intention. He obeyed a strong disposition to avoid injuring a child so that the skilled discursively structured 'moves' needed to enact that moment of his story were unhinged.

The core case of akrasia is where 'an agent … freely, knowingly, and intentionally performs an action A against his better judgement that an incompatible action B is the better thing to do' (Walker, 1988). It contrasts with an action where the relevant intention is held in place by an all-things-considered judgement and given effect by the agent's commitment to the reflective and evaluative balance he has struck. When that balance is upset, a less 'worthy' intention supported by objectively weaker and often less reflectively engaged and weighted reasons for action (<I must try this *apfelstrudel*>, <It's a child>) wins out. Despite their comparative weakness (in the light of the overall narrative integrity of the agent), the 'winning' reasons are rendered salient (by some contingent factor) at a strategic point where they derail the action that would be performed on the basis of an all-things-considered-best-judgement and the agent's reason fails him. Most of our intentions are not as strong as the bank robber's: a sticky pudding or freshly poured glass of Muscadet is all that is needed to unseat our 'firm' commitment to act as we should. 'Concentrating on—attending to—some statement of the reasons against the *akratic* course' (Peacocke, 1985, p. 73) is not enough: the will—the capacity to translate reason into action—must give effect to rationality in the battle that is self-control.

An irrational agent fails to maintain a commitment to an intention that fits his unfolding narrative. Competence in life skills or discursively shaped techniques of being somebody whom one wants to be determines whether one's 'best' intentions prevail so that more is involved that an 'attentional strategy' (Mele, 1987, pp. 87–88). The relevant competencies must inform one's psyche in such a way that it affects what one does and who one is. Knowing that an *apfelstrudel* is bad for me in certain ways and that it tempts me to act against my better judgement should therefore provoke me to train myself (or engage in a discipline conducive to the care of the self [Foucault]) so that I become the person I aspire to be. Similarly, knowing the signs of love, and that the signs I am seeing are not among them, must be matched by skills of self-care if I am to draw a conclusion that I would rather not. In each case, (discursive) techniques of the self configure one's thoughts and actions so that they are responsive to argument and reflection.

Foucault (1994) mentions a critical function, the struggle, a curative or therapeutic function, and the help of others in the care of the self (p. 97). One such technique is to rehearse strategies for dealing with various possible 'temptations' or 'challenge points' so that one acts well in the real-life situation that co-creates the truth of one's being. The bank robber, facing an unrehearsed challenge—the little child—found his action structure disarticulated in favour of an instinctive, and therefore robust, reason (here, a moral claim). In more usual cases, the usual suspects do the same—appetites, wishes, yearnings, romantic fancies—and as a result, the agent does A in spite of his or her settled intention to do B (or not-A). His or her action is 'free and intentional' (Walker, 1988), but it is not the action dictated by his or her perfect mind because he or she does not have the skill to translate all-things-considered-best-intentions into practice when faced by such things as a liking for *apfelstrudel*, or the bank robber's feeling for little children.

The present account holds that an intention is an actively maintained construction enacted by an agent and vulnerable at various points (such as the appearance of the child, the muscadet, or the *apfelstrudel*) where the complex or balanced strategy one has formed can be disrupted in such a way that (all-things-considered) weak reasons win out solely because they do not depend on the reflective and intentional competence of the subject. The recognition of the skills of care of the self finesse more elaborate accounts of the mind as a propositional machine enacting functional relationships.

Church (1987) draws a distinction between reflective and unreflective intentional states, allowing her to treat certain reasons for action as 'presentational' in that they are de facto effective despite being less open to discursive reflection and evaluation than 'representational' or reflectively accessible motives or reasons (p. 359). Representational reasons have an inferential richness and structure provided by the mastery of language (permitting rational evaluation and hypothetical assessment). She argues that the contents of subconscious and conscious states play similar roles in mental explanation although, because the former are not open to conscious reflective judgement, they are not moderated like their conscious cousins. Thus, if I desire that A loves me at the conscious level, but at a subconscious level am beginning to think that A does not love me, then these stand in opposition although their status vis-à-vis consciousness is quite different. The thought that she does not love me is never made fully explicit and conscious because to do so would bring it into full reflective awareness and engagement with my conscious and therefore critical faculties. But the cognitive significance or meaning it would have if it were conscious causes me to gather all the evidence I can to prove it wrong (e.g. she goes to the same corner store as me because she wants to have contact with me, she waves to me to indicate that she really likes me, and so on). What has slipped from view here is the integrative self who uses techniques to craft himself or herself in the face of a challenging world.

The interpretive and reconstructive work on an ongoing brain–world (subjective being-in-the-world) stream of interactions surfaces in the current account. Events inscribe one's brain pathways according to their inchoate content, and by discursive work and reflective articulation, their significance becomes explicit. The stream of interaction has signifier-related effects on me without their signification being fully determined or engaged with my conscious narrative self until I so engage it. The psyche, however, responds to the implicit and potential links between events and significations, and is prone to be influenced by those connections even when the contradictions that follow from a clear and fully explicit assignment of signification would alert it to cognitive conflicts needing attention. Being rightly linked, as a subject, to the truth is therefore the result of mastery of techniques of the self articulating the touch of the world in terms of the world of discourse and that mastery does not come easily or without the benefit of 'argument' (Foucault 1994, p. 101).

Akrasia is as discussed by Aristotle in that one might not command the techniques of the self required to translate one's intentions into actions that are fitting in the light of one's values and the actual relation between the self and the truth (Foucault).

Theoretical analyses of action and its failures are, however, best evaluated by applying them to real situations in which various kinds of irrationality are evident.

13.3 Why am I doing this operation?

I sometimes find myself operating on a manipulative patient who has got me to agree to operate on their lumbar spine when the findings and magnetic resonance imaging (MRI) scan are inconclusive as regards any significant pathology. One asks, 'Why am I doing this operation?' or 'How did I ever get into this situation?' That this happens to others is evident from the patients with, for instance, multiple laparotomies and a diagnosis of 'bowel spasms' or a coccygectomy as a result of refractory coccodynia. The akrasia usually dawns on one with a slightly sinking feeling as you take up the scalpel and the cold light of reflection tells you that it is an operation you wish you were not doing, you will find hard to justify in your audit or review meeting with your colleagues, and on which you would justifiably pour scorn if it was done by somebody else. What is more, rueful reflection usually exposes the faulty reasoning.

You may have 'Sir Galahad' syndrome, as happens when the patient tells you that you are the only doctor who has really understood them. They may say that anything would be better than the agony they are presently in or that if there is any chance at all of helping them, they would like to take that chance. You may have assured them (quite realistically) that the operation will not make them worse. Finally, there might have been some other factor making you vulnerable at the time: you are tired and at the end of a long clinic, your bank account is a bit thin that month, the patient has played upon a sense of rivalry with some other doctor who has attended them, and so it goes on.

None of these are good reasons to take scalpel in hand, but that is the nature of akrasia. We do that which we have less good reason to do than the alternatives open to us and, when we reconstruct how we have got ourselves into the unenviable position, we find various points at which a rational and professional approach to the patient's problem has been derailed. The Sir Galahad appeal creates a strong desire to help and to validate one's noble rescuing persona (it works much better with those subscribing to male stereotypes and with younger rather than older clinicians, excepting always those who satisfy the aphorism 'There is no fool like an old fool.') The clinical instinct to be a caregiver and to show it by buying into the patient's story and your role in it as rescuer, who 'takes the patient's predicament to heart' rather than weighing it against a considered judgement about efficacy and future probabilities works against professionalism. The patient's desperation and their apparent confidence that you will be able to help them discount any misgivings you might have and obscure your perfectly clear apprehension of the fact that, at the other end of this game, the same patient will be implying that you were promising what they hoped for and projected into the situation, that if they had only known they would be so bad afterwards they might not have chosen the operation, that the pain and disappointment is so much worse than anything they ever imagined, and so on. You know beforehand, according to your best and most detached professional judgement, that that is how things are most likely to go, but you are hooked by a multiplicity of tempting conversational moments (devices and desires internal to the transference in play). The crucial moments are easy to miss: the lingering collusion, in thought at least, to the idealized image of yourself; the secret thought that maybe you can do better than your colleagues; the hope that maybe this manipulative patient has a genuine problem and you will be the one who does the trick and relieves her suffering. The moment they are articulated these thoughts are shown for what they are, but the akratic intention as it forms surreptitiously immobilizes the arguments of realism and hard-won clinical experience and you are seduced by the lure of yet another success; you pronounce the fateful words and the patient has got your guarantee that you will rescue her. Akrasia strikes again.

13.4 I knew I shouldn't do that

There are some even less comprehensible varieties of akrasia. In surgery, it is an injudicious snip of the scissors producing a gush of blood or the extra bit of dissection that causes damage to an important structure that one was trying to spare. Often, such a slip follows an explicit thought that it would not be wise to snip or extend the dissection, or the equally prudent thought that one has taken as much of the tumour as it is safe to remove. It is just after that lucid moment that one is seized by a surgical *djinn* or demon saying 'Go on, just cut it' or 'Just take that little bit there; you can probably get away with that.' This last phrase is always the giveaway that the act is akratic. You think you will get away with it and, even though almost nothing speaks for the act and any reasoned thought would speak against it, you do it. One of my surgical mentors used to say, 'Surgery is not about what you can get away with; it is about what you can do safely every time.' A pinch of his conservatism adds balance to any surgical recipe for success. Elsewhere in the clinic, the voice of reason and experience urges caution against the promptings of the demon of adventure or the headstrong romantic quest of complete cure. The more temperate voice of skill, restraint, humility, and self-control is part of phronesis and keeps us from well-intentioned hubris that can seriously mess up the lives of patients.

Particular skills of acting and care of the self evince general styles of being-in-the-world and inculcate in oneself habits of argument whereby reason informs action and draws widely on reflective experience. Those skills save one from the excesses of therapeutic chutzpah and self-inflated judgements about one's own powers; they link one's subjective life to the truth, even if at times that is expressed in ways that are quite zany, joyful, and creative.

13.5 'But I never get infections'

Self-deception is the epistemic partner of practical irrationality or akrasia. It is, of course, never found in good clinics (well, almost never). If we are honest, most of us, in those reflective and melancholy moments when some operation or intervention has gone badly, become acutely aware of the cognitive devices we use to shield ourselves from the truth. 'I never get infections' is an example of the Dennis the menace style of reflection when he accused Mr. Wilson of having a bad memory. 'Why do you say that?' asked Mr Wilson. Dennis replied, 'Because you always remember the bad things I do.' Surgical memory is, in this sense, a 'good memory' (perhaps it needs to be, considering the challenges we deal with). Neurosurgeons make claims like 'All my aneurysms tend to go well' and lumbar disc surgeons claim success rates in the 90% range. Each discipline finds honest retrospective series or carefully monitored prospective series sobering in the light of the statistics of the clinical tearoom (particularly in relation to 'the new treatment'). But why are we so good at systematically fooling ourselves?

Doctors have to be sanguine about their abilities to do good. In surgery, one invades and damages a human body in the effort to improve on a distressing state of affairs. In medicine, one poisons people, and in psychiatry, one either poisons people or presumes that the light of one's countenance and the brilliance of one's conversation can relieve the maladies of the soul. Each requires a deep-seated feeling that one can do things successfully even though sometimes nature has so conducted itself that it is hard to see how the situation can be improved. For instance, whereas a neurosurgeon who finds a superficial meningioma in a young man can remove it and cure the problem, one more often finds a malignant glioma creeping through the glial interstices of the brain for up to 5 cm from the macroscopic edge of the tumour. A psychiatrist may one day see an intelligent 50-year-old who has fallen into a melancholy that responds brilliantly to electroconvulsive therapy (ECT) and on the next meet a 26-year-old with a personality disorder so profound and a social situation so awful that she seems to need a 'life transplant'. On other occasions, nature is doing its utmost to hold together a system gracefully degenerating into terminal dysfunction and we take it upon ourselves to do better. The surgeon may embark on an incremental replumbing of a marginal vascular system or the psychiatrist the imperious pharmaceutical adjustment of a cognitively impaired geriatric patient who is only just coping in a heavily structured everyday environment. All this mortality and morbidity is fertile ground for despondency and impressionistic sampling of the data, so is it any wonder that doctors, sanguine creatures that they are, are apt to look on the bright side?

Aristotle relates phronesis and right thinking to the 'golden mean' in a way that is quite apt for clinical life. Thus, true courage is neither foolhardy recklessness in the face of all or any odds nor is it timid and cowardly. True generosity involves striking the right balance between rash indulgence and meanness. So the optimism that allows one to persist in taking up cold steel (or dire poisons) against the ravages of time and nature has to be tempered by a realistic sense of what is achievable based on a clinical experience. The grounded soul refuses to inhabit castles in the air and keeps itself in touch with what has happened in the past and with the ways of the world. How should one deal with the abused and manipulative borderline patient, the somatizing and demanding drug addict, and the passive aggressive hysteric. Psychiatrists, one might hope, are much more savvy than surgeons in negotiating the discourses and relationships in play (even though statistics about boundary violations suggest otherwise).

The lessons of the clinic, similar to the therapies of the soul, do not change us overnight and, just as insight does not cure deep-seated problems in the psyche, rational resolve cannot replace the passage of time and the transforming effect of care for others (and the self) on the healer. Often, what is unspoken and irrational incline us to do what we do. In surgery, as in everyday life, those irrationalities recede in their power under the pressure of reality because at an even more fundamental level we are designed to be linked to the truth and respond to its contingencies. The mind, we could say, is a world detector and a behaviour adapter in the light of our engaged and subjective being-in-the-world.

Some of us are not as connected to the truth as others are and yet the fact that we are, of necessity, intentional and engaged with the world entails that we can become adapted to it. Perception is the first component of Aristotelian moral competence, followed by right dispositions and the skill of reflecting on the outcomes of our actions. This triad, allied to the techniques of care of the self, is therapy against folly of all sorts.

13.6 I am sure he will be better when he wakes up

Wishful thinking in all its guises is also to be found among surgeons even though they know as well as anybody else that the wish that a certain thing be thus and so has no bearing on the likelihood of its being so. But we hear ourselves saying, against the plain clinicopathological evidence, that 'The injury is not so bad' or 'If only I operate, he has a chance of pulling through.' This variety of therapeutic optimism is a necessary antidote to fatalism or defeatism, but it can also mean that we persist with heroic attempts to save life when careful reflection would show that what we are saving is perhaps not a life worth living.

This struck me most forcefully when a friend was admitted having suffered a catastrophic aneurysmal haemorrhage into the brain associated with a large blood clot. He was probably brain dead when I first saw him and, deep down, I knew that nothing I nor anyone else could do would bring him back from death. Fortunately, although called by the family, I was not the surgeon receiving acute patients that evening and a wiser head than mine took the decision not to operate. But before that decision was taken, the thought was there: if only I could open the brain and decompress the haematoma, the aneurysm would be able to be clipped and he would pull through. This was quite beyond the realms of probability or even possibility, but such seductive images that fly in the face of realistic assessment sometimes beset us, particularly as young doctors. Unfortunately, it has a downside—the self-blame when one fails to live up to the impossible ideal. It is natural for instance that a psychiatrist should believe that he or she could have prevented a patient from committing suicide even though the statistics may tell a different story. The failure of reason that makes us hope against hope is, however, as important as the critical reflection that teaches us the true lessons.

And here we can see some of the crucial ingredients of irrationality in general and wishful thinking in particular. In a case like that of my friend, the fact that he is my friend means that the desire that things come out well is strong and disposes one to form the belief that things will go well. The evidence is, to some extent, ambiguous especially when the situation is more unclear than in fact it was. In that situation, neither belief is rational because both go beyond the evidence at hand. Given the suspended state of belief that is consistent with an all-things-considered-best-judgement, the desire can influence the psyche in its attitude towards the facts, and all one needs to fuel wishful thinking is indeterminacy about the warranted conclusion and a little 'fudging' one way or another. These tendencies are widespread and arguably a part of that flexible rationality we all use to keep us going through life's turmoil. If the evil conclusion can be staved off, at least until the jury has to be called in, so to speak, then there is a window of opportunity for the psyche to entertain and adjust itself to any of the range of scenarios that might eventuate.

Again, the discursive-autobiographical-narrative meets brain-world-information-flow view of the psyche allows us to understand why the information gathered does not fully determine its articulation in our mental life as beliefs, desires, expectations, and so on. Human subjects characteristically sketch a number of 'takes' on a situation until one of them settles in as an all-things-considered-best-judgement of the situation. The negotiability of that process illuminates the practical problem of clinical prognosis and clinical acumen.

A good diet of clinical audit and evidence-based medicine adjusts wishful thinking, but it is an uphill battle because clinicians in general and surgeons in particular are great anecdotalists and 'there be dragons' and all manner of miracles. An individual story can be remembered in such a way as the details that make the case special are forgotten and the miraculous outcome is produced like a rabbit from a hat in an act of triumphant surgical or clinical prestidigitation. This is great stuff for dining out on or for 'puffing yourself up', but it is not a good belief-forming strategy.

13.7 Foibles and slips of the tongue

The psyche is built on the meeting of narrative and the stream of brain–world interactions subject to *meconnaissance*. We could, with Freud, talk of the censor operating between the unconscious and the preconscious but also, in a phenomenologically very real sense, between what one thinks and what one is inclined to say such that:

(i) There is a complex interplay between the network of signifiers and the flux of brain activity in dynamic contact with a context; and

(ii) There is an interplay of what it is legitimate to say in this discourse and what is thrown up from the network of signifiers as a result of the dynamics of subjectivity. This is beautifully illustrated by slips of the tongue.

> The vicar was coming to tea. The vicar was renowned for the size of his nose. Mrs. Bennett was therefore extremely careful to emphasize to her 8-year-old son, James, equally well-known for his candid comments, not to say anything about the vicar's nose. The vicar duly arrived. He politely engaged young James in conversation while Mrs. Bennett nervously got the tea, approvingly noting that James was taking pains not to fix his gaze on the vicar's nose. She entered the room with the afternoon tea tray and poured the vicar a cup

of tea. Then, in her most genteel voice, she asked, 'Vicar, would you like some milk with your nose?'

This is a classic slip of the tongue. The vicar's nose is salient in Mrs. Bennett's psyche even though her speech and actions are carefully structured not to lead to it being mentioned. Unfortunately, the associative structure underlying her speech activates the resonating but suppressed node and its signifier. Notice that we do not need to posit an unconscious to explain the phenomenon in this case nor do we, I suggest, in most of the slips that spring to mind (or tongue). I could have pursued the case of the aversive road near my grandmother's house by providing the following example.

> I am speaking to my grandmother and intend to say to her, 'I was thinking so intently about why I might feel uncomfortable about that road when I almost hit a car' but instead say 'I was thinking so intently about why I might feel uncomfortable about that road when I almost hit a dog.'

Here, the signifier 'dog' displaces the conscious 'car' in the classic way. On the present account, we need opt neither for a conscious-but-suppressed nor subconscious explanation for slips of the tongue because the signified content is lurking in the stream of signification (associatively), and at a moment when one's attention wavers or is not tightly controlling one's speech, that content informs speech other than that consciously intended. Behaviour, here speech behaviour, is a stratum of manifestation associated, as de Saussure (1972) noted, with a stratum of signification (p. 111).

13.8 Phronesis, experience, and character

Judicious action and reflection upon one's own action are, according to Aristotle, two features of practical wisdom that are closely entwined with experience and the development of character. In clinical training, we attend to the first but sometimes not sufficiently to the other (although supervision and mentoring are starting to become more widespread in all clinical disciplines). For many, the most vivid lessons about character are learnt in a very unpleasant way when we see someone acting as we hope we never will ourselves. The irony is that we inherit and absorb not only skills but also attitudes and habits from those who train us and, whereas deficient skills can and are usually surpassed, the habits are harder to correct. The same lessons carry over to everyday life.

There is no doubt that well-honed surgical skills are the right ground on which to breed good attitudes as are good social and interpersonal skills are in the wider world. Defensive and insecure personal attitudes are antithetical to both open-mindedness and the appropriately grounded self-confidence that underpins good interpersonal relations. What is more, the person who is constantly trying to prove himself or herself is *driven* in a way that is ultimately destructive both to self and to close personal relationships. The weight of personal insecurity and inadequacy is a kind of heaviness in the soul that clogs the footsteps of personal and intellectual life. A certain lightness of being comes with the irony and humility of openness to the lessons of experience and is a prophylaxis against the repetition caused by unforgotten and forgotten wounds.

Reflection and the care of the self connect one to the truth in thought and action so as to move on from one's personal failings and share that 'gay science' (though not necessarily the death of God) with others. Sound, flexible, responsive, dispositions are the basis of more or less successful adaptations to life's challenges, and to supplement sound habits with humour lightens the soul by detaching one from an overly serious attitude to oneself. It holds up to reflection the things that we become too serious about and allows them to be seen for what they are so that humour, friendship, wry commentary on the faults and failings of oneself and others, and a positive caring attitude towards oneself shape one's persona. Plato's 'know thyself', Aristotle's view that friendship is important in a virtuous life, and Christ's commandment to love God and our neighbours as ourselves all foster well-being and a harmony of the lively demons.

Unconscious foibles, the psychopathologies of everyday life, are quirks of personality and as much part of human individuality as epistemic commitments, character traits, patterns of relationship, values, allegiances, and so on. By contrast, those deep wounds in the psyche that distort our reactions, responses, and relationships with others require transformation through the techniques of care for the self. A human being is inscribed by the reflections of self in the mirror of discourse such that most significant revisionary projects are cooperative, undertaken with the aid of trusted companions on the journey of life. The result is an imago and a lived subjectivity differently configured with respect to the world of meaning that frames one's being-in-the-world.

It remains to try and draw together the strands of the present account by recounting the journey of a life.

Chapter 14

Concluding autobiographical postscript

'Who do people say that I am?'

Let me tell you the story of a little boy. This little boy was conceived as the result of a shipboard romance and born about 1900. His mother was unmarried and he lived with the stigma of illegitimacy and no father. He was educated in the state school system but left school aged fourteen, too young to go to the First World War. He then became a piano tuner's apprentice, but by the time he had finished that apprenticeship the age of the wireless had begun, so he had no trade to follow. He trained as a tram conductor and married a woman who was better educated than he was and had, to some extent, taken the role of matriarch in a family of 9 of which she was the oldest sister. After our hero had pursued his occupation for a few years, the trams were replaced by buses.

He did unskilled work and had three children, all girls. None of them entered tertiary education and he held various jobs in various factories, always working hard and honestly as a loyal, even devoted, employee. He visited his mother faithfully and regularly although she had been a somewhat strict woman, but always introduced her to his daughters as his older sister and, until he died, they did not know that she was their grandmother. He could not cope with emotional challenges and conflicts although he had had to show great resilience in making something of his life. He would absent himself from conflict situations or lose his temper but was never aggressive towards others. Every confrontation was like a threat to the self.

He provided well for his family but lived always in the shadow of his wife, who was a big woman in all but physical stature. His activities were always rigidly confined within the narrow bounds of his competencies, but within those he worked diligently and well. He was always respected by his relatives and did his best to be congenial to all.

When he was 50, he and his wife adopted an illegitimate male child. This child, his wife knew, was going to be intelligent; in fact, the lawyer who arranged the adoption said, 'If he is not a surgeon, I will eat my hat.' The adopted child was his (adoptive) mother's pride and joy. From the moment of his arrival in the home, he was nurtured, loved, cherished, and indulged, his achievements were acclaimed, and his serious character faults were excused. He became the focus of so much aspiration that his (adoptive) father gathered the crumbs left over from the feast of love enjoyed by the child.

It became obvious that this little boy was intelligent but there was something not right with him. He was manipulative and often felt emotionally detached from events that he knew should move him. He lied, stole, misbehaved, was irresponsible, and was lazy but, despite all that, he was always a high achiever. At school, he did well, but his father did not or could not play sports with him and neither could his father engage him in intellectual discussion. The reasons for this were complex but probably included the father's own modest education and lack of a father. The child's blend of scepticism, romanticism, and searching interrogations were unsettling and often rebuffed so that from the age of 14 the home was no longer a place of intellectual stimulation for the adopted son. He learnt to succeed with his peers by making clever use of his not inconsiderable discursive skills and was blessed with some good friends. He grew further apart from his father and had an odd dissociated attitude to his mother, whom he deeply loved but also felt superior to.

The romantic relationships of youth had a tendency to become very intense, often too intense for his partners. He suffered further hurts compounding the deep unsignified hurt of the primal wound that was repeating itself at a level more basic than discourse. He met and married an intelligent and deeply sensitive young woman who was naive, trusting, committed, utterly morally upright, and extremely perceptive. During this relationship, he made a Christian commitment, but there too the same subjective abjection often threatened his sense of spiritual belonging or peace. The wound lurked.

We traverse the years and find the child in his 40s with a history of serious failures but also startling successes. He is a surgeon, as predicted; his adoptive parents have had moments of great pride and his father has been at times overcome by his feelings although yet acutely aware of how much he himself has been surpassed. His mother's hopes have been realized, although she died towards the end of his rise from professional and academic strength to strength. But beneath the discourses (and there are many of them that he has successfully mastered), there is the perennial fear of abandonment, betrayal, the sense of rejection, and alienation.

His psyche returns again and again to lick his wound. He fears (and has odd recurring dreams of) rejection. In one dream, his wife invites someone else to live in the house, and one night, he finds himself locked out of the house or only tolerated in a room apart when she is obviously laughing and talking in a loving and intimate way with the other person. He has dreams in which his romantic partners transform into something threatening or disgusting and so betray the relationship developing in the dream. When there is conflict in the household, he handles it badly. He often deceives to avoid confrontation. He absents himself from arguments, he loses his temper, and he is verbally, emotionally, and even physically abusive although he knows it to be wrong and inexcusable. He learns, to his dismay, that his children have called him 'psycho'. He begins to learn about the inscription on his body of patterns of response and reaction birthed at a time before discourse allowed him to begin his narrative and to understand that there are skills of care of the self that he has never had modelled to him and has not even begun to master. His discursive and narrative facility scantily cloaks a Gemini subjectivity prone to defensiveness and well armed with devices to protect the self and deflect the injuries that the schizoid world is poised to inflict on him.

The world is not, of course, schizoid and he has slowly come to slow realize that. The rewards and challenges of helping others, through surgery and, increasingly, through his discursive interactions, in the presence of a rapidly expanding reflective understanding of the inscriptions on his body have begun to reshape his narrative. It begins to be a narrative in which he is OK, grounded in a deep-seated conviction that he belongs and that no one can take certain things away from him—good things. The unsignified conviction that he is liked (most importantly), appreciated, and skilled in various ways, despite his flaws, begins to be disclosed in his probing and restless reflections on life.

That is what this book is about. In it, the discursive roots of the human psyche (or soul), articulated and expressed in narrative reflections, have been explored and their varieties of discontent dissected. Subjective being-in-the-world-with-others (*dasein-mitsein*) has been taken seriously and related to contexts that inscribe our bodies. The fertile coming together of discourse and inscriptions on the body has been traced through a trajectory carrying many traces of others and the mirror glimpses they give of a soul, variously preserved in ramifying and divergent inspir(it)ations and discontents of the mind. This book has inscribed its author as well as being inscribed by him and to some extent reconnected him to the truth of his being, thereby liberating his narrative and rendering him less powerless to heal his psychic wounds. If that is all it ever does, it has therefore been worthwhile, but the kind words of readers suggest that it has a less narcissistic role.

Of his Concluding *Unscientific Postscript*, Soren Kiekegaard (1846/1968) wrote,

> In the end, all corruption will come about as a consequence of the natural sciences ... But such scientific method becomes especially dangerous when it would encroach also upon the sphere of spirit. (p. xv)

The human spirit and its profound relationship to the Divine spirit was, for Kiekegaard, a foundation of his being. A narrow and exclusive secular science that makes claims to completeness threatens constantly to obscure and weaken such foundations and thereby restrict philosophical thought about the human condition and create the discontents associated with alienation within the human soul.

My thesis explicitly concerning the human soul or psyche is that the pretensions of a narrow (and somewhat obtuse) pursuit of reductive science in the area of the human psyche and its discontents diminishes us all. Philosophical scrutiny or subjectivity linked in a certain way to the truth, communication, and empathic imagination (the hallmark of good phenomenology and ultimately good psychology) results in a more humane psychiatry and is, I believe, the right way to illuminate the afflicted psyche. Such an orientation seems to be needed more than ever in a climate where economic forces threaten clinical psychiatry and drive it towards a short-sighted biological conception of mental disorder and recipe book approach to the therapies of the soul.

This work celebrates the human psyche despite all its failings and discontents. The human psyche is a remarkable creation born of the interaction between word and flesh or, if you prefer, discourse and the situated body. As such, it is a unique metaphysical species that has given birth to both metaphysics and epistemology, creations with which it has become bewitched (in counter-Oedipal ways). Reason can, however, take a quasi-ironic or even gay (in Nietzsche's sense) attitude towards its epistemic offspring such as philosophy, psychiatry, and psychology, and the elusive relationship between an individual embodied subject and his or her relation to the mirror world, an attitude informing this book.

Metaphysics and the mind

Metaphysics concerns the real nature of things and ontology concerns what there is, two closely related inquiries, and philosophers who go in for that sort of thing are generally either realists or anti-realists.

Realism

Realism is the general view that the way things are is independent of our way of knowing them. Some people take realism to be a commitment to the fact that we are part of a real world, but that is an ambiguous view held by other philosophical camps as well (such as phenomenology, existentialism, and pragmatism). Others take realism to be opposed to idealism, which is slightly misleading because both claim that there is a (real) way the world is but one of them, idealism, claims that the world comprises mental entities (whether in the human mind or the mind of God, however construed).

Realists claim that ontology and metaphysics can be separated from epistemology—the philosophical analysis of knowledge—but Kant (1789/1929) remarks:

> Ontology that presumptuously claims to supply, in systematic doctrinal form, synthetic a priori knowledge of things in general (for instance, the principle of causality) must, therefore, give place to the modest title of a mere analytic of pure understanding. (B303)

Kant argues that once we have gone as far as possible in deepening our ways of knowing things, or undertaken an 'analytic of pure understanding', then we can go no further and that beyond all our ways of thinking of things, we cannot reason about them or their natures. That claim implies that the closest we can get to an understanding of what things really are (metaphysics) or what things there really are (ontology) is to analyse knowledge so as to discern those aspects of it that are indispensable in conceiving of there being a world to know. Knowledge, however, implicates epistemology so that Kant is deconstructing the separation of metaphysics and ontology from epistemology. In this, he is similar to postmodern thinkers, although his commitment to universal truths distinguishes him from them.

These thoughts can be clarified with a famous example. Consider the morning star and the evening star. Imagine that, as a medieval thinker, I am well acquainted with the evening star—the first light in the sky visible in the evening. Now snap me into the 20th century so that I learn that I am really seeing the planet Venus. But is this really what I am seeing or am I seeing a lump of stuff orbiting an obscure star in an undistinguished solar system. Or am I really seeing (and here follows an exhaustive physical specification of the object we call the planet Venus) or is it (and here follows an impossibly complex quantum description of a region of space-time specified relative to some arbitrary point). At a certain point, it becomes clear that we are not talking about actual knowledge or even possible knowledge but 'in principle' knowledge and that we have lost sight of the meaning of the phrase 'The first heavenly body visible in the evening' or any other meaningful description.

Which of these is the true or fundamental metaphysical description of the evening star? To argue for any of them is to miss the point that each only comes into contention within a system of discourse making certain things visible and obscuring others. Thus, Heidegger (1953/1996) observes, 'what is questioned is to be defined and conceptualized in the investigating' (H5), and agrees with Kant that (i) the tasks of epistemology and metaphysics cannot be separated and (ii) the descriptions we apply to reality are human creations framing the world in ways that make sense to us in the light of our need for rational coherence and generality. The mind or brain or the human subject in itself, or *simpliciter*, is a construct arising from a (Cartesian) way of interrogating our existence as beings-in-the-world and that interrogation has no Archimedean point (outside the world) but occurs from within as we try to find ways of articulating and dealing with ourselves in our complex engagement with our environment (or domain of adaptation). The 'view from nowhere' is an impossibility; we are always already situated and can only make evident to ourselves what is revealed and what is concealed by adopting some way of thinking of whatever it is we are thinking about (Nagel, 1986). With this in mind, we can investigate the so-called relation between the mind and the brain (bearing in mind the relationship between *the evening star* and *the planet Venus*).

The mind and the brain

Some philosophers call the relationship of the mind to the brain 'strict supervenience', and express that in the following claim: there is no 'mental event' (for want of a better term) that does not reflect a brain event (Heil, 1992, p. 58). Bolton and Hill (1996) use a similar notion in discussing the realization of mental activity in brain processes and talk about encoding meanings in brain states and events (pp. 76ff). But what does this mean?

The brain receives input from the sensory systems, transforms it in certain ways, and on the basis of its ongoing activity, programmes motor output. For instance, imagine that you see a fly upon the wall. A pattern of impulses arises in the retina, travels through the optic nerves, is processed in the thalamus (and collaterally sets up tracking and scanning routines in the tectum and cerebellum), and is then relayed to the occipital cortex where further processing results in an effect on cortical function as a whole. Imagine that the fly catches your attention. Information is passed through cortical assemblies (higher-order visual) linking it to (linguistically organized) activity allowing you to categorize what you are seeing as a fly and engage diverse other cognitive processes so that it achieves 'cerebral fame'. A number of possible reactions and responses are thereby potentiated ranging from interest, to anger, to aggression, to wonder (at, for instance, what-it-is-like-to-be-a-fly).

Why do the brain processes concerned carry information to do with flies? They do so because they make use of connections with patterns evinced by instances in which the term 'fly' was used (or could have been used). The use of the term 'fly' (and the practices in which the relevant rules are mastered) links this occasion to others involving small black flying insects of a certain type, discussions of hygiene, and so on. Thus, the connections determining that it is a fly, *qua* fly, that is the object of thought depend on activating just these links forged in the network of human practices in which flies are noticed and communicated about. But this network is constituted by people, their habits, habitat, and interests so that human activities and the network of conceptual rules structuring them are implicated in the explanation of any thought (such as <that is a fly>).

The importance of the human and interpersonal context of brain activity is underscored by neuroscience and information-processing theory that treats the brain as a complex, multilayered neural network (Clark, 1990; Macdonald & Macdonald, 1995b; Smolensky, 1988). Information is transmitted through the neuronal networks of the brain in ways configured by an individual's learning history. The brain begins with a certain (probably hardwired) 'associational skeleton', and has a vast network of possible connections in which associations and patterns of transmission are developed on that primordial base. Certain synaptic connections are strengthened (by processes such as long-term potentiation) and others weakened (perhaps even lost through dendritic pruning) so that the brain registers patterns indicating significant features (and events) in the subject's domain of activity. Therefore, genetically programmed brain pathways form their actual connections as a result of social experience (Eisenberg, 1995, p. 1563) mediated by speech (Dennett 1991; Luria, 1973).

Work in cognitive neuroscience confirms that we develop strategies of information selection from a potentially overwhelming stimulus milieu (Neisser, 1976; Young, 1986) and that the selective strategies, generated in higher centres of the brain, affect information processing in lower centres. But what do the higher centres tell the lower centres to 'look out for'?

Models of cognition

Approaches to human cognition are no longer dominated by computer-based models involving discrete representations whose syntax underpins transactions of the type found in an ideal language or system of logic (a strategy based on the theory that language is a calculus and thought comprises transformations of functionally specifiable representations). A functionalist position is appealing in that it pictures formal transactions (as in a code) captured by causal processes involving (syntactically) structured items of information so that mental states and processes are just a way of talking about the transformations between states and configurations of excitation in the brain, logically organized and connected according to a proposition-like calculus. But human thought does not fit this mould because various things that formal or propositional algorithms do very well we do not, and other things that they do very badly we find quite easy (Gillett 1989; Rumelhart et al. 1986; Smolensky, 1988). What is more, the importance of discourse (implicating culture and interpersonal relations) in understanding human thought and action undercuts the individualism of the functional-causal model (Fodor, 1975).

Connectionist systems, however, have a number of fascinating features suited to messy, complex domains, where they interact with other systems in ways that bedevil static and formal models of cognition:

- they have smooth degradation curves for stimulus recognition that cope with items of information based on (family or paradigmatic) resemblances rather than structural congruence;

- they allow workable 'content addressability' even for approximate or deviant samples of an input type unlike formal systems where aberrant inputs cannot 'tap in' to the information store unless they exhibit quasi-mathematical forms;

- they also deal with multiple interacting constraints in similar ways to human thought, where such constraints may carry the information needed to complete a task but in ways that involve complex interactions between different inputs and require a 'holistic' and dynamic weighting of many aspects of the presentation.

Classical computing strategies, faced with such problems, are paralyzed by combinatorial explosions because they proceed from one 'decision' to the next rather than weighing and balancing all the indeterminacies until a 'good-enough' solution emerges. Parallel Distributed Processing (PDP) systems can also learn to recognize and create 'classifications' for novel stimuli without requiring ready-made 'slots' into which the new item will fit. Finally, they evince considerable 'neural realism' in terms of the way they match human facility with informational tasks.

The fundamental arguments between classicists and connectionists tend to focus on the related issues of compositionality and syntax in thought. Regarding connectionism:

(1) It does not construe cognitive processes as involving symbol manipulation.

(2) The whole network is conceived of as a dynamic system which, once supplied with initial input to the input units, spreads inhibitions and excitations among its hidden units, eventually exciting certain output units and inhibiting others. (Macdonald & Macdonald, 1995b, p. 9)

Cynthia Macdonald notes that connectionists need to account for the systematicity of thought in the absence of explicit realizations (and therefore individual existence) of the semantic components forming the system (so that they cannot causally interact with each other and be combined and recombined).

Many argue that semantics is directly related to the world around the subject and not to internal variables (Millikan, 1993) and Smolensky (1995) rests semantics on (ecologically) 'relational descriptions and relational explanations of function' (p. 289) or 'intentional' (phenomenological sense) relations to objects and features in the world:

> The resulting connectionist model of mental processing is characterized by context-sensitive constituents, approximately (but not exactly) compositional semantics, massively parallel structure-sensitive processing, statistical inference, and statistical learning with structured representations.

> (Smolensky, 1995, p. 192)

Connectionist systems therefore realize patterns of excitation linked, on the one hand, to distributed patterns of neural activity tied to features and objects commonly encountered in the environment and, on the other, to the signifiers of natural language as they occur in human interactions. Therefore, the relevant signifiers reflect a dynamic interplay between the terms of natural languages, the verbal and non-verbal things people do to each other, and features of the world so that the human subject is, we could say, (neurocognitively) inscribed by signifiers, human practices, and the objects and events in the world where those practices go on so that our thought engages with the world through 'language games'. We can illustrate as follows.

Imagine I see a brown cow in one field and a black and white cow in another. The words apt to the first situation are 'brown cow in the field' and the second 'black and white cow in the field'. Now, given the points of congruence and distinction between these two utterances and some 'good-enough' rules about the structure of English, there are discernible associations (in Heidegger's sense, connections tied up with our dealings with things[1]) between the signifiers and what they signify. Compositionality arises from these associations so that multitracked dispositional links between the conditions of language use on different occasions can be made by the brain networks concerned.

The present account is congenial to Andy Clark's (1995) conciliatory arguments for the claim that 'any system complex enough to count as a believer will reveal (under some post hoc analysis) semantically clustered patterns of excitation' (p. 352) because most situations registered by the individual thinker are penetrated by the words and utterances of others in that or similar situations. Thus, the three kinds of input noted are

(i) The conditions of utterance;

(ii) The parsed utterance; and

(iii) The use of language by speakers to do things.

A distributed network sets up a dynamic interplay between the excitations preferentially activated in distributed areas of the brain dealing with these three types of information. Significations can then be assigned to components of the utterance and an actual-world, content-laden, significance assigned to the whole. Both satisfy two different sets of constraints (as noted): *first*, the semantic structure of the discourse currently framing the event, and *second*, the ecologically salient objects of attention and happenings in the situation. The constraints arise in distinct ways but have in common our engagement in the world (or dealings with things). The first arises from discourse and the influences (largely interpersonal and cultural) to be discerned there and the second from adaptation to the physical environment as it affects the body of the thinker. Problems in either (loss of attunement to the world or to others) can cripple the semantic engine.

---

[1] Heidegger talks of da-sein dwelling in the midst of associations or dealings with the world, which then form the basis of circumspection, a kind of engaged knowledge.

The upshot of this train of thought is reflected in a remark by Smolensky (1995) suggesting that functional encoding or structured brain states may be a will-o'-the-wisp in mental explanation, a conclusion with profound implications for theories of mental causality.

> From the point of view of the connectionist model builder, the class of networks that might model a cognitive agent who believes that dogs have fur is not a genuine kind at all but simply a chaotic disjunctive set. (p. 357)

Smolensky's scepticism echoes a remark of Wittgenstein's (1967).

> No supposition seems to me more natural than that there is no process in the brain correlated with associating or with thinking, so that it would be impossible to read off thought processes from brain processes. I mean this: if I talk or write, there is, I assume, a system of impulses going out from my brain and correlated with my spoken or written thoughts. But why should this system continue further in the direction of the centre? Why should this order not proceed, so to speak, out of chaos? ... It is thus perfectly possible that certain psychological phenomena cannot be investigated physiologically, because physiologically nothing corresponds to them. (¶608–609)

Wittgenstein discusses a seed and the plant it gives rise to as an illustration of his meaning. By so doing, he indicates that he does not question the idea that human mental life crucially implicates the brain and its processes but directs his comments at the idea of explanations of mental phenomena in general in terms of theory from the appropriate biological sciences (a topic for Appendix B). Such aspirations occur within biologically inspired accounts of the mind according to which physical–causal explanations are the only genuine explanations (for instance, Millikan [1993]). *If*, as he posits, the regularities and explanatory connections in semantics and mental life are much more ecological, reflecting the sociocultural history and context of the individual concerned (the kinds of explanation and description that are found in discursive psychology, for instance) and they have no clear analogue at the physical level, *then* the idea that all explanations (including the psychological or intentional) must be grounded in biology or physiology is mistaken. The point is noted often, but the implications for the metaphysics of the mind are also often neglected.

Implications for philosophy of mind

The idea that the mind operates according to contents (the cow is brown) and attitudes (such as belief, desire, intention, or doubt) towards them has been important since Hume. On this account, ideas, such as <that sheep is black> combine with a 'manner of our conceiving them' (Hume, 1739/1969, p. 144) to produce propositional attitudes (PAs) such as <the belief that tin roofs are red>, <the worry that there is tension in the air>, <the desire that things would be more relaxed>, <the intention to see my friend's husband 'put in his place'>, or <the expectation that the badger will shuffle out of the clearing>. Each conjunction comprises a state of affairs (characterized in some way or another) and an attitude adopted by the thinker and it involves concepts. It has intentional content in the sense that it is focused on something according to a way of thinking of it. PAs also explain behaviour, for instance, as follows.

(1) Anton thought the girls were laughing at him.

(2) When girls laugh at Anton, he wants them to believe he is indifferent to them.

(3) Anton is deeply disturbed by girls laughing at him.

(4) Anton feigns indifference to the girls.

The embedded PAs explain Anton's behaviour in terms of what he believes and intends, a kind of explanation called 'folk psychology' because of its widespread use in popular thinking about the acts and activities of other people (Fodor, 1968).

A realist about PAs (because of their explanatory role in human psychology) who also believes that real natural causes underpin explanations in general (e.g. Jaegwon Kim) infers that, in some sense, PAs are realized in the brain. Realist views come in weak or strong forms.

The strong form holds that a PA such as <the belief that that animal is a giraffe> is a distinct structural configuration of brain processes corresponding to some quasi-linguistic structure (perhaps in the 'language of thought'). Fodor (1987, 1990) has championed successive versions of such a theory for the last 40 years and inspired a large number of realist philosophers of mind who espouse some form of representationalism (e.g. Antony, 1989; Devitt & Sterelny 1987; Millikan, 1984) whereby PAs (as configurations in brain function) are suitably linked to sensory inputs, linguistic systems, and behavioural outputs and they computationally explain what we think, do, and say. Fodor's version, the language of thought (LOT) hypothesis, posits that thought is the manipulation of sentence-like entities functionally realized in the brain (Bolton & Hill, 1996, p. 80ff; Fodor, 1975).

The weak view (Clark, 1990; Dennett, 1981) accepts explanations using PAs but is more reserved about their realization in the brain. Such a position often appeals to neural networks and structures organized by and reflecting discursive formations and is sometimes interpreted as anti-psychological or eliminativist (it eliminates psychology in favour of neuroscience or 'cognitive neuroscience'). But mental structures and mental content could be as real as many things referred to in natural science such as species, magnetic fields, electron shells, photons, or energy levels, without corresponding to state analogues describable in physical or biological terms. Discursive reality may be reflected in brain structure in a connectionist way so that one cannot get an understanding of or even identify the connections involved by looking at the physical descriptions available in natural sciences such as biology or physiology (on causality and natural kinds, see Appendix B).

Appendix B

Causality, natural kinds, and psychological explanation

Contemporary metaphysics aims to provide logical specifications that constrain our thinking about the objects or kinds of things there are in the world. Wittgenstein (1922) referred to metaphysics as an artefact of the logical mirror reflecting the world (¶4121) and thereby converged with Kant, Heidegger, and their followers on the view that actuality and contingency (existence) is not reality as described by our conceptual structures, a human creation that is logically structured and far more orderly than the chaos of being.

Natural kinds are categories identified by our dealings with the world as being 'out there', independent of the human mind, so that we need only track them (or discern their nature) in order to understand the world (as it is objectively or 'in reality') and they are described in the objective (realist) terms of natural scientific disciplines.

Causality is 'the cement of the universe'—the mode of actual efficacy ordering reality and in terms of which we connect and explain what happens to things (Mackie, 1974).

These two entwined concepts express the basic commitments of metaphysics after Russell. They are undermined by Wittgenstein and others (including anti-realists of various kinds) who argue that the mirror held up to the world by logic always presents an idealization and configuration of what is (actually) 'going down'. They argue that such idealizations reflect what is significant to us (or intellectually tractable) and are discursive constructions. But what is causality—the force that actually makes things happen?

One contender for an account of causality is a counterfactual thesis that makes evident the role of the mind in discerning causal relations:

A caused B if and only if if A had not happened, then B would not have happened.

(Lewis, 1975)

It is known as the counterfactual analysis because it begins with a statement that is not true, viz. 'if A had not happened'. It captures what ordinary people often mean by a cause but relies on the powers of our imagination (not observation) to establish the relationship. That is problematic because something as basic to our understanding as causality surely should not rely so heavily on the imaginability of certain states of affairs. Reality, one might say, evinces a regularity fundamental to the order of nature and not one posited by flights of fancy.

Two other philosophical claims taken together yield a more appealing position:

(1) A successful causal claim identifies an actual physical relation between events.

(2) A successful causal claim identifies events related by some law of nature.

Jaegwon Kim (1993), a scientific realist, notes that the most straightforward explanatory account of mental activity, or any activity for that matter, is causal.

> If we think in terms of the divide between knowledge and reality known, explanation lies on the side of knowledge—on the side of the 'subjective' rather than of the 'objective', on the side of 'representation' rather than of reality represented. Our explanations are part of what we know about the world. (p. 228)

But he does not make any concessions to anti-realism or discursivism:

> Knowledge implies truth . . .
> Every bit of knowledge has an objective counterpart . . .
> The objective counterpart of an explanatory connection is a causal connection. (p. 233)

Thus, for Kim, a genuine explanation identifies an underlying *causal* connection between the *event doing the explaining and the event explained.* His claim seems persuasive for an actual physical phenomenon such as *the brick caused the window to break* because we can see and understand the singular or particular connection between the two events using an intuitive physics and mechanics (similarly, *the lever lifted the car, the jaws cut through the steel,* and so on). But it runs into serious philosophical problems in the case of mental phenomena.

First, there are no singular and identifiable realities (such as the brick, the lever, the cutter, and so on) in the case of mental phenomena and, in fact, the more we look, the more we are led away from realist (and especially reductive) claims in psychology (in the anti-realist direction of Wittgenstein and the connectionists). But an alternative conception of the relation between events might underpin a fairly realistic causal story for mental phenomena.

One popular account is the claim that a causal connection is an instance of a covering law: 'To explain an event is to exhibit it as occupying its (nomologically necessary) place in the discernible pattern of the world' (Salmon, 1993, p. 81). The claim echoes those who argue that the explanatory value of psychological predicates is both important and, in some sense, causal. Davidson (1980) puts the matter as follows: 'Where there is causality, there must be a law; events related as cause and effect fall under strict deterministic laws' (p. 208).

However, Davidson (1980) also offers a series of arguments to the conclusion that there are no laws (of the type found in a nomological account) available in the mental sphere.

(1) There are too many exceptions and *ceteris paribus* clauses to mental explanations for them to count as natural laws (p. 217). We can only gesture at psychological generalizations because all kinds of things undermine predictions and law-like regularities.

But perhaps, the fiendish complexity of the mental field, as in meteorology or some complex physicochemical field, is all that bedevils us here. Mental causation, on this view, merely confirms that any complex field of potentially interacting effects makes scientific predictions prohibitively difficult.

(2) Mental explanations are governed by reason and not just observed contingencies (p. 223).

This point is extensively discussed by Morris (1992) who notes that there is a way that things *ought* to go in mental explanation rather than it just panning out according to causal contingency. Thus, in evaluating an explanation of action, one asks 'Does it make sense?' and if it does not, even though the agent's thought is an accurately rendered, one would say 'That does not explain anything, he must have been temporarily deranged.' For instance, Jesse robs a bank and somebody explains that he did so because the teller was wearing a red shirt. Now, even if that is the thought preceding the intention to rob the bank, it does not explain anything because there is no rational connection between the teller's red shirt and robbing the bank. Things are entirely different in the physical world. I see a lightning flash and hear a peal of thunder and the claim 'That does not make sense because lights cannot cause sounds' cuts no ice. Instead, we set about trying to understand the causal connection by doing the scientific work to find the connection. The scientist might be *surprised* at the forces discovered in a way that does not and cannot occur in normal mental life. Mental explanations make sense because they operate according to standards of reason (however perverted and unusual the reasons in a given case). We do not change the rules to accommodate the inexplicable case; rather, we seek a story that does make sense or is meaningful, or else, we invoke abnormality (or the Ucs). Davidson contends that mental explanation explains behaviour according to the framework of meaning or rationality, one that cannot be assimilated to law-like causal prediction (*pace* Bolton & Hill, 1996, p. 204). But does this argument distinguish mental and physical types of explanation?

(3) The mental domain is open to effects not amenable to mental explanation, such as incidental stimuli, socio-historical conditions, and so on (Davidson, 1980, p. 224).

In the domain of physical law, by contrast, principles of the highest generality operate because, *ex hypothesi*, the domain is closed in that everything is part of it. Nature is everywhere structured according to natural laws. Non-physical incursions in the physical world are not permitted because the mathematical adequacy of any model of the universe depends on its being all encompassing so that events described in any other way can only be acknowledged to have physical effects if a physical explanation is forthcoming.

However, there are clear examples of things with no adequate physical or biological description that do have a profound effect on human minds. For instance, the French revolution and the thoughts and actions it occasioned is not capturable in any descriptions or laws found in the natural sciences. There is therefore a fundamental dissimilarity between mental and physical explanation unless one holds to a fairly extreme Berkeleyan type of theism in which all events hang together because of mental connections, many of which exist only in the mind of God. But that price is unacceptable to most philosophers.

Davidson (1980) himself thinks that mental descriptions are one way (but not the only way) of picking out states and events that explain other states and events by causal laws.

> If the causes of a class of events (actions) fall in a certain class (reasons) and there is a law to back each singular causal statement, it does not follow that there is any law connecting

events classified as reasons with events classified as actions—the classifications may even be neurological, chemical, or physical. (p. 17)

He therefore accepts a nomological account of causality (in which any causal connection must be an instance of a causal law connecting the events and states in question) but argues that such laws do not cover psychological explanations and that the laws allowing us to say that mental events are causal events actually relate to the physical events being denoted (to which they refer). So, for Davidson, psychological explanations must rely on biological laws and generalizations to provide ultimate explanations for the phenomena of human psychology and are not sufficient unto themselves? What is more, he needs basic entities, events, or states that appear in more than one guise (mental and physical) to make the ontology work. Well, 'It ain't necessarily so.'

It is plausible that the physical states, events, and laws connecting them are all incomprehensible and that there are no discernible states and events 'corresponding' to the mental states and events concerned at a physical (physiological or biological) level. Wittgenstein's (1967) analogy with the seed now resurfaces (pp. 208–209). Physiology (or DNA biology) connects a plant's phenotype to its history (of genesis) and cannot be regarded as a code from which phenotype can be read (absent the correlations being painstakingly made); the brain may be equally inscrutable (apart from some relatively non-specific though nevertheless useful generalizations within cognitive neuroscience).

His point is not that of Antony (1989) who takes Davidson to task because he gives too much away by arguing against the causal efficacy of the mental. Mental causality, on the seed/DNA/phenotype analogy, is not material or efficient (of the type investigated by empirical sciences such as mechanics) but is formal or teleological (of the type found in ecology or embryology). We are enlightened by a mental explanation but not because it names physical states whose state descriptions enter into principled (antecedent cause type) explanations. For instance, 'He unloaded the truck in the front garden because he wanted to repay the householder for his rudeness' explains the truck driver's actions in a way that 'The brain state called X caused the bodily movements clustered together under the term Y' does not. The first explanation encourages us to look at certain features of the human story connecting the truck driver, the householder, and the bricks, but the second tells us very little about the wider human life-world related significance of the brick-dumping behaviour. Mental explanation lays bare certain connections because of their significance rather than merely identifying physical states which, if we only understood them, would be shown to be causally connected to each other in biological ways. Davidson fails to explain why this 'laying bare of the connections' matters to us or is significant if it only rests on causal connections between physical states related in law-like ways—why should we bother, what's the point?

In any event, the prospects for the physical causal story are, in fact, quite bleak. Morris (1986) argues that causal accounts worthy of the name obey the 'non-a priori (NAP) requirement' and the 'independent existence (IE) requirement'. The thought is that the relationship should be genuinely discoverable by investigation rather than a pseudo-relationship (so sleep is not caused by the 'dormative virtue' of certain substances—an a priori relationship—but by an independently existing, biochemical species that interacts with the brain in such a way to cause it). Now consider, for instance, the intention that caused John to hit Keith. It vaguely corresponds to a configuration of brain activity that culminates in the hitting and arises from a complex pattern of excitation, seamlessly embedded in the holistic activity of the brain, moving dynamically over the brain areas involved in voluntary action. But the (neurophysiological) reality is only identifiable on looking for the neural precursors of an action (so violates the NAP requirement) and is part of the execution the action (so does not satisfy the IE requirement). Thus, to think of the intention and action as discrete events standing to one another as cause to effect is to misconstrue both of them.

We do better when we realize that explanations of the intentional type concerned serve to 'distinguish among events, to differentiate the networks and levels to which they belong, and to reconstitute the lines along which they are connected and engender one another' (Foucault, 1984, p. 56). An intentional explanation locates the agent's doings in a nexus of human meaning and relationships rather than in a network of physical processes (including neural activity)[2]. We can choose which descriptions and connections are the most revealing and, by so doing, enter what Bolton and Hill (1996) call the domain of decision, taking responsibility for the kind of knowledge we valorize in psychiatry, but we should not delude ourselves that to make a certain kind of choice is to render the contours of psychiatry and disordered human subjectivity in a more realistic way (where we are appealing to commonsensical realism and not some rarefied and unrealistic metaphysical variety).

Causal explanations in psychology are not really what we are after in psychiatry. They are fine for cognitive neuroscience but even there can often blind us to the patterns of adaptation that holistically fit an organism into its (ecological or interpersonal) setting. The human organism relies on its brain to develop routines that reiterate patterns of language-related activity structuring its relation to the human life-world. If the brain is malfunctioning in certain ways—for instance, it cannot narrow its attention on the basis of human techniques of response transmitted between individuals around here—then the human being will become a misfit in our life-world. If the brain malfunctions in other ways, for instance, because it cannot 'tune in' to the rhythm of human activity and give and take in our life-world, then the human being will fail to fit as a being-in-the-world-with-others in a different way. If the brain does not make the connections with emotional and interpersonal responses that others make, then the terms of engagement between that individual and fellow members of the kingdom of ends are changed (in a more calculating and self-serving direction).

Each of these is a disorder or discontent of the mind with causal underpinnings perhaps discoverable in neurophysiological (or cognitive neuroscientific) terms. But the significance of what is going on is registered and articulated with our life-world in terms of the behaviour, conversation, and relationships of the person concerned and how those aspects of being human become configured in the context of the individual's life history, a result that is singular and not general and colourfully

---

[2] I shall return to this issue in Appendix F.

narrative rather than colourlessly scientific. Thus, each malady of the soul is not a natural kind with a causal configuration but is unique or particular to the person concerned, and each suffering patient is an enigma who is more than a code to be cracked by the dispassionate analyst because he or she is a soul who cries out to other souls for recognition, witness, and a hand of compassion (or even healing).

Appendix C

Consciousness, thought, intentionality, and language

Thoughts involve telling how things are with the world. When a person can tell how things are in the world, then she can act on that information. But the ambiguity of the word 'tell' highlights the close relationship between knowledge and language. It is important in the current context that 'tell' has its primary use in narrative and I have argued that consciousness is a narrative spun on the basis of one's engagement with the world (through inscriptions, of two types, on the brain).

The traditional view is that human beings have thoughts that may or may not be expressed in language, which is an 'add-on' to the capacity to think. But is that the case?

> William James, in order to show that thought is possible without speech, quotes the recollection of a deaf-mute, Mr. Ballard, who wrote that in his early youth, even before he could speak, he had had thoughts about God and the world. What can he have meant? Ballard writes: 'It was during those delightful rides, some two or three years before my initiation into the rudiments of written language, that I began to ask myself the question: How came the world into being?' Are you sure, one would like to ask, that this is the correct translation of your wordless thought into words?

> (Wittgenstein, 1953, ¶342)

Wittgenstein notices the clarity of thought that is achieved by articulation. Arguably, as one of my supervisors in Oxford remarked (after Chesterton), 'How do I know what I think until I have written it down?' Even if this is not true of every thought, it is plausible that the capacity to think certain thoughts is internally or conceptually linked to mastery of a certain fragment of language. Dummett (1981) remarks: 'The basic tenet of analytic philosophy ... may be expressed as being that the philosophy of thought is to be equated with the philosophy of language' (p. 39). But what is the relationship between thought and language?

Knowledge involves true thoughts and a person thinks in order to get to know about (or discursively engage with) things around him or her. He or she gathers information so as to derive some truth (or signification) from his or her situation that is framed in terms of concepts obeying certain rules. For instance, if one sees a green giraffe, then the concepts <green> and <giraffe> apply to your encounter and <red>, <square>, and <lion> do not. Truth, we might say, is arrived at by the correct (legitimated) use of certain concepts (according to the praxes in which they are used to reveal and order the significance of things encountered).

Concepts enter into desires, questions, strategies, hypotheses, and all our discursively structured orientations and enactments. In the thought <I would like to see

a green car>, one uses the first person (as distinct from <you> or <he>), <like> (rather than e.g. <fear> or <hate>), and so on for <see>, <green>, and <car> according to the relevant discursive skills so that, in signification, we deploy skills formed in some discourse or other.

Wittgenstein (1953, ¶570) remarks: 'Concepts lead us to make investigations are the expression of our interest and direct our interest.' Concepts organize experience by ordering and systematizing our contact with the world through ways of responding to or classifying things according to rules (Gillett, 1987, 1992) that link different experiences and give them meaning by connecting what is present and available in the present situation to what one has learnt to do at other times and places. When one thinks, for example, <that is a house>, one relates what one is seeing to a rich fabric of knowledge that resides in the rules governing the use of the concept <house>. Such rules

(i)   Are taught and learnt in human interactions;

(ii) Record a pattern of responding in conformity to a rule;

(iii) Allow one to reason about the world and guide one's actions in it;

(iv) Are highly informal and flexible.

Concepts, one might say, are the tools of cognitive adaptation and the rules governing them articulate skills for their deployment by those of us living around here.

Intentionality and private language

A phenomenological path provides us with a naturalistic understanding of the content and significance of experience for human consciousness and action. Brentano argued that the essential feature of the mental was *intentionality* or *aboutness* (1924/1973; 1929/1981, p.58) and noted the selectivity and holistic richness of consciousness:

> A person who hears a chord and distinguishes every single note that it contains is conscious of the fact that he hears them. But a person who does not distinguish the various notes is only indistinctly conscious of them, since he hears them all together, and is conscious of hearing the whole, which includes hearing every individual note. His consciousness, however, does not distinguish every part of the whole.
>
> (Brentano, 1929/1981, p. 25)

Thus, consciousness is more than having the world impinge on one: it involves attention and focusing on conditions shared by the current experience and others related to it so as to delineate what is to be found in a situation through active and dynamic engagement with significant things in the world (Neisser, 1976). The interactive cycle of perception, the selective gathering of information related to those objects relevant for adaptive behaviour, the gestalt nature of figure-ground differentiation, the difference between subliminal consciousness and focused attention, the intentionality of perception (things are seen as being thus and so), and so on are all part of any adequate account of experience and thought (given that conscious experience cannot simply be read off underlying brain events).

The active nature of consciousness recalls Brentano's account of intentionality whereby the conscious mind actively differentiates a focus of attention from the array of information in front of it so that it structures experience by distinguishing a topic or object of thought according to the concepts grasped by the subject (Brentano, 1924/1973). Brentano observed that the objects of which one is conscious are differentiated from other objects. Thus, when I notice the fly on the wall, I must notice it *as something* (e.g. a black speck, a piece of dirt, or a fly) and the contents of consciousness depend not only on the object as a physical stimulus but also on the way in which I am thinking of that object and have differentiated it from context or ground in my conscious experience so that it becomes a meaningful object of perception (Anscombe, 1981). To specify the intentional object is to say what I apprehend it as or what it signifies to me—to reveal the signification in play (Wittgenstein, 1953, II. xi).

Intentionality, by relating features of the world to signification, enables a subject to develop structures for mapping the world so that he or she can plan and organize her activity (thus, *re-presentation*, a way of recovering for present use the significant and meaningful features of an object or situation with which one has, in the past, been presented). Signification is (importantly) conceptual; it involves a recoverable characterization of the object (e.g. as a fly or, in a different case, as the man from next door) in a way that leads us to Husserl's (1962) discussion of noetic content (pp. 235ff).

Husserl (1962) followed Kant in holding that the subject, from contact with the world, received information of a primitive undifferentiated sort (*hyle* or sensile matter; sensory matter [Kant]). The subject then makes sense of this information by imposing detailed *noetic content* (conceptual or meaningful content) elaborating the primitive noema—<something out there>. The ideal forms or *noemata* are objective and normative for the signification in question; for instance, the judgement <that is an apple> is evaluated against the noematic standard for being an apple. But this strong, indeed essential, relationship between a given noema and the object or condition in the world intended by it requires an essential link between something ideal (in the mirror-world of logic)—a *noema*—and the world. Wittgenstein forges the missing connection (as does Kant [Gillett, 1997a]).

There is a pervasive structure of rules governing discourse that, *inter alia*, prescribes what conditions in the world warrant the application of any concept. Such shared rules, defined in terms of conditions mutually accessible by more than one thinker, forge the link between a subject and the world because the rule is articulated and used by the subject. They are world involving in that correct use must be conveyed through what Cavell (1993) calls 'triangulation' as part of a shared praxis (language-related activity). Think, for instance, of the concept <cat>. The rules governing its application must link my use of the concept <cat> to the usage of others, and if I cannot access the conditions responded to by my teacher or interlocutor, then it is unclear how I could be corrected when I make mistakes, track the conditions it is tied to, or know that I am using it as it ought to be used on any subsequent occasion; hence the famous 'private language argument' (Wittgenstein, 1953, ¶201ff).

Wittgenstein argues (as does Kant) that I could not learn the use of any word if the conditions of use were hidden in the mind and inaccessible to others by inviting us to imagine a situation in which a totally private sensation is followed by a resolution to mark it for future use by fixing a sign 'S'. He then observes that the only criterion for thinking that I am encountering S again is that it seems to me that I am. But *it seems to me that I am right* is not the same as being right, and so the criteria for correctness cannot be private in this way and 'An inner process stands in need of outward criteria' (1953, ¶580). Our concepts are given their content by rule-governed skills developed in a shared world in which human beings invent various techniques, use signs to mark them, and teach them through training in their use in the context of intersubjective discourse in a shared domain of activity.

Millikan (1993) also discusses rule following, as a natural or biological function, and argues that the purpose of meaningful communication is to share thoughts on objects equally available to other thinkers so that the objects that are the focus of the discourse must be out in the world and not in the mind of either thinker. The discourse and associated training are, on the present view, prescriptive and normative, located in a sociocultural setting, and not the result of a purely natural or biological mechanism in the head (Baker & Hacker, 1980, p. 336; Wittgenstein, 1953, ¶196). That fact means that intersubjectivity is central in understanding intentional adaptation and the development of cognition immerses each of us in a normative context, which we learn to articulate and think about in terms conveyed by speech and to which we must adapt to become a human subject.

Consciousness and the gap

A further problem in the discussion of consciousness is the so-called 'gap' problem. The gap is the incomprehensibility of what it is like to be me in the face of a detailed specification of neurobiological processes. I have argued that the gap is an artefact of the private theatre view of consciousness in which there is an inner array (including qualia, qualitative features of experience) that makes up one's autobiographical world. But the gap can also be accounted for in terms of (i) the difference between being in the world and thinking about being in the world; (ii) the whole story of my life trajectory as a being-in-the-world-with-others; and (iii) the difference between an informational state and the engaged experience of a critter like me.

The first is graphically illustrated by the difference between a brick hitting your foot and being told about a brick hitting your foot (you don't get a bruise for a start).

The second is the Othello in a nutshell problem—How do you sum up Othello as a one-liner and convey the richness and complexity of the play?

The third is the suspicion that attaches to a silicon humanoid (call him Hugo) who picks up all the information from an alien setting, who makes the right kinds of reflexive moves and ejaculations that would accompany the kind of information it is sending back ('Ouch, that feels hot!'), but who is not a *critter like me*—so, what does it really feel like to Hugo?

Articulating these things draws on all the ills that flesh is heir to and our engagement in practices and forms of life which unite us as human beings (so that if a lion could talk, we could not understand him). In that milieu, one learns to compare, connect, and evoke the many shared situations in the human life-world that add nuance and colour to one's current experience and so convey to others what it is like to be placed as one is at that moment.

Varieties of alienation

Alienation (*Entfremdung* in German) refers to the separation of things that naturally belong together, or to the antagonism between things that should be in harmony. Its most important use is in relation to the alienation of people from aspects of their 'human nature' (*Gattungswesen*, usually translated as 'species-essence' or 'species-being') and it arises from various kinds of social arrangement or structure. Marx sees it as a systematic result of capitalism in which the state authorizes certain individuals to alienate from others the natural products of their labour under terms that amount to exploitation and reduce all human relations to marketplace transactions (Marx & Engels, 1845/1970).

I want to distinguish four types of alienation relevant to psychiatry (and the philosophy of medicine in general).

(1) Alienation from one's illness

(2) Alienation from oneself

(3) Alienation from one's culture

(4) Collective alienation—'How can we sing the Lord's song in a strange land?'

Alienation from one's illness

This form of alienation occurs when an illness is described and reconfigured by what I have called 'the basilisk-like gaze' of contemporary scientific biomedicine (Gillett, 2004). That gaze, based on anatomy, the study of cadavers ('fixed' or 'petrified' human beings), objective scientific measurements, 'fixes'(choose your own sense) the suffering individual in terms based in the biomedical model of health and disease and its scientific categories. The discourse framing that discussion may be quite unfamiliar to the patient and have the effect of distancing their illness from them as something that is beyond their understanding because the way it is constructed and reflected back to them is so arcane and inaccessible (Hunter, 1991). The patient therefore devalues or discounts his or her own intuitions and observations about the illness and can conceal a great deal that would be of clinical importance on the basis that it is not legitimate knowledge of the type that should be part of medical treatment or their own adaptation to their illness.

Alienation from oneself

Alienation from oneself is produced when one's imago (image-ego) is so distorted by discursive forces that one cannot recognize oneself or feel at home in one's subjective body as one's mode of being in the human life-world. It could happen through various processes, some biological and some discursive. The problem happens in psychosis when the subject's ongoing informational contact with the world is thrown out by a failure of the smoothly articulated processes of perception, cognition, and action that engage one with the world and fashion one's lived, signified trajectory in it as a coherent 'self'. This is the failure of ipseity, discussed by Sass and phenomenological theorists, and it makes the psychotic's conscious life radically solipsistic and fractured from the competencies that one normally gains through using shared meanings to structure one's life and experience and to guide one's actions. The alienation of dissociative disorders is otherwise: in it, the meanings that articulate life are not properly grounded in what is happening between oneself as an embodied subject and the human life-world. That results in one miscalling what is going on between the self and world so that the legitimacies and connections of the mirror-world of discourse are not linked in the right kind of way to one's own being-in-the-world-with-others.

Both types of alienation from self represent a breakdown of the normally smoothly negotiated matching of the world of meaning and the world of actual physical engagement with things and people around one.

Alienation from one's culture

This again is a breakdown in the ability of the individual to structure his or her life according to the language games and forms of life around here. It may happen because one is a stranger in a strange land or because one has been cut off from the ability to value and identify with one's own culture (perhaps because that culture is repressed, despised, or dispirited, no longer being a place of living and energetic activity, so that its demons—enlivening informing forces and entities—have died).

Collective alienation—'how can we sing the Lord's song in a strange land?'

This can occur to a whole culture when its language and the forms of life structured by that language are allowed to die or become marginalized and devitalized. That death leaves whole groups of human beings lacking a place to stand where they belong and can have their traditional identity affirmed. In a sense, it cuts them off from the roots or ground of their being and disconnects them from the sources of value that normally go along with lineage, heritage, tradition, heroes of the past, myths, and a solidarity and identity that transcends the current era.

Appendix E

Epistemology and other minds

There are two strands to epistemology: the first concerns the justification of knowledge claims (philosophical epistemology) and the second our method of gaining knowledge (a psychological or cognitive-developmental account). Naturalism in epistemology undermines this distinction because a story about how we get knowledge embeds an understanding of its natural function in our adaptation to a domain of action and thus its status as the kind of thing endorsed by epistemic norms (warrant and reliabilist accounts take this form [Plantinga, 1993]). The phenomenological and hermeneutic perspectives (and therefore, post-structuralist views) note that the natural events and processes (allowing the psyche to take frames or horizons of meaning and apply them to being-in-the-world) are shaped by social and cultural factors producing second nature as the basis of human adaptation. These approaches concur with contemporary developmental psychology in placing primary (or primordial) intersubjectivity (always already being with others) as a fundamental human condition.

Classical empiricist theories

Most epistemologies share a commitment to experience as the basis of knowledge (Berkeley, 1710, 1713/1969; Hume, 1739/1969; Kant, 1789/1929; Locke, 1689/1975) so that 'I am looking at something red' is justified on the basis of its connections to current experience (usually construed in terms of [causal] processes within the individual).

I have noted that psychotic phenomena such as hallucination and delusion are best understood according to a different theory in which consensual validation and shared modes of constructing experience are deficient in the psychotic's mental world. Autism reinforces that argument by prompting a radical revision of the foundations of an adequate and plausible account of human knowledge. A human being interacts within a meaning-giving environment (a discursively structured life-world) embodying norms that both shape and provide a framework of justification for the skills that comprise epistemic virtue.

Traditional empiricist epistemology lays its foundations on the physical organs of human sensation (lower-level components of a causal system) and works upwards from them to 'representations' and the quasi-computational processes comprising cognition (an approach called methodological solipsism [Fodor, 1968]). Thus, knowledge is a complex product of work done on 'stimuli', 'sensory input', 'simple impressions' (Locke, 1689/1975), or 'sense data' (Russell, 1959) where the 'input' is generally defined by reference to physical receptors and their functions (i.e. patches of coloured light, sounds, smells, and so on) and forms the building blocks of more complex experiences (or representations) such as the perception that one is looking at a starling, hearing a Beethoven sonata, or passing a coffee shop. The obvious analogy is with the periodic table in which atoms are combined to form molecules exhibiting a rich variety of chemical properties, but the atoms themselves come in only a limited range of basic types. Indeed, one might see psychophysics and perceptual physiology as an attempt to begin this systematic building of a psychology of perception (and therefore, as doing the scientific work predicated on the empiricist approach to epistemology).

Empiricist epistemology and the associated Empiricist Representational Theory of Mind (Gillett, 1992) treats complex constructions (such as the idea of Paris or the idea of human beings as a distinct type of thing in the world) as constructions. Thus, in discerning that one is dealing with a human subject, the theory implies that we construct representations of bodily movements from simpler (though still fiendishly complex) patterns of impressions and then infer from those complex ideas (of bodily movements) the inner states and events causing them (according to a 'theory of mind'). This is the classic 'theory theory' (Morton, 1980) of other minds using inference to the best explanation 'Inference to the Best Explanation' (IBE) as its cognitive modus operandi.

On the theory-theory account, one attributes beliefs, desires, and intentions to others through deploying (possibly tacit) theoretical knowledge. One uses connecting links (such as those between line of vision, attention, and perception, and/or between perception, background knowledge, and belief, and/or between belief, desire, and intention, and/or between perception, intention, and action) and predicts and explains the actions of others (Carruthers, 1996, p. 24). The 'theory theory' thus claims, 'What I will recognize when I recognize that I have M is a state having a particular folk psychological characterization' (Carruthers, 1996, p. 26). The theory is usually modified so that implausible conscious inferential moves are not required by having the embedded inferences not at the personal conscious level but rather subpersonal (or tacit).

Thus, an empiricist (or even a post-empiricist) regards perceiving a human being as a highly complex epistemic attainment based on the article of faith that a realistic naturalized epistemology must begin with physically, causally, or biologically specifiable inputs to our receptors and the way in which combinations of these provide input into higher circuits (Dretske, 1988, Millikan, 1984; Pinker, 1997). Devitt (1990), for instance, remarks, 'In psychology, we are concerned to explain why, given stimuli at her sense organs, a person evinced certain behaviour' (p. 377), a thesis that holds sway even when the role of language (and therefore, implicitness, intersubjectivity, and a shared world) in cognitive content is explicitly acknowledged.

> Our perceptual experience (what we ordinarily refer to as the look, sound, and feel of things) is being identified with an information-carrying structure—a structure in which information about a source is coded in analog form and made available to something like a digital converter for cognitive utilization.
>
> (Dretske, 1988, p. 162)

The child, according to this approach, is an epistemic individual—'the scientist in the crib' (Bruner, 2000) confronting a blooming, buzzing confusion. He or she distils certain regularities out of that 'flux' and derives meaningful patterns with adaptive value in the world, a form of solipsism, the more sophisticated and cognitively plausible versions of which (such as post-empiricism) note the active and exploratory nature of that phenomenon (but the computational and physicalist approach to human knowledge is far more applicable to autism than normal human epistemological development).

Post-empiricism embraces, for instance, views such as those of Piaget (and Pinker) who follows Kant in emphasizing the need for the thinker to approach experience already equipped with certain rules (the conservation of matter, the interaction of coincident bodies, and so on) that operate on the sensory flux in such a way as to yield ideas about objects, events, and causes, in accordance with 'an intuitive mechanics'. Piaget's (1972) developmental theory links the orderly and progressive elaboration of observations and inferences into a system of epistemology to the developmental stages of childhood in which a cognitive individual explores the world to discover, from its own observations, the patterns and regularities existing there.

Given such a theory, some of the most complex patterns that the child must unravel are the patterns associated with other human beings. The child must derive knowledge not only that this is a complex animate being but also that it is a being of the same type as itself and is as conscious of the world as the child finds itself to be (or even more so). This truly outstanding inference (underlying the argument from analogy to the existence of other minds) becomes more implausible the more one questions it (Malcolm, 1958; Zahavi, 2004, p. 149).

The central tenet of 'the argument from analogy to the existence of other minds' (common to both hot [simulation theory] and cold [IBE], forms) is that the child uses the analogy between himself or herself and others to infer that they are conscious minds.

(1) The child only perceives physically detectable and describable patterns of stimuli.

(2) The child has an experience of self as conscious agent.

(3) The child notices patterns of stimuli emanating from the other similar to those arising from himself or herself.

(4) The child concludes that the other person is a conscious agent.

(I shall defer attending to premise 2 until we discuss what we might call empathy—or *verstehen*-based approaches to the problem.)

Premise 3 states that the child sees certain patterns of movement and thinks <Aha, that being moves like me, so possibly is in other respects like me and so has conscious experiences>. But this is too quick. The movements of the other are, according to the epistemic constraints accepted by the theory, no more similar to my actions than an alien experience of my arm going up is similar to my raising my arm. What is more, the most salient, *subjective* features (conscious accompaniments or mental associations) of the situation are missing when another interacts with the world. How do I ever conclude that that object over there, in the path of an oncoming dog, is in the same situation as I am when I face an oncoming dog if the situations are totally different? There is no fear or impression of being approached unless I already have some empathic tendency and some predisposition to mobilize it to inform the scene played out before me. Thus, on the basis of stimulus conditions (only some aspects of which are comparable), I am supposed to conclude that a being over there is similar to me. But it is only similar if I already feel the empathy that is supposed to follow from my inference; truly, an impasse.

Imagine that I, Child Robinson, abroad in a world of complex and strangely animate objects, see one of those objects, A, approach another, B. If A approached me, I would feel fear. This event does not cause me any detectable fear, but I nevertheless conclude that there is a fear-making internal organ (the mind) involved because the manifestations evident in B look similar to manifestations arising in myself (note that they only look this way to someone who is in a position I have never occupied in relation to myself). 'But how do I know they look like that?' If I were to perform the imaginative feat of occupying the position where I observe the head of the other to be and the further imaginative feat of conceiving that the other might be the kind of being who could be *appeared to*, then there might be an analogy. A moment's thought should suggest that what is going on here is so unlike anything that happens to me (it does not feel the same, the movements do not look the same, and so on) that it could not be the same. To grasp the sameness, I would have to grasp the possibility of and instantly appreciate what it would be like to be me in another place, that is, to be another minded being. Thus, the argument from analogy suggests that I must be in the epistemic position I am supposed to arrive at before I come to the conclusion that leads to that position. We are left with an impossible dilemma:

Either I empathize and thus realize that this is the kind of situation I might be in and so the conclusion is redundant: I am already thinking of the other as similar to me—conscious, or being-appeared-to, and acting in or responding to the world;

Or I view this phenomenon as I would any other and notice that it does not have any of the apparent and salient features that accompany consciousness and therefore that the inference flies in the face of all the methods I normally use.

Apart from the fact that the child is supposed to arrive at the conclusion required as a premise in the argument, an additional source of implausibility is the fiendish complexity of such a theory and the early stage in cognitive development at which it is posited (Leslie, 1987). Thus, the account fails in both of the aims of a theory of knowledge of other minds: it fails to justify the claim to know that someone else is conscious or has a mind in that the conclusion is unsound on the basis of the premises and evidence available; it also fails to explain the knowledge of other minds because the theory is implausible when faced with real data from real children. Give me an intuitive awareness of intersubjectivity or a natural tendency to mirror or feel with others (such as might lead to an ability to empathize) and I find myself surrounded by other subjects; refuse me that position and I have no reason to arrive at it. The prospects are not good for the other minds inference as a plausible account of how we come to know that other minds exist (whether I do it by simulation or theory).

This difficulty haunts any epistemic individualist trying to understand human life in a world inhabited by other creatures with whom it has no primordial mode of 'feeling with' or identification. But we are not like that: we have mirror neurones that attune us to the thoughts, feelings, and intentions of others. We are linked to others in exactly the (subjective) respects that inform my own behaviour (the manifestations of my imago). I read the meanings in what others do and use our shared discourse to frame myself against the same horizon of meaning and value. Thus, the 'other minds' inference fits the experiences of autistic people but seems hopelessly awry when applied to the normal child intuitively connected to others as a being-in-the-world with them.

Empathic or verstehen theories

The two different attempts to overcome the other minds puzzle within empiricism (theory-theory and simulation-theory) are distinct from one another despite their similarities in form (data [internal recognition] and cognition [analogical inference]).

> According to theory-theory, as I use the term, autism is centrally a deficiency of knowledge or at any rate of belief. Simulation-theory says that autism is a deficiency of imaginative capacity—the capacity to project the self imaginatively into a situation other than its own current, actual position.

> (Currie, 1996, p. 243)

Currie (1996) distinguishes between 'having a theory of mind, engaging in simulative or empathetic role taking, and understanding other minds' (p. 245) where the first two are proposals about how we do the third. Currie likens the contrast to that between *knowing that* and *knowing how* in that the first concentrates on beliefs and inferences and the other on skills and mental capacities. The interactive or intersubjective view based on praxis, attunement, and discursive interactions contrasts with both.

The underlying individualist thesis in the argument from analogy (in general and theory-theories of knowledge of other minds in particular) also affects 'empathic', *verstehen*, and 'simulation' theories so that they all fail when subject to the criticism of traditional epistemology arising from a searching reflection on the problems of autism. Simulation theory (or empathic- or *verstehen*-based theories) avoids the implausibilities of theory-theory by invoking a special kind of knowledge with a basic role in one's understanding of the world and what happens in it. Goldman (1993), for instance, conceives of introspective knowledge as follows:

(1) I have awareness of my own mental states by introspectively categorizing them.

(2) I categorize my mental states on the basis of their qualitative features.

(3) When I observe another person, I simulate their current mental states by imaginatively projecting myself into their situation.

(4) This simulation allows me not only to predict what they will do but also to feel what they feel.

He illustrates as follows: 'To estimate how disappointed someone would feel if he lost a certain tennis match or did poorly on a certain exam, you might project yourself into the relevant situation and see how you would feel' (Goldman, 1993, p. 27).

This 'hot' theory implies that I use my emotive and introspective recognition and categorization of mental states in my own case and project that into the situation of another. As an individualistic theory, it falls foul of the basic objection to the argument from analogy that we have already discussed (inferring analogy in the face of startling dissimilarity) but also of Wittgenstein's proscriptions against private language as a basis for meaningful rule-governed use of categories (see Chapter 1 and Appendix A).

Firstly, the argument depends upon my identifying the other person as a being like me. How do I form this view? If it is just innate or instinctive to feel this way about others, as the phenomenologists suggest, it gives infants a real evolutionary advantage that can overcome their 'specific prematurity' (Lacan, 1977). It enables children to affiliate themselves to competent and well-adapted 'critters like me around here' and learn the tricks they have developed to organize their experience and activity. But that evolutionary trick cannot be offered as a solution to the traditional problem of other minds.

According to Goldman's account, a subject categorizes his or her own mental states on the basis of their qualitative or subjective features. In doing this categorization job, as Wittgenstein (1953) notes, 'whatever is going to seem right to me is right; and that only means that here we can't talk about "right"'(¶258). I can stand to be corrected and indeed, in cognitive development, must learn to differentiate and correctly judge the states I am in. Ask oneself a cognitive-developmental question: 'Has he known from birth and incorrigibly that just this state is anger?' Note that, were he French, he would always have known something different, viz. that just this state is *colere*. This innate incorrigibility about the meaning of a word which, by happy coincidence, seems to be given the same meaning by every other co-linguistic speaker seems just too miraculous to underpin a good philosophical theory of mind.

Second, notice the difficulty he has with the question 'How do you know that what you refer to as anger is exactly the same as what another person refers to as anger?' There are two possible answers, both of which are problematic.

The first answer would be as follows:

(1) He recognizes conditions C1, C2, C3 and the reactions R1, R2, R3 in person B.

(2) He imaginatively identifies with the person concerned.

(3) He feels state X—a state he calls 'anger'.

(4) He concludes A must be in the state X, called 'anger'.

But the mirror neurone system makes this inference otiose. Wittgenstein's account of mind holds that anger refers to whatever people feel when a set of manifestations (critical conditions and reactions) enable us to discern when a critter like oneself is in a certain state and again converges with what we know about the mirror neurone system making the internal 'hot' 'posit' and inference redundant. Thus, simulation theory fares little better than theory-theory by suggesting that we neither perform complex (albeit cognitive operations) nor do we spark inferential chains from classifying our own inner states (by incorrigible introspective faculties of self-knowledge) but rather we resonate with others and learn to place ourselves against the shared structures of meaning that pervade the human life-world.

This shared practice view of mental life recognizes the idea that a developing human thinker latches on to skills defined and refined in discourse with others when that thinker begins to articulate his or her mental life so as to exploit regularities and inter-active expectations to kick-start the difficult process of self-knowledge (a complex of descriptions and evaluations). *Second*, noting certain common human tendencies (first nature), it relativizes the discourse about the mind to the language in which the developing thinker is immersed (thus English—'anger', French—'colere') as they are formed (develop a second nature). *Third*, it forges an internal link between the meanings of intentional terms used by different thinkers and thus incorporates the essentially shared nature of meaning. Hence, as already noted, to say 'I am angry' is to say 'I am in the state characteristic of human beings when certain conditions impinge on them and they react in characteristic ways' and to say this because one has picked up the appropriate use of 'anger' from those competent in one's natural language. *Fourth*, it relativizes the ascription of mental states to the culture in which one has grown and learnt to know oneself (Harre & Gillett, 1994).

Therefore, a mental categorization (or ascription of, say, 'depression', 'joy', or 'anger') refers to 'the state that creatures like me tend to be in when they find themselves in certain conditions'. On this view, the inner feeling is naturally tied to the meaning of the mental term and our tendency to categorize similar situations by using techniques associated with shared linguistic terms becomes pivotal. This, in turn, implies that our language about the mind is based on a primitive and shared recognition that each of us is surrounded by creatures of the same type. But this then finesses the need for each of us to develop internalized theories about other minds and inserts the engagement with others (as minded or subjective beings) as a fundamental aspect of human experience.

The empiricist approaches begin with behaviour and context and miss the primary intersubjectivity that attunes us to others so, even though in their developed form, they forge conceptual connections between self and other attribution (of mental states) they do not quite catch the closeness of that relation. Thus, we are still left with some form of inference to the mental life of others as the basis of interpersonal knowledge. On the other hand, phenomenological theories justify a substantial emphasis on intersubjectivity as primary (or primordial) in the human condition as a being engaged with others in a shared life-world.

Action explanation, free will, and moral responsibility

Explaining action

I have argued (in Appendices A and B) that mental explanation or the explanation of behaviour in terms of the thoughts, attitudes, and other aspects of an individual's mental life is not a kind of causal explanation but is rather a way of understanding the meaning of the act performed and the way in which it is enacted at a particular moment in the story of the individual concerned. Therefore, it maps the individual onto the structure of meaning and human practices that articulate the human life-world of the individual and 'folk around here' (something that autistic children find impenetrable). Traditional discussions of intentional action explain the bodily movement that is the agent's action in terms of states within the agent that causally determine that movement through the will or the volition of the person.

The will and disorders of volition

A classically insane patient has psychotic disorders of thought and may, as a result, have hallucinations, disruption of thought form and content, and delusions (see Chapter 5). In such patients, the ability to reason about, formulate, and act upon a coherent plan is disordered, and although the patient undertakes a course of action that appears intentional, logically sound, and rational in some sense (as in the case of the infanticidal mother), we often recognize that there is a disorder of belief or reasoning sufficient to undercut our normal judgements of motive, intention, and responsibility. Why is this?

The crucial connection between reasoning, character, and intention is undermined in psychosis because the person *qua* rational, willing agent has through a causal process (the disease) become caught up in a range of thoughts and images over which he or she does not have control and which are not properly connected to his or her usual personality and patterns of thought. It is only when the agent is in the normal ownership or authorship relation to the act he or she performs that we are able to attribute moral responsibility.

An intention is a decision to act as a result of beliefs, attitudes, and reasoning and the will is the ability to translate reasoning into actions. An agent with willpower (or volitional integrity) does it consistently and well, and is appropriately responsive to the situation in which he or she acts. Imagine two people, Mat and Nat, faced by a situation involving offensive provocation (such as sledging in a cricket match).

Each of them knows that self-control is an advantage. The first, Mat, finally loses it, gets into a slinging match, is cautioned, and soon after gets bowled out, but the other player, Nat, remains cool and collected, despite the insults he is enduring. Nat clearly has a stronger will than Mat because he is able to act reasonably, forming a settled resolve not to be rattled, and recognizing that a loss of temper would cause him to play rashly, controls his behaviour. He exercised *phronesis* (practical wisdom or developed virtue).

The psychotic cannot do this because his mind and thought is often fragmented and his reasoning and associations so disrupted that he does not act with the consistency of a person in control of what he does. We can attribute the disordered intention or failure of the will to an 'illness' disrupting his ability to think and act with relatively consistent, coherent, and controlled intentions because psychotic thought and experience is marked by bizarre and unfathomable turns poorly integrated into the person's character and thus disconnecting action from his or her responsibility. But no such disorder of thought undermines the actions of a psychopath whose volition is differently impaired.

Volition and rules

The will is the fount of actions and volition is the ability to act as one chooses. In the case of Mat and Nat, Mat's outburst could be explained in more than one way. Mat could say, 'The insults and remarks I had to endure became so offensive that eventually I thought, *Hang it all, nothing is worth putting up with this!*' or perhaps 'I knew I shouldn't but eventually I just lost it and exploded.' In the first case, there is a shift in the balance of reasons; in the second, he lacks the ability to enact the conclusion of his all things considered 'best judgement' (Davidson, 1980). A third possibility is that he is overcome by an uncontrollable urge to do the wrong thing. These three possibilities can be explored in the light of the neurophilosophy of the will.

Practical reasoning and the will are beset by a range of notoriously difficult philosophical problems beginning with the famous is–ought dispute. Many follow Hume, believing that a judgement of fact—what is the case—is quite different from a judgement of value—what ought to be the case. But *oughts* or prescriptions discursively underpin judgements of what is the case in that judging that a state of affairs is thus and so one assigns a significance to it according to how one thinks one *ought* to see it (as a result of training and perhaps conversations with others). For instance, imagine an unequal exchange of goods, Jo, and Bro. You remark, 'Jo seems to have made a bad deal.' Your friend, somewhat more knowing says, 'That, my boy, is extortion under threat.' You learn that some relevant aspects of the situation are not evident to you and realize that you need a correct view of the facts. So '*is*'s' (here <that is extortion>) and '*oughts*' (<you ought to see it as such>) are interwoven in our thoughts, intentions, and actions.

What is more, a lot of important beliefs—for instance, that one is disliked—are based on reactive attitudes. We perceptually track moral, emotive, and other factors in our experiences with others and reason about moral affectations as much as we do about anything else we perceive; both contribute to a sound view of the world and the personal and social realities within it (Bruner, 1990). Philosophers focused on perceptual beliefs such as <the cat has tortoise-shell colouring> neglect beliefs such as <he is angry> or <that is extortion> in which the sensitivity or recognition involved in judgements such as <he is cruel>, a moral belief, or <he doesn't like me>, a reactive belief, comes into play. Beliefs of that kind are common in practical and moral reasoning (figuring out what I should do) as distinct from speculative or theoretical reasoning (figuring out what is the case) but they help us to track significances, affordances, opportunities, and other clues to the human life-world. There is therefore a sense of 'rational' or 'sound' thinking that draws on an all-in or balanced ability to make judgements about life events and what a person should do (Spitzer, 1990c, p. 46).

There is also a significant link between what I do and who I am. Consider the implausibility of a libertarian doctrine of intentional action in which behaviour has a capricious or unpredictable relationship to a person's character. If Xavier acts violently or deceitfully when he is normally gentle, sensitive, patient, considerate, and honest, we look for some explanation. Why has he suddenly 'lost the plot' or acted 'out of character' and is he responsible for the change? If some causal disruption of the narrative pattern that is his (more or less) integrated character (such as a personal betrayal that is deeply wounding or a psychotic illness) has occurred, we make the necessary allowances. Notice that we fit his behaviour in an account of his adaptation to the world as a being of a certain type and we reckon that most of us, most of the time, enact the cumulative repertoire of (normatively structured) meaning making skills that form character and inform one's lived narrative.

The idea that in each of us there is a Cartesian (extensionless and unconfigured by historical contingency) point of willing unconnected to preceding conditions (as implied by some construals of the idea of free will) is non-sensical. Sartre, for instance, relates human action to the 'nothingness at the heart of being' that is human consciousness so that an action manifests a moment of consciousness informed by the person's apprehension of the way that things could be (even they are not presently that way). This *negation* (or counterfactual), constituted by the judgement that things are *not* thus and so, motivates action rather than any antecedently existing conditions (including inner states of my psyche) and it reflects the value conferred on the non-existent state of affairs by a choice of the agent: 'Thus, the being of value *qua* value is the being of what does not have being' (Sartre, 1958, p. 93). The freely conferred value is fundamental in action and therefore an intrinsic feature of being human: 'Human reality does not exist first in order to act later; but for human reality to be is to act, and to cease to act is to cease to be' (Sartre, 1958, p. 476).

Sartre (1958) argues that any situation is radically subject to one's willed choices because an act of apprehension is also involved in conferring significance upon any situation.

We choose the world, not in its contexture as in itself, but in its meaning …

This means that we apprehend our choice as not deriving from any prior reality but rather as being about to serve as foundation for the complex of significations which constitute reality. (pp. 463, 464).

Sartre (1958) denies that psychic mechanisms or states deterministically produce action (and therefore opposes all psychodynamic accounts) because the key to understanding action is the free apprehension by the individual of the modifiability of the current situation into something it is not. 'The free project is fundamental for it is my being' (p. 479) and experiencing a situation as being thus and so is therefore a matter of one's choices about the significances and meanings informing it; 'there is freedom only in a situation, and there is a situation only through freedom' (p. 489).

Sartre's view implies a non-causal story about meaning and the psyche and embeds the claim that character is cumulative action, so that a person is constituted by what he or she does. Therefore, the 'inner self' causing a person to act thus and so is a myth or an excuse offered when our behaviour falls short of some ideal or expectation. The 'inner self', 'the real me', and 'my character' or personality, for Sartre, provide a refuge for cowards because they seem to diminish one's immediate responsibility for acting in a certain way here and now. For instance, 'I would go for a run every day but I just get absorbed in my work' is a kind of excuse for preferring to sit around than to go jogging; 'I am the kind of person who cannot resist pudding' blames an inner disposition rather than admitting, 'I often take more pudding although I know and believe I should not.' One should own one's actions and take responsibility for them because even if one has a disposition, a present choice, here and now, translates it into action.

Sartre's existential libertarianism, despite its philosophical and phenomenological support, ignores the reality that we all live and act on the basis of a myriad dispositions and commitments. We resonate with Luther's cry 'Here I stand, I can do no other!' The evident connections between psychic attributes and intentional action become a pressing topic in philosophical analyses of unconscious and extraconscious factors in the genesis of psychic states. But the metaphysics of the world of meaning entails that the connections cannot be causal; so we need a better story to tell about human action.

Hume (1739/1969), in an attempt to take account of character in the genesis of human action, coined the term 'liberty of spontaneity' (p. 455). By this, he meant that a free action, or an act for which the agent is responsible, is properly called so because it is caused by the desires and beliefs (inner states) of the agent. However, prior causal events form a series and the causal chain producing the mental events (in principle or theoretically) link mental states and events to what affects the mind (which one is inclined also to think of in causal terms). Thus, a causal link between intentional action and states and events in the mind leads beyond those events to the states and events producing them so that the story of any action becomes the story of a series of events causing a human being to act as he or she does, and there is no place for the agent, in it (except as the actual conduit for the relevant causal chains). In short, the causal account is in danger of implying that my behaviour is produced by events not under my control with little hope of distinguishing acts caused by an abnormal process (as is posited in psychopathy and other 'disorders of volition') from 'normal' acts morally attributable to the agent.

The account is not easily fixed in any way compatible with our deeper intuitions about responsibility and human action. Some theorists argue that intentional acts are just acts caused by the agent and that 'agent causality' makes them intentional

(Morris, 1992, pp. 126ff) so that I am responsible for those acts I bring about through a prior act of the will. But if that prior act of the will is also an act which I must bring about, we have a further problem of explanation. Why would the psychic movement—the act of the will—causing my overt act not itself be a caused event? If that is itself something I bring about, a regress of 'acts of the will' then looms (Morris, 1992, p. 135). We therefore need to go beyond the obscure 'brought about by me' or 'agent causation' condition.

An adequate account of willing should explain why doing something freely or willfully rests moral responsibility for the act on the agent. I have argued that intentional action, say stealing a car, involves rule following because (rule-governed) concepts structure meaningful action in the human world. Therefore, because rules (including moral rules) might be obeyed or not obeyed, following a rule is not (essentially) compelled or automatic. A rule does not force you to obey it; on the contrary, you must adopt the practice of obeying it (if it is to structure your behaviour). For instance, if I want to make a cake, just any old set of ingredients combined in any old way will not do; there are limits to what will pass. One can refuse to follow a rule to shock others ('That is not a fur, that is a dismembered living creature!'), because one cannot be bothered ('Finesse, schminesse, I don't do subtlety'), to make a point ('Why should $-1 \times -1 = +1$, not -2?') or through sheer bloody-mindedness ('It is not tax, it is theft and extortion'). Mastering a practice and sticking to it are aspects of a skill or ability that some have and others do not, and even if an agent possesses the skill, it can be exercised or not according to the agent's attitude. Thus, finding out why a certain person did not have the skill (or had not cultivated the ability), or chose not to use it on a particular occasion, may tell us more about him than any battery of brain imaging results.

Notice that rules and rule following result in an agent developing skills or techniques that are adaptive around here and use the significance of things (that is a handle) to exploit those things (if I turn it, something might open up) and solve puzzles or problems in the domain (Aha, so that is how we get out of here!). Such techniques aid in both short- and long-term social and general adaptation (I told you guys I would show you the way; now do you trust me?). As a result, one learns to operate effectively and in a way that fits one into the activities and projects of others as a participant in the human life-world (So how are we supposed to find this thing?)

A significant set of problems for critters like us are moral problems in which we negotiate our being-in-the-world-with-others in ways that show reciprocity and allow us to build relationships. In those problems, the moral 'ought' is an important guide and we ignore it at our peril (You ought not to lie like that if you want to work with other people and you want them to trust you!)

A strong will reflects a person's ability to translate reason into action (through self-control and application to a task) and a good will conducts itself in the light of reasons formed in relation to moral oughts (i.e. one fulfils one's duties and acts with appropriate sensitivities in relation to others). The relevant skills are related to but not coextensive with skills of linguistic and cognitive manipulation combined (minimally) with motor coordination, emotional competence, and interpersonal regard, any or all of which can be more or less developed in a given individual.

We can condense this *ubersicht* of action by reflecting on Nietzsche's (1886/1975) remark:

'Unfree will' is mythology; in real life, it is only a question of strong and weak wills. (¶21)

Nietzsche regards the idea that prior cause is the determinant of human action as an illusion 'according to the prevailing mechanistic stupidity' (¶21), noting that animals in general take control over their environment so that it does not push and pull them around like the inert objects of Newtonian mechanics. He remarks:

It is almost always a symptom of what is lacking in himself when a thinker detects in every 'causal connection' and 'psychological necessity' something of compulsion, exigency, constraint, pressure, unfreedom; such feelings are traitors, and the person who has them gives himself away.

(Nietzsche, 1886/1975, ¶21)

Freedom, is, therefore, a product of life skills that broaden one's horizons, enable one to devise promising ways of acting in diverse situations, and make one able to enact one's thoughts where reason (or cognitive skills generally) enables one to anticipate and not merely be 'bushwhacked' by contingencies. Intentions, as the determinations of the will that guide and shape our actions, spring from one's life story. In this way, human intentions are a sophisticated expression of the will to power rather than causal impulses arising within me that move me to behave in certain ways[3]. The will to power seeks, through anticipation, to control environmental contingencies rather than merely being subject to them and it works, in the human case, through shared cultural techniques and meanings that organize experience. Life stories should be seen as lived narratives built by using the techniques or disciplines that have formed me and allowed me to develop the powers commanded by my human group; our lives are therefore infused by cultural meanings and our bodies (and brains in particular) are the medium in which modes of enacting one's values are inscribed.

With freedom and power over the environment comes responsibility, but as one responds, at least for the ethical soul, self-directed and self-interested freedom is cast in the light of the truth of our being-in-the-world-with-others and the values that flow from that. Thus, Foucault remarks that ethics should link together truth and the subject so as to 'arm the subject with a truth it did not know' and make that truth 'a quasi-subject that reigns supreme in us'

If the brain is inscribed with the values that one embraces and is the medium that enables us to enact those values in the world, what then of the idea that brain events and not subjects (beings of meaning and value) cause human behaviour?

Brain events and moral responsibility

Even though the contribution of brain events to discussions of moral responsibility is not straightforward, a discussion of brain events (thus 'neurophilosophy') deepens the present analysis of action and intention.

---

[3] Hence, Nietzsche's protest that the unfree will is a myth.

Weakness of the will or *akrasia* (discussed in Chapter 13) is an inability to translate 'all things considered best judgement about what to do' into action (Davidson, 1980). An *akratic* person does what he or she knows is not the best thing to do (for prudential or moral reasons). The psychopath may have weakness of the will (there is a high incidence of addiction and fecklessness) but also has two other problems: first, an *inability to appreciate the moral force of certain considerations*, such as the suffering of his victim or the rightful claims of others on property; second, *an inability to judge what is prudent or in his own long-term best interests*. The psychopath does, however, know how to get what he wants in the short term (consequences be damned!) and therefore shows cleverness (in Aristotle's sense). But human beings must negotiate a world structured by complex social rules and features that ought to moderate what one does about short-term goals and satisfactions so that practical wisdom requires perception, response, and reflection in relation to what in social and personal life counts as something (and in particular, the effect of the action on others or one's own deferred [future] self). To act well in a human life-world, whether for one's own purposes or in relation to moral obligations, is to take account, among other things, of the actions, interests, and attitudes of others so that the psychopath's inability to succeed in relation to these complexities may indicate an important feature of such a mental disorder. Of course, we may still be left with a 'fuzzy boundary' between those individuals who cannot (on the basis of some constitutional defect) and those who do not (for morally reprehensible reasons) do what is right in relation to others.

An adequate philosophical theory of action and the will should therefore

(i) Exhibit the link between action and character;

(ii) Pay due attention to the nature of rule following;

(iii) Account for the effect of social context on behaviour; and

(iv) Demonstrate the conceptual foundations of moral responsibility.

These features are often neglected in the neurophilosophy of intention and action.

A variety of psychological experiments have been held to show that unconscious cerebral events precede and give rise to intentions to act so that the agent does not consciously initiate the events constituting an action. The thesis casts doubt on the idea of freedom of the will in that if unconscious brain events do precede intentions to act, then the operation of the mind on the world, through action, would be explained by physical events and their causes rather than the conscious thoughts of the agent (Spence, 1996). The problem recalls the metaphysical questions concerning the 'mental' and the 'physical' but focuses on the causation of mental events by (brute) physical events.

The debate begins with Libet (1985), whose work is interpreted as demonstrating that physical events in the brain precede the mental events associated with action when he related *the subject's first awareness of an intention to make a movement* to *the first detectable indication of this movement in the brain*—that is, the 'readiness potential' (see also Brunia & Haagh, 1986). 'Libet and his collaborators have now been able to show that this readiness potential change in the brain occurs up to half a second *before a subject mentally decides that he intends to make a movement*' (Young, 1986, p. 73).

Libet timed the events by making the subject, when he first became aware of his intention to move, report the position of a spot on an oscilloscope screen. The time of 'the conscious intention' was then taken to be the time the spot was actually in the reported position. This time was then related to the averaged electroencephalograph (EEG) record showing the readiness potential (RP) and it emerged that the time of initial conscious awareness, as reported by the subject, was 300–500 ms later than the RP. He then argued:

(i) The mental event of intending to act causes the act.

(ii) The physical event precedes the mental event of conscious intending, and is unconscious; therefore,

(iii) The physical event *causes* and is explanatorily prior to the mental event.

(iv) Conscious intentions are not the events which initiate human action.

(v) Unconscious brain events really explain human behaviour.

Call i to v *the argument to physical priority* (APhP). Three problems bear on it:

(1) The general relationship between brain events and conscious events;

(2) The relationship between conscious experience and human action;

(3) The concept of simultaneity in the context of mental experience—that is, between two mental experiences and between a mental experience and a physical event.

We also need to revisit the causal theory of action informing APhP. The thesis is that an action is a bodily movement produced by a preceding mental event—an intention; that event can then be timed relative to the brain events preceding the bodily movement. One ought to be critical of this model in that an intentional action is, paradigmatically, a move structured by a conscious technique underlying which there is a tract of brain activity such that there is not any one-to-one relation between brain events and conscious events (Dennett, 1991; Gillett, 1993a; and Appendix A&B above). The subject uses his or her skills to make a meaningful response to the situation he or she is in and sticks to it through various challenges. When the response is complex, involving difficult cues and considerations, some agents do not command the requisite skills (e.g. where there is moral sensitivity and restraint or self-control required, psychopaths seem particularly bad at doing what is called for).

The continuous and dynamically unfolding nature of normal action looks unsuited to the action theory at the heart of Libet's analysis, but premises i, ii, and iii of APhP (viz. that *there is a mental event—the intention*, that *the brain event is a cause antecedent to that mental event*, and that *the brain event is unconscious*) are directly based on that thesis about conscious experience, action, and the nature and timing of brain events.

The naive identification between 'mental events' and 'brain events' has been discussed in Appendix A, but the following three assumptions are also suspect:

(a) A conscious experience is potentially reportable on the basis of introspection.

(b) Such reports are the *only* means of identifying conscious experiences.

(c) The (reported) conscious experiences prior to an action are its mental 'causes'.

Libet (1985) needs temporally locatable conscious events and comparable brain events to make his case, but (see Appendix A) this assumption is metaphysically unsustainable. Libet worries about (a) when he considers the possibility of 'a non-recallable phase of a conscious urge … so that the reported time would apply only to a later, recallable phase of awareness' (p. 535), but a conscious experience involves narrative (re)construction of what is going on between oneself (or one's body and brain) and the world at a given time so as to relate that to one's being-with-others and unfolding life story. Libet assumes (as a Cartesian might) that the posited intentional event is transparently introspectible by the agent, but the recognitional skills pervading mental life arise in public discourse and shared significations based on the responses of others to one's own responses (e.g. 'I see you resented his blaming you for the accident') so that they relate to completed actions manifest to those witnessing them, a conception that then frames one's interpretation of the intention behind it (Dennett, 1991).

Therefore, contra (a) and (b), conscious experience is partly constituted by the reports one formulates (they are the way one 'tells' what is going on) and it may have shades and nuances in experience not fully exhibited in what is reported (to self and others), so that any introspective report is a selective (and contestable) signification of the state of one's psyche at a particular time, in a particular context. The currents and eddies of the psyche do not merely amount to information about oneself apt for transmission to others but use shared techniques of signification in the light of 'the imperatives' (Lacan) operating between people around here to present what one did in a certain light.

Because conscious experience outstrips discursive reports of it and our dynamic interactions with the environment cannot be parsed into staccato moments of intention and action (*do I intend every step I take or just to walk to the door?*), the subjective timing of a report (in whatever form) does not 'fix' the time of any discrete event corresponding to the conscious intention to act (thus, Libet's assumptions are false). Premise ii of the APhP holds that the physical event preceding the reported 'intention' is unconscious (i.e. it preceded the subjects' reports of the *earliest* 'awareness' that they intended to move). But the 'awareness' is not instant and complete; so, the recognition and signalling of an impending movement or report is (most plausibly) a conscious and explicit summary of something taking shape over (microneuro-) time corresponding to activity (of the multimodal, informationally complex, all-things-considered kind) typical of the 'organs of civilization' (i.e. the frontal lobes and their ramifying connections).

A second objection to the temporal claims of APhP arises from Libet's own work. Libet attempts to get around the problem that reports or indications must follow what they report or indicate (so that actual conscious intentions predate their being reported or indicated) by asking his subjects to relate their first awareness to the time of *another mental event*—'a visual sensation' from tracking a spot on an oscilloscope screen—and to pick the point apparently coincident with the awareness (by assuming constant patency between actual awareness and indication or report). But there are (quite apart from the mistaken metaphysics) two serious problems in the method.

First, it is not clear that the time at which a subject experiences a spot in a particular position is identifiable with the time of the spot actually being in that position. Libet (1985) carried out a control experiment (using the oscilloscope spot) to gauge the accuracy of subjects' timing of stimulus events using the method; 'a skin stimulus was delivered at an irregular, randomized time after the start of each trial and the subject reported the time of his awareness of that stimulus ... [thus] the discrepancy between the subject's reported timing and the actual stimulus time could be objectively determined.' (p. 534). He found that the time at which the spot was actually in the position in which it was reported to be (for three of the five subjects employed) *preceded* the time at which the skin stimulus was applied (p. 534) by about 100 ms. This is nonsensical in that it looks that a perception may precede the physical event perceived and Libet describes it as an 'error', commenting that 'the amount of error found in the stimulus series did not qualitatively alter the difference between onset of RP [readiness potential] and W [ostensible time of volition]; in fact, it generally enlarged the differ-ence' (p. 534). It would be more plausible to suggest that his control experiment undermines confidence in the 'moving spot' method in general and generates consid-erable uncertainty about time relations between the introspectively identified 'mental events' and the physical events to which Libet and others attempt to relate them.

Dennett's thesis (that consciousness is a narrative summation of what happens between the brain and the world) explains these results and supports the claim that 'conscious control of a process is not the same as becoming aware of the volitional intent' (Stephens, 1996, p. 95). Conscious reporting is quite unrelated to the time scale of neurophysiological processes preceding actions even though the way that I tell my story affects what I think and do about myself, others, and the world.

Phenomenological or *verstehen*-based analyses offer further support. The subject is likely to think something such as 'I think I am aware of an intention to make a movement; is that really definite enough for me to register? Yes it is; now where is that damned spot?' Such thoughts would compound the indeterminacy of time relations in Libet's experiments.

Second, that the relationship between conscious mental events and reports of them is not as Libet's model implies is demonstrated in an experiment involving brachial compression where subjects were able to move their anaesthetized hand as instructed by the experimenter, while firmly denying that they were doing so (Laszlo, 1966). That implies that introspected 'intentions' reflect the functioning of a sensory–motor loop implicated in action rather than indicating the initiation of movements in the brain. In short, Libet seems to be trying to measure aspects of an extended process called intentional action as if it were a discrete causal event when the intention is a guiding structure for sensorimotor activity retrospectively reconstructed for consciousness (and reporting to others) from good-enough indicators of what is going on (as suggested by Dennett's [1991] 'multiple drafts model'; Gillett, 2008). Thus, 'nineteenth-century psychology and twentieth-century electrophysiology do not mix' (Vanderwolf, 1985) because there are no precisely determinable mental events in consciousness but rather episodes (some of which are momentary) in my lived conscious narrative. Neither are there clear-cut, meaningfully parsed, brain events but rather a stream of neural activity with diverse relations to moments of conscious experience. Thus, the posit of a one-to-one correspondences between brain events and mental events is based on a metaphysical mistake.

In fact, given the holistic nature of cerebral activity (especially in the frontolimbic systems), the concept of 'simultaneous mental events' is inherently problematic. Relations that are determinate in space and time require individuation of the *relata* in those terms (thus, this cube exploded 2 s before and 25.1 cm away from the other one). But is it meaningful to say that thought Th_1 occurs after or at the same time as thought Th_2? Was each thought an instantaneous whole or did it take time to unfold? Where did each occur? If they were brain events, then what distance were they from each other? The fact that 'brain events' form a seamless stream of shifting activation patterns should make us quite suspicious of any dogmatic claims. How does the before–after relationship apply to distributed events and activation vectors in brain networks? And what does that mean in terms of the causal ordering of the complex events forming a narrative whereby the subject 'tells' what he is doing?

The idea of neatly packaged brain events corresponding to identifiable mental events is therefore implausible and scepticism (or at least anti-realism) about the ontology and metaphysics of mental and physical events (strengthened by connectionist models and the multiple ways that informational transactions are mediated in patterns of brain events) is the only sustainable attitude for philosophical psychology.

Thus, Libet's conclusion (shared by his commentators) that physical events precede their mental counterparts is wrong-headed because of the inherent uncertainty in determining the time of mental events, and the highly detailed arguments for physical precedence in the explanation of human behaviour adduced to support 'the illusion of free will' thesis betray naivety about neurophysiology and the metaphysics of the mind (Wegner, 2002). In fact, 'an unfree will is a myth' (as Nietzsche rightly concluded) and we are discussing the skills (that a person may or may not possess) required to translate reason into action.

One might diagnose the problem as a failure to realize that mental attributions focus on people in discursive relations and on their various physical, interpersonal, and moral commitments to certain modes of being of which actions are moments. Therefore,

(i) The will or volition is the skill to translate the results of argument or reason into action suitably adapted to the situation in which one finds oneself.

(ii) The will is continuous with the range of skills involved in learning to judge rightly or accurately how things are in the world.

(iii) The will is part of one's life as a thinking being.

(iv) Conversation and reasoning also form part of one's life as a thinking being.

(v) As one learns to make good judgements of fact, one also imbibes a sense of how things are for other people in shared situations.

(vi) That sensibility or knowledge can influence one's reasoning about how to act but is not directly self-serving.

(vii) Moral sensibility registers that (empathic) knowledge.

(viii) Instrumental reasoning may or may not find a place for empathic knowledge.

(ix) Prudential and moral reasoning do respond to empathic knowledge because both are affected by one's history of dealings with others.

(x) There is a defect in volition (that impairs one's ability to act appropriately as a being-in-the-world-with-others) caused by a lack of sensibility to how it is with others and an over indulgence of one's own desires.

(xi) Freedom of the will—a good and strong will—allows one to conduct oneself in the light of reason because it is the light of reason and to enact the good.

(xii) A good will is alert to the full reality of one's being-in-the-world-with-others and shows consideration for those affected by what one does.

On the present account, the will is a faculty allowing one to translate the results of conversation (or argument, in a broad sense) into action, or to enact one's own life story in a way that takes account of the possibilities in the world around one. One can fail to do this because one has a weak will and one can be morally defective when one pays no regard to the needs, vulnerabilities, and ends of others. Both defects of volition may be evident in psychopathy (and more widely).

Appendix G

Structuralism and post-structuralism

Structuralism is an influential current in contemporary continental thought, where thinkers such as Claude Levi-Strauss, Roland Barthes, and Jacques Lacan would regard themselves as either structuralists or heavily influenced by structuralism. Thinkers such as Michel Foucault and Jacques Derrida are often termed post-structuralists because they have gone beyond structuralism and they have certain evident affinities with Wittgenstein.

Structuralism originates with the linguist Ferdinand de Saussure (1857–1913) who elaborated his structural linguistics at the University of Geneva. Two years after he died, his students gathered and published lecture notes under the title *Course in General Linguistics* (1972). For de Saussure, language and thought are not separate because language itself has two integrally related and inseparable aspects—sound and ideas—such that without language thought can only be 'a shapeless and indistinct mass' (p. 9). Sound and ideas reciprocally delimit linguistic units. If we picture language as having two interacting layers of reality, one is sound and the other mental activity and the distinctions created in either affect both.

The linguistic unit is the sign, roughly equivalent to a word, carrying multiple significations and with two axes fundamental to its function as the sign: the *horizontal* and the *vertical* (p. 11).

> *The vertical axis* represents the two aspects of the sign—the signifier and the signified. *The horizontal axis* is the (structural) role of the sign within a language as a whole. The 'value' of the sign is given by its relation within a system of differences and distinctions and different languages divide things differently. There can be no necessary connection between the signifier and the signified because the meanings in play depend on the system or structure of significations and the relation to a signification is (to some extent) arbitrary. The arbitrary nature of the sign, for de Saussure, implies that it is only within a conventional, social space that a linguistic term can be created.
>
> The arbitrary nature of the sign explains in turn why the social fact alone can create a linguistic system. The community is necessary if values that owe their existence solely to usage and general acceptance are set up; by himself, the individual is incapable of fixing a single value.

(cf Wittgenstein, 1953)

Because the value of a sign is totally determined by its place in the system of differences constitutive of language, the value or meaning of a term comes negatively from the sign's differences within a system of differences and the binary nature of the differential system defines the basic structure (red, not red, etc.) Because the sign cannot be removed from the structural context in which it has value, meaning and language form an organic structure in which all the terms reciprocally determine each other just as the signifier and the signification reciprocally determine one another in the vertical register and together make up the sign.

Traditional linguistics, such as the kind of analysis which Wittgenstein (1922) gives in the *Tractatus*, is atomistic. Meaning has self-sufficient positive values as atoms tied to objects and words too are conceived as atomic units divorced from other units. De Saussure's holism together with the social context of language use take us to post-structuralism where we consider the practices and sociopolitical context within which language functions. That is a step towards the 'postmodern' whereby consciousness is seen as completely delineated by language, and is *dispersed* across a field of conventionally constituted difference situated in the human life-world.

In fact, we end up close to Wittgenstein's emphasis on structures of rules that are intricately connected with one another and with the language-related activities in which they come into play. What is added by postmodernism is, among other things, an acknowledgement of the workings of power and the situation of the body in a milieu that inscribes it with skills, techniques, modes of relatedness, positions, institutional expectations, and so on. In the face of such diverse forces acting on the situated subjective body, the thought that there is a substantial essence or core-person at the heart of the psyche is somewhat effaced and so the psychological subject (of much traditional phenomenology and metaphysics) becomes decentered or problematized and concepts such as authenticity and character are, to some extent, deflated.

Philosophical problems of personal identity

The metaphysics of mind has been discussed in the preceding, but to deal with the metaphysical problems of identity, we need to clarify the role of essentialism in metaphysics.

The essence of a thing is that set of properties (usually sorted into necessary and sufficient) that entail that a given substance (or thing) is a thing of a certain type or kind. We can see the link (between essentialism and metaphysics) at work in the following questions:

(H1) What makes a person a person?

(H2) What makes this the same person as X?

The second question particularizes the essence and applies it to a numerical individual, and a variant of it is especially relevant for human beings and their interests.

(H3) What makes this person the one I care about (i.e. myself)?

None of these questions are straightforward and they are closely connected. The problem of growth and change affects all of them in that a specification of present properties or features does not correspond to the future or past properties and features of the organism.

Contrasting with these forms of essentialism is existentialism and real-world conceptual analysis of the being-in-the-world of a human being whose existence precedes his or her essence. H1 is answered by Locke (1689/1975) in the following terms: '*Person* stands for ... a thinking intelligent being that has reason and reflection, and can consider itself as itself, the same thinking thing at different times' (XXVII.9). One strand of interpretation of this remark is dualistic and asks: 'What happens to personal identity if there is a disruption of the normal one-to-one relationship between person (as psyche or soul) and animal?' Our intuitions are revealed by a thought experiment similar to Locke's (1689/1975) prince and pauper case (XXVII.15).

> Imagine that two individuals, Jose and Mario, are in an accident. Fortunately, both have had 'brain information downloads' (BIDs) before this happened so that, although their brains were hopelessly scrambled, the BID read-out could be read back in to restore their mental function after brain recovery. But the brain care institution doing the BID read-in is staffed by a worker who is bad with foreign names and reads Mario's mind into Jose's brain and vice versa. So who wakes up when Mario's body becomes conscious? We should note that we are going to encounter a person who has Jose's memory, attitudes, subjective relationships, moral commitments, desires, idiosyncrasies of character, tastes in music,

and so on through all the (non-physical) personal attributes you can think of. Therefore, the person who wakes up in Mario's body thinks he is Jose, loves Jose's girlfriend, is an atheist (like Jose) and not Roman Catholic (like Mario), remembers things from Jose's youth as if he had lived through them, and so on.

As the full picture sinks in, many think that a body switching has occurred and Mario's body is now inhabited, for all intents and purposes, by Jose. So, in this case, where the psychological constitution has come apart from the normal bodily continuity, we are inclined to think that personal identity depends on the mind.

Parfit's (1971) imaginative extensions of the observation that a person with a split brain might give evidence of both knowing and not knowing what stimuli he had perceived in an experimental situation follow some of the more lurid philosophical writings on such cases to posit radical fragmentations (Sperry, 1979) that break the connection between personal identity and a single autobiographical consciousness. Parfit concurs with Locke that autobiographical consciousness and memory are key features of the 'unity' of mental life and that each can occur in degrees unlike metaphysical or ontological identity, and argues that, were it possible (by various brain or other manipulations) to divide a person so that they became two streams of conscious experience (or fuse two people such that they became one), neither of the cases is the same as death (in that the person would seem to themselves to be continuous). These cases represent a loss of the one-to-one identity relation, but in each case, the person seems considerably better off than they would be if they were dead— they might even think of themselves as surviving (after a fashion). Thus, Parfit and others conclude that there is nothing very important that we are one of and that the problem of split brains (along with the thought experiments based on it) shows that psychological continuity and not identity is what we should care about.

This (neo-Lockean) strand of thought seems telling against the dualist thesis that personal identity (PI) rests on the existence of a single mental substance having the properties that make one the type of being who is a person (i.e. forming the essence of a person such that what happens to it settles questions about identity) and is held by some to favour an analysis of PI in terms of psychological properties.

The resulting theories argue that PI is no more than the continuity, configuration, and interconnectedness of various mental functions. They are therefore reductive in that PI comprises a set of (causally or otherwise) linked psychological states and they come in both *strong* (iconoclastic) or *weak* (nothing changed) forms.

The weak conclusion is that there is no more or less to PI than can be derived from an analogy with a woven tapestry cord so that even though there is no single entity underpinning identity (just as there is no single thread running the length of the cord, a core or substantial basis for the unity of the whole), what there is suffices for what we ask of PI. It is clear that the woven cord has certain emergent properties which are other than any properties of the coloured strands making it up: for instance, the cord might hold a person's weight where a single thread would not. If we call this property *Strength* (St), then St is a reducible property in the sense that it is mathematically (or logically) derivable from a property of the component threads even though its magnitude is greater. A more interesting property is something similar to *longitudinal continuity for more than one metre* in that it only comes into being through the combining of and the interconnections between the threads and cannot be accounted for by a straightforward sum of parts (so we might call it an *emergent property*).

But its dimension (length) is not radically emergent: it is just a greater magnitude of a property already instanced in the world. Therefore, more interesting as an emergent property is the pattern woven into the cord in that it is dependent on, but clearly different in kind from, any property of any of the monochromatic threads contributing to it. Such a radically emergent property creates a type of reality not evident in the components contributing to it (the monochromatic threads) and therefore requires a language (of patterns and harmonies of colour) and categories peculiar to the cord level. The emergent realities require us to take account of a new feature of the world introduced by the cord as a whole so that the holistic entity has an explanatory role not corresponding to any attribute of the threads making it up. In an analogous way, one might say that a PI comes about as a set of psychological properties and elements are combined in a connected series with a particular (e.g. narrative) character that does not appear in the world until the whole in which they are instanced appears. One can then object to a reduction (of PI to psychological states) in that the psychological states (in and of themselves) depend for their properties on the whole of which they are part (so that the whole—the person concerned—cannot merely be a posterior—or secondary—reality as required by a reductive view, whether weak or strong).

The strong conclusion about PI takes the cord to be analogous to a bundle of rags. Rags can come and go but the bundle remains more or less the same (as does a heap in the face of losses and gains). More importantly, the bundle is just a bundle without interestingly new emergent properties. If developed in relation to PI, the analogy can lead to a loosening of moral and personal ties between different moments of a life history and ground a 'thin' view of PI whereby identity becomes just a shorthand way of referring to a collection of certain psychological characteristics qualitatively distinct, in sum but not in essential constitution, from the bundle constituting another person. But if any reductive view ignores constitutive features whereby the whole forms or shapes its parts, the thin view grossly neglects that aspect of persons and their subjectivities. In fact, the more holistic view of a person as a being whose psyche takes shape over time and affects what happens to it seems indispensable in psychiatric theory and practice.

The strong version of the bundle theory relies heavily on psychological connectedness (of which a prominent feature is the links forged by memory) implying that an autobiography is a number of events and experiences connected to one another by the causal links between a historical episode in the person's life and the current trace of that experience in the memory store. Coincidence in the same physically realized 'library' of stored memories is then theorized as being what constitutes a continuous life story. This view of the psyche and the philosophical accounts of memory on which it relies are, however, inadequate (see Chapter 10).

Kant identified a deep problem with the bundle-of-psychological-events-and-states theory of PI that could be derived from Hume's skeptical observations on PI: 'When I turn my reflection on *myself*, I never can perceive this self without some one or more perceptions; nor can I ever perceive any thing but the perceptions. 'Tis the composition of these, therefore, which forms the self' (Hume, 1739/1969, p. 676).

Kant (1789/1929) invoked the logical principle of unity that integrates the mental life of a person and argued that a theory potentially fragmenting the psychological subject undermines a person's cognitive unity as an integrated thinking thing who has gained their cognitive competencies through intersubjective dealings with others (and who is therefore morally responsible and engaged in a shared world). Hume's empiricism led him to conclude that 'we have no impression of self or substance, as something simple and individual,' so that there could be nothing to PI apart from some far-from-obvious (but perhaps causal) principles of connection between conscious states. Kant observed that Hume starts from a faulty dichotomy, viz. that the self is either posited to be a distinct thing or substance (and therefore should be perceptible as such) or it does not exist. He argues that the Cartesian 'mental substance' is a mistake caused by reifying or hypostasizing what is in fact a logical principle by thinking of it as a 'noumenal' substance (Kant, 1789/1929, pp. B406–432). What unifies consciousness and reason and is indicated by the *I think* is the rational activity of discursive cognition and not a substance at all. The relevant cognitive activity (of synthesis)

(i) Assigns conceptual content to moments of experience; and

(ii) Makes rational connections between different thoughts.

The first of these recalls the fact that the faculty of the understanding, in its work of conceptualizing experience, deploys skills in judgement developed over time and in diverse experiences so that the *I think* implies a longitudinal continuity in cognition whereby present experiences and judgements are built on past encounters and the conceptual activity developed and refined within them. That, in turn, implies the biographically integrated (or narrative) identity of the thinker doing the cognitive work (I discuss this in Gillett, 2008).

If Kant is correct, then the lack of a perceptual impression corresponding to the self is not to the point because the *Transcendental Unity of Apperception* is a principle of cognitive life and not a substance at all. That principle can be enriched into the principle of narrative or authorial unity currently discussed by a number of authors (Harre & Gillett, 1994; Shechtman, 1996; Taylor, 1989). Metzinger's (2004) attack on the idea of PI has a neo-Lockean form in that it focuses on the impossibility of the sense of self capturing a single unified essence or substance with all the features that Cartesian mental substance-based identity theories need a self to have (2004). Kant (and the current narrative theorists) therefore evades his attack in pointing to the cognitive unity of a coherent thought life and its variably skilled attachment to a real-world trajectory of encounters. Metzinger also misses the point in that the inscribed body is the (situated) occasion for one's subjective experience that takes on cognitive characteristics shaped by one's trajectory through the human life-world. In this sense, one's self is a construction one makes on the basis of one's being mirrored in and through one's dealings with others (or through intersubjectivity), and as with any other construction, it is subject (as Lacan so intriguingly explores) to meconnaissance and all the evaluative influences that shape our ways of being human. The lived

PHILOSOPHICAL PROBLEMS OF PERSONAL IDENTITY | 393

subjectivity that is oneself is therefore not a something but not a nothing either. It is based on one's existence as a being-with-others and it reads into one's being articulations of self that arise for oneself from the mirror-world created by being-in-the-world-with-others-around-here, a lived socio-historico-culturally located reality that articulates the psyche and experience of those who engage in it.

To bring this discussion right up to date and take account of the literature on embodied subjectivity informing contemporary discussions of identity, we can point to the located inscribed body as a subjective sense maker tracing a singular path through the world and forming (and being formed by) relationships with others, the view that underpins the present work. Knowing oneself, on this account, is a matter of relating the significations that go into one's *imago* to the truth of one's being-in-the-world-with-others so as to understand any meconnaissance involved and to have the skills to be able to critique and struggle with the inadequacies associated with that.

References

Akinci, M.K. and Johnston, G.A.R. (1993) Sex differences in the effects of acute swim stress on binding to GABAa receptors in mouse brain. *Journal of Neurochemistry* **60**(6); 2212–2216.

Allison, R.B. (1982–83) The multiple personality defendant in court. *American Journal of Forensic Psychiatry* **3**; 181–192.

Andorfer, J.C. (1985) Multiple personality in the human information-processor: a case history and theoretical formulation. *Journal of Clinical Psychology* **41**(3); 309–324.

Andreason, N.C. (1987) Creativity and mental illness: prevalence rates in writers and their first-degree relatives. *American Journal of Psychiatry* **144**; 1288–1292.

Andreason, N.C. and Glick, I.D. (1988) Bipolar affective disorder and creativity: implications and clinical management. *Comprehensive Psychiatry* **29**; 207–217.

Anscombe, E. (1981) The intentionality of sensation: a grammatical feature. In *Metaphysics and the Philosophy of Mind*. Oxford: Blackwell.

Antony, L. (1989) Anomalous monism and the problem of explanatory force. *Philosophical Review* **98**; 153–187.

APA (1978) Electroconvulsive Therapy Task Force report no. 14. Washington: American Psychiatric Association.

APA (1994a) *Diagnostic and Statistical Manual of Mental Disorders IV*. Washington: American Psychiatric Association.

APA (1994b) *Diagnostic and Statistical Manual of Mental Disorders IV: Case Book*. Washington: American Psychiatric Association.

Appelbaum P.S. and Zoltek-Jick, R. (1996) Psychotherapists' duties to third parties. *American Journal of Psychiatry* **153**; 457–465.

Arendt, H. (1963) *Eichmannn in Jerusalem: A Report on the Banality of Evil*. London: Faber.

Aristotle (1925) *The Nicomachean Ethics* (D. Ross, tr). Oxford: University Press.

Aristotle (1984) *The Complete Works of Aristotle*, vol. I (J. Barnes, ed). Princeton: University Press.

Aristotle (1986) *De Anima* (H. Lawson Tancred, tr). London: Penguin.

Armstrong, D. (2004) *Truth and Truthmakers*. Cambridge: University Press.

Asperger, H. (1944/1991) Autistic psychopathy in childhood. In *Autism and Asperger Syndrome* (U. Frith, ed). Cambridge: University Press, pp. 37–92.

Baars, B.J. (1988) *A Cognitive Theory of Consciousness*. Cambridge: University Press.

Baier, A. (1985) *Postures of the Mind*. London: Methuen.

Baker, G.P. and Hacker, P.M.S. (1980) *Wittgenstein: Meaning and Understanding*. Oxford: Blackwell.

Barnes, J. (1982) *Aristotle*. Oxford: University Press.

Barthes, R. (1972) *Mythologies*. New York: Hill and Wang.

Bazelon, D.L. (1974) Psychiatrists and the adversary process. *Scientific American* **230**(6); 18–23.

Beadle, M. (1970) *The Child's Mind*. New York: Doubleday.

Bekerian, D.A. and Bowers, J.M. (1983) Eyewitness testimony: were we misled? *Journal of Experimental Psychology: Language, Memory and Cognition* **9**(1); 139–145.

Benjamin, B.S. (1967) Remembering. In *Essays in Philosophical Psychology* (D.F. Gustafson, ed). London: Macmillan.

Berger, P. (1967) *The Sacred Canopy: Elements of a Sociological Theory of Religion*. New York: Random House.

Berkeley, G. (1710/1969) *A Treatise Concerning the Principles of Human Knowledge*. London: Everyman.

Berkeley, G. (1713/1969) Dialogues between Hylas and Philonous. In *A New Theory of Vision and Other Writings*. London: Dent and Sons.

Berrios, G.E. (1993) European views on personality disorders. *Comprehensive Psychiatry* **34**(1); 14–30.

Bhaskar, R. (1979) *The Possibility of Naturalism*. Brighton: Harvester Press.

Biederman, J., Milberger, S., Faraone, S.V. *et al.* (1995) Family environment risk factors for attention-deficit hyperactivity disorder. *Archives of General Psychiatry* **52**; 464–470.

Birkett, P., Brindley, A., Normal, P., Harrison, G., and Baddeley, A. (2005) Control of attention in schizophrenia. *Journal of Psychiatric Research* **40**(7); 579–588.

Blackburn, R. (1975) An empirical classification of psychopathic disorder. *British Journal of Psychiatry* **127**; 456–460.

Blackburn, R. (1988) On moral judgements and personality disorders: the myth of psychopathic personality revisited. *British Journal of Psychiatry* **153**; 505–512.

Blackburn, R. and Lee-Evans, J.M. (1985) Reactions of primary and secondary psychopaths to anger-evoking situations. *British Journal of Clinical Psychology* **24**; 93–100.

Blackburn, S. (1984) *Spreading the Word*. Oxford: Clarendon.

Blair, R.J. (2003) The neurobiological basis of psychopathy. *British Journal of Psychiatry* **182**; 5–7.

Blank, M.A. and Foss, D.J. (1978) Semantic facilitation and lexical access during sentence processing *Memory and Cognition* **6**; 644–652.

Block, N. (1995) On a confusion about a function of consciousness. *Behavioural and Brain Sciences* **18**(2); 227–247.

Bolton, D. and Hill, J. (1996) *Mind, Meaning and Mental Disorder*. Oxford: University Press.

Boorse, C. (1977) Health as a theoretical concept. *Philosophy of Science* **44**; 542–73.

Bordo, S. (1985) Anorexia nervosa: psychopathology as the crystallization of culture. *Philosophical Forum* **17**(2); 73–103.

Bower, T.G.R. (1977) *A Primer of Infant Development*. San Francisco (Cal.): Freeman and Co.

Bowers, J.M. and Bekerian, D.A. (1984) When will postevent testimony distort eye witness testimony. *Journal of Applied Psychology* **69**(3); 466–472.

Bragan, K. (1987) Janet Frame: contributions to psychiatry. *New Zealand Medical Journal* **100**; 70–73.

Braude, S. (1991) *First Person Plural*. London: Routledge.

Braude, S. (1996) Multiple personality and moral responsibility. *Philosophy, Psychiatry, and Psychology* **3**(1); 37–54.

Bremner, J.D., Krystal, J.H., Charney D.S., and Southwick, S.M. (1996) Neural mechanisms in dissociative amnesia for childhood abuse: relevance to the current controversy surrounding the 'false memory syndrome'. *American Journal of Psychiatry* **153**(7); 71–82.

Bremner, J.D., Randall, P., *et al.* (1997) MRI-based measurement of hippocampal volume in posttraumatic stress disorder related to childhood physical and sexual abuse. *Biological Psychiatry* **41**; 23–32.

Brentano, F. (1924/1973) *Psychology from an Empirical Standpoint* (L. McAlister, ed). London: Routledge.

Brentano, F. (1929/1981) *Sensory and Noetic Consciousness* (L. McAlister, ed). London: Routledge and Kegan Paul.

Brett-Jones, J.R., Garety, P., and Helmsley, D. (1987) Measuring delusional experiences: a method and its application. *British Journal of Clinical Psychology* **26**; 256–257.

Brewin, C.R. (1996) Scientific status of recovered memories. *British Journal of Psychiatry* **169**; 131–134.

Brockington, I., Perris, C., and Meltzer, H.Y. (1982) Cycloid psychosis: diagnosis and heuristic value. *Journal of Nervous and Mental Diseases* **170**; 651–656.

Bruch, H. (1978) *The Golden Cage: The Enigma of Anorexia Nervosa*. Cambridge (Mass.): Harvard University Press.

Bruner, J. (1990) *Acts of Meaning*. Cambridge (Mass.): Harvard University Press.

Bruner, J. (2000) Tot thought. *New York Review of Books* **47**(4); 27–30.

Brunia, C.H.M. and Haagh, S.A.U.M. (1986) Preparation for action: slow potentials and EMG. In *Generation and Modulation of Action Patterns* (H. Heuer and C. Fromm, eds). Berlin: Springer-Verlag.

Buber, M. (1970) *I and Thou* (W. Kaufmann, tr). Edinburgh: T & T Clark.

Bulik, C.M., Sullivan, P., Joyce, P.R., and Carter, F.A. (1995) Temperament character and personality disorder in bulimia nervosa. *Journal of Nervous and Mental Disorders* **183**(9); 593–598.

Burge, T. (1995) Individualism and Psychology. In *Philosophy of Psychology: Debates on Psychological Explanation* (McDonald and McDonald ed). Oxford: Blackwell, I pp. 173–205.

Burnyeat, M. (1980) Aristotle on learning to be good. In *Essays on Aristotle's Ethics* (A. Rorty, ed). Berkeley: University of California Press, pp. 69–92.

Bursten, B. (1972) The manipulative personality. *Archives of General Psychiatry* **26**; 318–321.

Butler, J. (1989) Foucault and the paradox of bodily inscriptions. *The Journal of Philosophy* **86**(11); 601–607.

Butterworth, G. (1991) What minds have in common is space: spatial mechanisms serving joint visual attention in infancy. *British Journal of Developmental Psychology* **9**; 56–72.

Byatt, A.S. (1984) *Still Life*. London: Chatto and Windus.

Cahill, L. Prins, B. Weber, M. & McGaugh, J. B. (2002) Adrenurgic activation and memory for emotional events. *Nature* **371**; 702–704.

Cameron, J.L. Laing, R.D. and McGhie, A. (1955) Patient and nurse: effects of environmental changes in the care of chronic schizophrenics. *Lancet*.

Carr, C. (1994) *The Alienist*. New York: Random House.

Carruthers, P. (1996) Simulation and self-knowledge: a defence of theory. In *Theories of Theories of Mind* (P. Carruthers and P. Smith, eds). Cambridge: University Press, pp. 22–38.

Carruthers, P. and Smith, P., eds. (1996) Introduction. In *Theories of Theories of Mind*. Cambridge: University Press.

Carter, C.S., Robertson, L.C., and Nordahl T.E. (1992) Abnormal processing of irrelevant information in chronic schizophrenia: selective enhancement of Stroop facilitation *Psychiatry Research* **41**; 137–146.

Cavell, M. (1993) *The Psychoanalytic Mind*. Cambridge (Mass.): Harvard University Press.

Cesaroni, L. and Garber, M. (1991) Exploring the experience of autism through firsthand accounts. *Journal of Autism and Developmental Disorders* **21**(3); 303–313.

Chalmers, D. (1996) *The Conscious Mind: In Search of a Fundamental Theory*. Oxford: University Press.

Chodoff, P. (1987) Effects of the new economic climate on psychotherapeutic practice. *American Journal of Psychiatry* **144**; 1293–7.

Chodorow, N. (1978) *The Reproduction of Mothering: Psychoanalysis and Sociology of Gender*. Berkeley: University of California Press.

Chomsky, N. (1972) *Language and Mind*. New York: Harcourt Brace.

Church, J. (1987) Reasonable irrationality. *Mind* **XCVI**; 354–366.

Churchland, P.M. (1986) *Matter and Consciousness*. Cambridge (Mass.): MIT Press.

Clark, A. (1990) *Microcognition*. Cambridge (Mass.): MIT Press.

Clark, A. (1995) Connectionist minds. In *Debates on Psychological Explanation: Connectionism* (C. Macdonald and G. Macdonald, eds). Oxford: Blackwell.

Clark, S. (1996a) Minds, memes, and multiples. *Philosophy, Psychiatry, and Psychology* **3**(1); 21–28.

Clark, S. (1996b) Commentary on 'Multiple personality and moral responsibility'. *Philosophy, Psychiatry, and Psychology* **3**(1); 55–57.

Clarke, D. and Smith, G. (1994) Disorders of somatic function or perception. In *Foundations of Clinical Psychiatry* (S. Bloch and B.S. Singh, eds). Melbourne: University Press.

Cleckley, H. (1941/1976) *The Mask of Sanity: An Attempt to Clarify Some Issues About the So-called Psychopathic Personality*, 5th edn. St. Louis (Mo.): Mosby and Co.

Code, L. (1996) Commentary on 'Loopholes, gaps and what is held fast'. *Philosophy, Psychiatry, and Psychology* **3**(4); 255–260.

Comm, M. (1994 Dec) Letter. *Our Voice*, pp. 5–6.

Confer, W.N. and Ables, B.S. (1983) *Multiple Personality: Aetiology, Diagnosis and Treatment*. New York: Human Sciences Press.

Conway, M.A. (1990) *Autobiographical Memory*. Milton Keynes: Open University Press.

Coons, P.M. (1991) Iatrogenesis and malingering of multiple personality disorder in the forensic evaluation of homicide defendants. *Psychiatric Clinics of North America* **14**(3); 757–768.

Cooper, R. (2007) *Psychiatry and Philosophy of Science*. Stocksfield: Acumen.

Copjec, J. (1996) *Radical Evil*. London: Verso.

Currie, G. (1996) Simulation-theory, theory-theory and the evidence from autism. In *Theories of Theories of Mind* (P. Carruthers and P. Smith, eds). Cambridge: University Press, pp. 242–256.

Curzer, H. (2002) Aristotle's painful path to virtue. *Journal of the History of Philosophy* **40**(2); 141–162.

Cutting, J. (1990) Relationship between cycloid psychosis and typical affective psychosis *Psychopathology* **23**; 212–219.

Czynewski, A. (2007) Theoretical reasoning enhanced in schizophrenia. *British Journal of Psychiatry* **191**; 453–454.

Danzer, G., Rose, M., Walter, M., and Klapp, B. (2002) On the theory of individual health. *Journal of Medical Ethics* **28**; 17–19.

David, A.S. (1990) Insight and psychosis. *British Journal of Psychiatry* **156**; 798–808.

Davidson, D. (1980) *Essays on Actions and Events*. Oxford: Clarendon.

Davidson, D. (1982) Paradoxes of irrationality. In *Philosophical Essays on Freud* (R.Wollheim and J. Hopkins, eds). Cambridge: University Press.

Davidson, D. (1984) *Inquiries into truth and Interpretation*. Oxford: Clarendon.

Davidson, D. (1985) Donald Davidson responds. In *Essays on Davidson; Actions and events* (eds. B. Vermazen & M. Hintikka) Oxford: University Press, pp. 195–254.

Dawson, J. (2007) Concepts of liberty in mental health law [Online]. Available at: http://podcast.otago.ac.nz/weblog_humanities/UPL - Audio/2007/09/06/conceptsoflibertyinmentalhea.html (accessed 2008 Jul 7).

Dennett, D. (1981) *Brainstorms*. Brighton: Harvester.

Dennett, D.C. (1991) *Consciousness Explained*. London: Penguin Press.

De Saussure, F. (1972) *Course in General Linguistics* (R. Harris, tr). Chicago (Ill.): Open court.

Devitt, M. and Sterelney, K. (1987) *Language and Reality*. Cambridge (Mass.): MIT Press.

Devitt, M. (1990) A narrow representational theory of mind. In *Mind and Cognition* (W. Lycan, ed). Oxford: Blackwell.

Devonshire, P.A., Howard R.C., and Sellars, C. (1988) Frontal lobe functions and personality in mentally abnormal offenders. *Personality and Individual Differences* **9**; 339–344.

Dewey, M.A. (1992) Autistic eccentricity. In *High Functioning Individuals with Autism* (E. Schopler and G. Mesibov, eds). New York: Plenum.

Diaz, J.L. (1997) A patterned process approach to brain consciousness and behavior. *Philosophical Psychology* **10**(2); 179–196.

Diller, L.H. (1996) The run on Ritalin: attention deficit disorder and stimulant treatment in the 1990s. *Hastings Centre Report* **26**(2); 12–18.

Donaldson, M. (1979) *Children's Minds*. London: Fontana.

Donley, C. (1997) What makes an action the kind of thing one is responsible for? Essay for graduate class in Bioethics, Case-Western Reserve University.

Doring, F. (1990) The limits of irrationality. In *Philosophy and Psychopathology* (M.Spitzer and B.Maher, eds). New York: Springer-Verlag.

Dresser, R. (1997) Criminal responsibility and the 'genetics defense' [Unpublished manuscript].

Dretske, F. (1988) *Explaining Behavior*. Cambridge (Mass.): MIT Press.

Drury, M. O'C. (1996) *The Danger of Words and Writings on Wittgenstein*. Bristol: Thoemmes Press.

Dummett, M. (1981) *The Interpretation of Frege's Philosophy*. London: Duckworth.

Durham v. United States, 214 F.2d 862 (D.C.Cir.1954).

Eckert, E.D., Halmi, K.A., Marchi, P., Grove, W., and Crosby, R. (1995) Ten-year follow-up of anorexia nervosa: clinical course and outcome. *Psychological Medicine* **25**; 143–156.

Editorial (1990) Real insight. *Lancet* **336**; 408–409.

Ehrenzweig, A. (1976) Unconscious scanning and dedifferentiation in artistic perception. In *The Creativity Question* (A. Rothenberg and C.R. Hausman, eds). Durham (N.C.): Duke University Press.

Eisenberg, L. (1995) The social construction of the human brain. *American Journal of Psychiatry* **152**; 1563–1575.

Elliot, C. (1991) Moral responsibility, psychiatric disorders and duress. *Journal of Applied Philosophy* **8**(1); 45–56.

Elliot, C. (1994) Puppetmasters and personality disorders. *Philosophy, Psychiatry, and Psychology* **1**(2); 91–100.

Elliot, C. (2004) Six problems with pharma-funded bioethics. *Studies in the History and Philosophy of Science Part C* **35**(1); 125–129.

Esman, A.H. (1994) 'Sexual abuse', pathogenesis, and enlightened scepticism. *American Journal of Psychiatry* **151**(8); 1101–1103.

Eysenck, H. (1965) *Fact and Fiction in Psychology*. London: Penguin.

Eysenck, H. (1987) Extraversion-introversion. In *The Oxford Companion to the Mind* (R.L.Gregory, ed). Oxford: University Press.

Fahy, T.A., Abas, M., and Brown, J.C. (1989) Multiple personality: a symptom of psychiatric disorder. *British Journal of Psychiatry* **154**; 99–101.

Fairburn, G.C., and Brownell, K. (2002) *Eating Disorders and Obesity*. London: Guildford Press.

Fowles, D. (1993) *Electrodermal Activity and Anti-social Behaviour: Empirical Findings and Theoretical Issues* New York: Plenum.

Fields, L. (1996) Psychopathy, other-regarding moral beliefs, and responsibility. *Philosophy, Psychiatry, and Psychology* **3**(4); 261–278.

Fischer, J.M. and Revizza, M. (1998) *Responsibility and control: a theory of moral responsibility.* Cambridge University Press.

Fisher R.P. and Cuervo, A. (1983) Thematic construction versus trace retrieval operations in memory. *Journal of Experimental Psychology: Learning, Memory and Cognition* **9**(1); 131–138.

Flannery, M. and Glickman, M. (1996) *Fountain House.* Center City (Minn.): Hazelden.

Fodor, J. (1968) *Psychological Explanation: An Introduction to the Philosophy of Psychology.* New York: Random House.

Fodor, J. (1975) *The Language of Thought.* New York: Thomas A. Crowell.

Fodor, J. (1987) *Psychosemantics.* Cambridge (Mass.): MIT Press.

Fodor, J. (1990) *A Theory of Content.* Cambridge (Mass.): MIT Press.

Foucault, M. (1954/1987). *Mental Illness and Psychology* (A. Sheridan, tr). Berkeley: University of California Press.

Foucault, M. (1973) *Madness and Civilization.* New York: Random House.

Foucault, M. (1984) *The Foucault Reader* (P. Rabinow, ed). London: Penguin.

Foucault, M. (1994) *Ethics; Subjectivity and Truth.* London: Penguin.

Frame, J. (1961/1980) *Faces in the Water.* London: The Women's Press.

Frame, J. (1989) *An Autobiography.* Auckland: Century Hutchison.

Freckleton, I. (1996) Repressed Memory Syndrome: counterintuitive or counterproductive. *Criminal Law Journal* **20**(1); 7–33.

Freeman, C.P.L., Barry, F., Dunkeld Turnbull, J., and Henderson, A. (1988) Controlled trial of psychotherapy for bulimia nervosa. *British Medical Journal* **296**; 521–525.

Frege, G. (1892/1952) On sense and reference. *Translations from the Philosophical Writngs of Gottlob Frege* (P. Geach and M. Black, eds). Oxford: Blackwell.

Freud, A. (1986) *The Essentials of Psychoanalysis*. London: Penguin.

Freud, S. (1921/1985) Civilized sexual morality and modern nervous illness. In *Civilization, Society, and Religion*. Harmondsworth: Penguin.

Freud, S. (1922) *Introductory Lectures on Psychoanalysis* London: Allen and Unwin.

Freud, S. (1940) An outline of psychoanalysis. *International Journal of Psychoanalysis* 21; 27–84.

Friedman, J. and Meares, R. (1979) Cortical evoked potentials and extraversion. *Psychosomatic Medicine* 4; 279–289.

Fukuda, M., Hata, A., Niwa, S.I. *et al.* (1996) Event-related potential correlates of functional hearing loss: reduced P3 amplitude with preserved N1 and N2 components in a unilateral case. *Psychiatry and Clinical Neurosciences* 50(2); 85–87.

Fulford, W.K.M. (1987) In *Persons and Personality* (A. Peacocke and G. Gillett, eds). Oxford: Blackwell.

Fulford, W.K.M. (1989) *Moral Theory and Medical Practice*. Oxford: University Press.

Gallagher, S. (2004) Understanding interpersonal problems in autism: interaction theory as an alternative to theory of mind. *Philosophy, Psychiatry, and Psychology* 11(3); 199–218.

Gallagher, S. (2005) *How the Body Shapes the Mind* Oxford: Clarendon.

Ganaway, G.K. (1989) Historical versus narrative truth: clarifying the role of exogenous trauma in the etiology of MPD and its variants. *Dissociation* 2; 205–220.

Gardner, H. (1974) *The Shattered Mind*. New York: Random House.

Gardner, H. (1993) *Creating Minds*. New York: Harper Collins.

Gates, R. and Hammond, R. (1993) *When the Music's Over*. Armidale: University of New England Press.

Gelder, M., Gath, D., and Mayou, R. (1983) *Oxford Textbook of Psychiatry*. Oxford: University Press.

Gibson, J.J. (1966) *The Senses Considered as Perceptual Systems*. Boston (Mass.): Houghton Mifflin.

Gillett, G. (1987) Concepts structures and meanings. *Inquiry* 30; 101–112.

Gillett, G. (1988) Consciousness and brain function. *Philosophical Psychology* 1; 327–342.

Gillett, G. (1989) Representations and cognitive science. *Inquiry* 32; 261–276.

Gillett, G. (1990a) Neuropsychology and meaning in psychiatry. *Journal of Medicine and Philosophy* 15; 21–39.

Gillett, G. (1990b) Multiple personality and irrationality. *Philosophical Psychology* 4(2); 173–184.

Gillett, G. (1990c) Consciousness, the brain and what matters. *Bioethics* 4; 181–198.

Gillett, G. (1990d) An antisceptical fugue. *Philosophical Investigations* 13; 304–321.

Gillett, G. (1991) Language, social ecology and experience. *International Studies in the Philosophy of Science* 5(3); 195–204.

Gillett, G. (1992) *Representation, Meaning, and Thought*. Oxford: Clarendon.

Gillett, G. (1993a) Actions, causes, and mental ascriptions. In *Objections to Physicalism* (H.Robinson, ed). Oxford: Clarendon, p81–100.

Gillett, G. (1993b) Free will and mental content. *Ratio* VI(2); 89–108.

Gillett, G. (1993c) Social causation and cognitive neuroscience. *Journal for the Theory of Social Behaviour* 23; 27–45.

Gillett, G. (1993d) 'Ought' and well-being. *Inquiry* 36(3); 287–306.

Gillett, G. (1993e) Explaining intentions. *British Journal of Philosophy of Science* 44(1); 157–166.

Gillett, G. (1995) Humpty Dumpty and the night of the Triffids: individualism and rule following. *Synthese* **105**; 191–206.

Gillett, G. (1997a) Husserl, Wittgenstein, and the Snark. *Philosophy and Phenomenological Research* **LVII**(2); 331–350.

Gillett, G. (1997b) A discursive account of multiple personality disorder. *Philosophy, Psychiatry, and Psychology* **4**(3); 213–222.

Gillett, G. (2001) Intention and agency. In *Intention in Law and Philosophy* (N. Naffine, R. Owens, and J. Williams, eds). Burlington: Ashgate, pp. 57–69.

Gillett, G. (2004) *Bioethics and the Clinic: Hippocratic Reflections.* Johns Hopkins University Press.

Gillett, G. (2005) The unwitting sacrifice problem. *Journal of Medical Ethics* **31**; 327–332.

Gillett, G. (2008) *Being Somebody: Subjectivity, Identity and Neuroethics.* Exeter: Imprint Academic.

Gilligan, C. and Wiggins, G. (1988) The origins of morality in early childhood relationships. In *Mapping the Moral Domain* (C. Gilligan, J. Wood, and J. Taylor, eds). Cambridge (Mass.): Harvard University Press.

Giordano, S. (2005) *Understanding eating disorders.* Oxford: University Press.

Glass, A.L. and Holyoak, K.J. (1986) *Cognition,* 2nd edn. New York: Random House.

Gleitman, H. (1991) *Psychology,* 3rd edn. New York: Norton.

Glowinski, H., Marks, Z., and Murphy, S. (2001) *A Compendium of Lacanian Terms.* London: Free Association Books.

Goffman, E. (1968) *Stigma.* London: Penguin.

Goldman, A.I. (1993) The psychology of folk psychology. *Behavioral and Brain Sciences* **16**; 15–28.

Gordon, R. (1996) 'Radical' similationism. In *Theories of Theories of Mind* (P. Carruthers and P. Smith, eds). Cambridge: University Press, pp. 11–21.

Grandin, T. (1992) An inside view of autism. In *High Functioning Individuals with Autism* (E. Schopler and G. Mesibov, eds). New York: Plenum.

Green, C. and Gillett, G. (1995) Are mental events preceded by their physical causes? *Philosophical Psychology* **8**(4); 333–340.

Greenhill, L.L. (1992) Pharmacologic treatment of attention deficit hyperactivity disorder. *Psychiatric Clinics of North America* **15**(1); 1–27.

Griffiths, P. (1997) *What Emotions Really Are.* Chicago: University Press.

Guze, S. (1989) Biological psychiatry: is there any other kind? *Psychological Medicine* **19**; 315–323.

Hacking, I. (1995) *Rewriting the Soul.* Princeton: University Press.

Hacking, I. (1998) *Mad Travellers: Reflections on the Reality of Transient Mental Illness.* London: Free Association Books.

Hampshire, S. (1969/1979) Some difficulties in knowing. In *Philosophy As It Is* (Honderich, T. and Burnyeat, M. eds). London: Penguin.

Hare, R.D. (1970) *Psychopathy: Theory and Research.* New York: Wiley.

Hare, R.D. (1980) A research scale for the assessment of psychopathy in criminal populations. *Personality and Individual Differences* **1**; 111–119.

Hare, R.D. (1983) Diagnosis of antisocial personality disorder in two prison populations. *American Journal of Psychiatry* **140**(7); 887–890.

Harlow, H.F. and Harlow M.K. (1972) The young monkeys. In *Readings in Psychology Today*, 2nd edn. Albany: Delmar Publishers.

Harpur, T.J., Hare, R.D., and Hakstian, A.R. (1989) Two-factor conceptualisation of psychopathy: construct validity and assessment implications. *Psychological Assessment: A Journal of Consulting and Clinical Psychology* **1**(1); 6–17.

Harre, H.R. (1983) *Personal Being*. Oxford: Blackwell.

Harre, H.R. and Gillett, G. (1994) *The Discursive Mind*. Thousand Oaks (Cal.): Sage.

Harris, V. (2006) Electroconvulsive therapy: administrative codes, legislation, and professional recommendations. *Journal of the American Academy of Psychiatry and the Law* **34**(3); 406–411.

Havens, L. (1966) Charcot and hysteria. *Journal of Nervous and Mental Diseases* **141**(5); 505–516.

Health Department Victoria (1990) Report of a board of investigation appointed by Mr. T. Daly, Chief General Manager, Health Department Victoria, to enquire into certain clinical and management practices at Lakeside Hospital Ballarat, with specific reference to the death of patient X and the Ward Twenty-Two outing of August 30, 1990.

Heidegger, M. (1953/1996) *Being and Time* (J. Stambaugh, tr). New York: SUNY Press.

Heil, J. (1992) *The Nature of True Minds*. Cambridge: University Press.

Helson, R. (1976) Women and creativity. In *The Creativity Question* (A.Rothenberg and C.R.Hausman, eds). Durham (N.C.): Duke University Press.

Hemsley, D.R. (1977) What have cognitive deficits to do with schizophrenic symptoms. *British Journal of Psychiatry* **130**; 167–173.

Hemsley, D.R. (1992) Cognitive abnormalities and the symptoms of schizophrenia. In *Phenomenology, Language, and Schizophrenia* (M. Spitzer, F. Uehlein, M. Schwartz, and C. Mundt, eds). New York: Springer-Verlag.

Hershman, D.J. and Lieb, J. (1988) *The Key to Genius: Manic Depression and the Creative Life*. New York: Prometheus.

Hill, J.C. and Schoener, E.P. (1996) Age-dependent decline of attention deficit hyperactivity disorder *American Journal of Psychiatry* **153**(9); 1143–1146.

Hinshelwood, R.D. (1995) The social relocation of personal identity as shown by psychoanalytic observations of splitting, projection and introjection. *Philosophy, Psychiatry, and Psychology* **2**(3); 185–204.

Hobson, R.P. (1990) Concerning knowledge of mental states. *British Journal of Medical Psychology* **63**; 199–213.

Hobson, R.P. (1991) What is autism. *Psychiatric Clinics of North America* **14**(1); 1–17.

Hobson, R.P. (1994) On developing a mind. *British Journal of Psychiatry* **165**; 577–581.

Holmes, C.A. (1991) Psychopathic disorder: a category mistake. *Journal of Medical Ethics* **17**(2); 77–86.

Hornsby, J. (1985) Physicalism, events and part-whole relations. In *Actions and Events* (Lepore and McLaughlin, eds). Oxford: Blackwell.

Howard, R.C. (1986) Psychopathy: a psychobiological perspective. *Personality and Individual Differences* **7**; 795–806.

Howard, R.C., Fenton, G.W., and Fenton, P.B.C. (1982) *Event-Related Potentials in Personality and Psychopathology: A Pavlovian Approach*. Letchworth (Herts.) UK: John Wiley & Sons.

Howard, R.C., Fenton, G.W., and Fenwick, P.B.C. (1984) The contingent negative variation, personality and antisocial behaviour. *British Journal of Psychiatry* **144**; 463–477.

Hume, D. (1739/1969) *A Treatise of Human Nature* (E.C. Mossner, ed). London: Penguin.

Hunter, K.M. (1991) *Doctor's Stories.* Princeton: University Press.

Husserl, E. (1950/1999) *Cartesian Meditations* (D. Cairns, tr). Dordrecht: Kluwer.

Husserl, E. (1962) *Ideas* (W.R. Boyce Gibson, ed). New York: Collier.

Husserl, E. (1970) *The Crisis in European Sciences and Transcendental Phenomenology* (D.C. Evanston, tr). Evanston (Ill.): Northwestern University Press.

Ikebuchi, E., Nakagome, K., and Takahashi, N. (1999) How do early stages of information processing affect social skills in patients with schizophrenia. *Schizophrenia Research* **35**; 255–262.

Investigative Task Force (1991) The Investigative Task Force's findings on the Aradale Psychiatric Hospital and Residential Institution. Health and Community Services, Health Department. Victoria.

Jamison, K.R. (1993) *Touched by Fire.* New York: Free Press.

Jamison, K.R. (1996) *An Unquiet Mind.* London: MacMillan.

Janet, P. (1901/1983) *The Mental State of Hystericals* (C.R. Corson, tr). New York: Putnam.

Jaspers, K. (1913/1974) Causal and meaningful connexions between life history and psychosis. In *Themes and Variations in European Psychiatry* (S.R. Hirsch and M. Shepherd, eds). Bristol: John Wright and Sons.

Jaspers, K. (1923/1997) *General Psychopathology* (J.Hoenig and M.W.Hamilton, trs). Baltimore (Md.): Johns Hopkins University Press.

Jaynes, J. (1990) Verbal hallucinations and preconscious mentality. In *Philosophy and Psychopathology* (M. Spitzer and B. Maher, eds). New York: Springer-Verlag.

Jensen, P.S. Hinshaw, S.P., Swanson, J.M. *et al.* (2001) Findings from the NIMH Multimodal Treatment Study of ADHD (MTA): implications and applications for primary-care providers. *Journal of Developmental and Behavioural Pediatrics* **22**(1); 60–73.

Jensen, P.S. Hinshaw, S.P., Swanson, J.M. *et al.* (2007) Three-year follow-up of the NIMH MTA study. *Journal of the American Academy of Child and Adolescent Psychiatry* **46**(8); 989–1002.

Jodelet, D. (1991) *Madness and Social Representations.* Berkeley: University of California Press.

Jolliffe, T., Lansdowne, R., and Robinson, C. (1993) Autism: a personal account. *Communication* **26**(3); 12–19.

Kafka, F. (1953) *The Trial.* London: Penguin.

Kant, I. (1788/1956) *The Critique of Practical Reason* (L.W. Beck, tr). Indianapolis (Ind.): Bobbs Merrill.

Kant, I. (1789/1929) *The Critique of Pure Reason* (N. Kemp Smith, tr). London: Macmillan.

Kant, I. (1790/1951) *Critique of Judgement* (J.H. Bernard, tr). New York: Hafner.

Kant, I. (1793/1960) *Religion within the Bounds of Reason Alone* (T.M. Greene and H.H. Hudson, trs). New York: Harper and Row.

Kant, I. (1798/1978) *Anthropology from a Pragmatic Point of View* (V.L. Dowdell, tr). Carbondale: Southern Illinois University Press.

Kaplan, A. (2002) Psychological treatments for Anorexia. *Canadian Journal of Psychiatry* **47**; 235–242.

Karmiloff-Smith, A. (1986) From meta-process to conscious access: evidence from children's metalinguistic and repair data. *Cognition* **23**; 95–147.

Karmiloff-Smith, A. (1992) *Beyond Modularity.* Cambridge (Mass.): MIT Press.

Kelly, G.A. (1955) *The Psychology of Personal Constructs*. New York: Norton.

Kemp, R., Siew, C., McKenna, P., and David, A. (1997) Reasoning and delusions. *British Journal of Psychiatry* **170**; 398–405.

Kendall-Tackett, K.A., Williams, L.M., and Finkelhor, D. (1993) Impact of sexual abuse of children: a review and synthesis of recent empirical studies. *Psychological Bulletin* **113**(1); 164–180.

Kierkegaard, S. (1843/2001) *Johannes Climacus: A Life of Doubt* (T.H. Croxall, tr). London: Serpent's Tail.

Kierkegaard, S. (1846/1968) *Concluding Unscientific Postscript* (D. Swenson, tr). Princeton: University Press.

Kim, J. (1993) Explanatory realism, causal realism, and explanatory exclusion. In *Explanation* (D. Hillel Rueben, ed). Oxford: University Press.

Kim, J.J., Foy, M.R., and Thompson, R.F. (1996) Behavioural stress modifies hippocampal plasticity through N-methyl-D-aspartate receptor activation. *Proceedings of the National Academy of Sciences* **93**; 4750–4753.

Kim, M-C., Lee, T-K., and Choi, C-R. (2002) Review of long-term results of stereotactic psychosurgery. *Neurologia Medico-Chirurgica* **42**; 365–371.

Klein, R.G. (1995) The role of methylphenidate in psychiatry. *Archives of General Psychiatry* **52**; 429–433.

Klein, R.G., Abikoff, H., Klass, E., Ganeles, D., Scese, L., and Pollack, S. (1997) Clinical efficiency of methylphenidate in conduct disorder with and without attention deficit hyperactivity disorder. *Archives of General Psychiatry* **54**; 1073–1079.

Kleinig, J. (1985) *Ethical Issues in Psychosurgery*. London: Allen and Unwin.

Kocan, P. (1980) *The Treatment and the Cure*. North Ryde: Angus and Robertson.

Koch, C. (2004) *The Quest for Consciousness*. Englewood (Col): Roberts and Co.

Kolers, P.A. and von Grunau, M. (1976) Shape and colour in apparent motion. *Vision Research* **16**; 329–335.

Kovel, D. (1988) A critique of DSM III research. *Law Deviance and Social Control* **9**; 127–146.

Kripke, S. (1982) *Wittgenstein on Rules and Private Language*. Oxford: Blackwell.

Kristeva, J. (1995) *The New Maladies of the Soul*. New York: Columbia University Press.

Lacan, J. (1977) *Ecrits*. New York: Norton & Co.

Lacan, J. (1979) *The Four Fundamental Concepts of Psycho-analysis* (A.Sheridan, tr). London: Penguin.

Laing, A. (1994) *R.D. Laing: A Biography*. London: Peter Owen.

Laing, R.D. (1962/1965) *The Divided Self*. London: Penguin.

Laing, R.D. and Esterson, A. (1970) *Sanity, Madness and the Family*. London: Penguin.

Landry, D. (1989) I believe in God and integration. *The Advocate* **21**(3); 6–7.

Laszlo, J. (1966) The performance of a simple motor task with kinaesthetic sense loss. *Quarterly Journal of Experimental Psychology* **18**; 1–8.

Leslie, A.M. (1987) Pretence and representation: the origins of a theory of mind. *Psychological Review* **94**; 412–416.

Leslie, S. (1988) Diagnosis and treatment of hysterical conversion reactions. *Archives of Disease in Childhood* **63**; 506–511.

Levinas, E. (1996) *Basic Philosophical Writings*. Bloomington: Indiana University Press.

Levy, N. (2007) The responsibility of psychopaths revisited. *Philosophy, psychiatry and psychology* **14**(2); 128–38.

Lewis, A. (1934) The psychopathology of insight. *British Journal of Medical Psychology* **14**; 332–348.

Lewis, D. (1975) Causation. In *Causation and Conditionals* (E. Sosa, ed). Oxford: University Press.

Lewis, D.O. and Bard, J.S. (1991) Multiple personality and forensic issues. *Psychiatric Clinics of North America* **14**(3); 741–756.

Lewis-Fernandez, R. and Kleinman, A. (1995) Cultural psychiatry: theoretical, clinical, and research issues. *The Psychiatric Clinics of North America* **18**(3); 433–448.

Libet, B. (1985) Unconscious cerebral initiative and the role of conscious will in voluntary action. *The Behavioural and Brain Sciences* **8**; 529–566.

Locke, J. (1689/1975) *An Essay Concerning Human Understanding* (P. Nidditch, ed). Oxford: Clarendon.

Loewenstein, R.J. (1991) Multiple personality and child abuse. *Psychiatric Clinics of North America* **14**(3); 741–756.

Loftus, E.F. (1993) The reality of repressed memories. *American Psychologist* **48**(5); 518–537.

Lovibond, S. (2002) *Ethical Formation*. Cambridge (Mass.): Harvard University Press.

Ludwig, A.M. (1994) Mental illness and creative activity in female writers. *American Journal of Psychiatry* **151**; 1650–1656.

Ludwig, A.M., Brandsma, J.M., Wilbur, C.B., Benfeldt, F., and Jameson, D.H. (1972) The objective study of a multiple personality. *Archives of General Psychiatry* **26**; 298–310.

Luria, A.R. (1973) *The Working Brain*. Harmondsworth: Penguin.

Luria, A.R. (1976) *Cognitive Development*. Cambridge (Mass.): Harvard University Press.

Lynn Stephens, G. (1996) Commentary on 'Free will in the light of neuropsychiatry'. *Philosophy, Psychiatry, and Psychology* **3**(2); 97–98.

McCarthy and Thomson. (1996) *The Hungry Heart*. Auckland: Hodder, Moa Beckett.

Macdonald, C. and Macdonald, G., eds. (1995a) *Debates on Psychological Explanation: Philosophy of Psychology*. Oxford: Blackwell.

Macdonald, C. and Macdonald, G., eds. (1995b) *Debates on Psychological Explanation: Connectionism*. Oxford: Blackwell.

Mackie, J. (1974) *The Cement of the Universe*. Oxford: University Press.

MacLean, C. (1977) *The Wolf Children*. London: Allen Lane.

MacLeod, S. (1972) *The Art of Starvation*. London: Allen and Unwin.

Maden, A. (2007) England's new mental health act represents law catching up with science: a commentary on Peter Lepping's ethical analysis of the new mental health legislation in England and Wales [Online]. *Philosophy, Ethics, and Humanities in Medicine*, **2**: 16doi:10.1186/1747-5341-2-16. Available at: http://www.pubmesdcentral.nih.gov/articlerender.fegi?artid=1963448 (accessed 2008 Jul 19).

Maher, B. (1990) The irrelevance of rationality in adaptive behaviour. In *Philosophy and Psychopathology* (M.Spitzer and B.Maher, eds). New York: Springer-Verlag.

Malcolm, N. (1958) Knowledge of other minds. *Journal of Philosophy* **55**(23); 969–978.

Malcolm, N. (1959) *Dreaming*. New York: Humanities Press.

Manschrek, T. (1992) Clinical and experimental analysis of motor phenomena in schizophrenia. In *Phenomenology, Language, and Schizophrenia* (M. Spitzer, F. Uehlein, M. Schwartz, and C. Mundt, eds). New York: Springer-Verlag.

Manshour, G.A., Walker, E.E., and Martuza, R.L. (2005) Psychosurgery: past, present, and future. *Brain Research Reviews* **48**; 409–419.

Martin, C.B. and Deutscher, M. (1966) Remembering. *The Philosophical Review* **75**; 161–196.

Martin, G., Powrie, R., and Ashforth, P. (1997) ADHD in children and adolescents. *New Ethicals* **34**(3); 45–54.

Marx, K. and Engels, F. (1845/1970) *The German Ideology* (C. Arthur, tr). New York: International Publishers.

Massarotto, A. (1996) When is it ethical to administer behaviour altering drugs to children? [Unpublished student essay]. University of Otago Medical School.

McCarthy, A., and Thomson, M. (1996) *The Hungry Heart*. Auckland: Hodder, Moa Beckett.

McEvoy, J.P. Frater, S., Everett, G. *et al.* (1989) Insight and the clinical outcome of schizophrenic patients. *The Journal of Nervous and Mental Disease* **177**; 48–52.

McGhie, A. (1969) *The Pathology of Attention*. London: Penguin.

McIntyre, A.C. (1958) *The Unconscious: A Conceptual Study*. London: Routledge and Kegan Paul.

McMillan, W.T. (1982) Insanity as a defence in a criminal trial [Unpublished manuscript].

McNeish, J. (1997) *The Mask of Sanity*. Wellington: David Ling Publishing.

Meares, R., Hampshire, R., Gordon, E., and Kraiuhin, C. (1985) Whose hysteria: Briquet's, Janet's or Freud's? *Australian and New Zealand Journal of Psychiatry* **19**; 256–263.

Mednick, S.A. (1976) The associative basis of the creative process. In *The Creativity Question* (A. Rothenberg and C.R. Hausman, eds). Durham (N.C.): Duke University Press.

Megone, C. (1998) Aristotle's function argument and the concept of mental illness. *Philosophy, Psychiatry, and Psychology* **5**; 187–201.

Mele, A. (1986) *Irrationality*. Oxford: Clarendon Press.

Mele, A (1987) *Irrationality*. New York: Oxford University press.

Mental Health Review Tribunal (1993) SRT 28/93. *In re J.*

Merleau Ponty, M. (1964) *The Primacy of Perception* (K.Edie, ed). Evanston (Ill.): Northwestern University Press.

Merskey, H. (1995) Multiple personality disorder and false memory syndrome. *British Journal of Psychiatry* **166**; 281–283.

Merskey, H. (1999) Ethical aspects of the physical manipulation of the brain. In *Psychiatric Ethics* (S. Bloch, P. Chodoff, and S. Green, eds). Oxford: University Press, pp. 275–300.

Metzinger, T. (2003) *Being No-one—The Self-Model Theory of Subjectivity*. Cambridge (Mass.): MIT Press.

Metzinger, T. (2004) The subjectivity of subjective experience: a representationalist analysis of the first-person perspective. *Networks* **3**(4); 33–64.

Meyer, D.E. and Schvanenveldt, R.W. (1971) Facilitation in recognizing pairs of words: evidence of a dependence between retrieval operations. *Journal of Experimental Psychology* **90**; 227–234.

Mickley, D.W. (1999) Medical dangers of Anorexia Nervosa and Bulimia Nervosa. In *Eating Disorders: A Reference Sourcebook* (R.Lemberg & L.Cohn eds). Phoenix: Oryx press.

Milberger, S., Biederman, J., Faraone, S.V., Murphy, J., and Tsuang, M.T. (1995) Attention deficit disorder and co-morbid disorders: issues of overlapping symptoms. *American Journal of Psychiatry* **152**(12); 1793–1799.

Miller, L. (1987) Neuropsychology of the aggressive psychopath: an integrative review. *Aggressive Behavior* **13**; 119–140.

Millikan, R. (1984) *Language, Thought, and Other Biological Categories*. Cambridge (Mass.): MIT Press.

Millikan, R. (1993) *White Queen Psychology and Other Essays for Alice*. Cambridge (Mass.): MIT Press.

Millikan, R. (1995) Reply: a bet with Peacocke. In Debates on Psychological Explanation: Philosophy of Psychology Macdonald and Macdonald (eds.) Oxford : Blackwell.

Minuchin, S., Rosman, B.L., and Baker, L. (1978) *Psychosomatic Families: Anorexia Nervosa in Context*. Cambridge (Mass.): Harvard University Press.

Moncrieff, J. (1997) Lithium: evidence reconsidered. *British Journal of Psychiatry* **171**; 113–119.

Montgomery, B. (1996 Nov 24) The very ordinary monster. *Sunday Star Times*, Auckland, New Zealand, p. A13.

Moore, A., Hope, A., and Fulford, W.K.M. (1994) Mild mania and well-being. *Philosophy, Psychiatry, and Psychology* **3**(1); 165–178.

Moray, N. (1987) Attention. In *The Oxford Companion to the Mind* (R.L. Gregory, ed). Oxford: University Press.

Morris, M. (1986) Causes of behaviour. *Philosophical Quarterly* **36**; 123–144.

Morris, M. (1992) *The Good and the True*. Oxford: Clarendon.

Morton, A. (1980) *Frames of Mind*. Oxford: University Press.

Mullen, P. (2004) The autogenic (self-generated) Massacre. *Behavioural Sciences and the Law* **22**; 311–323.

Mullen, P.E. (1992) Psychopathy: a developmental disorder of ethical action. *Criminal Behaviour and Mental Health* **2**; 234–244.

Mullen, P.E. (2007) On building arguments on shifting sands. *Philosophy, Psychiatry, and Psychology* **14**(2); 143–148.

Mullen, P.E., Martin, J.L., Anderson, J.C., Romans, S.E., and Herbison, G.P. (1994) The effect of child sexual abuse of social, interpersonal and sexual function in adult life. *British Journal of Psychiatry* **165**; 35–47.

Mullen, R. (2003) Delusions: the continuum versus category debate. *Australian and New Zealand Journal of Psychiatry* **37**; 505–511.

Nagel, T. (1986) *The View from Nowhere*. New York: Oxford University Press.

Neisser, U. (1976) *Cognition and Reality*. San Francisco (Cal.): Freedman and Sons.

Neisser, U. (1988) What is ordinary memory the memory of? In *Remembering Reconsidered* (U. Neisser and E. Winograd, eds). New York: Columbia University Press.

Nelson (1988) The ontogeny of memory for real events. In *Remembering Reconsidered* (U. Neisser and E. Winograd, eds). New York: Columbia University Press.

Nemiah, J.C. (1989) Janet redivirus: the centenary of *L'automatisme psychologique*. *American Journal of Psychiatry* **146**; 1527–1529.

Nietzsche, F. (1878/1994) *Human All Too Human* (M. Faber and S. Lehmann, trs). London: Penguin.

Nietzsche, F. (1886/1975) *Beyond Good and Evil* (R.J. Hollingdale, tr). London: Penguin.

Nietzsche, F. (1887/1956) *The Genealogy of Morals* (F. Golffing, tr). New York: Doubleday

Nordenfelt, L. (1994) A response to 'Mild mania and well-being'. *Philosophy, Psychiatry, and Psychology* **3**(1); 179–184.

Nussbaum, M. (1990) *Love's Knowledge*. Oxford: University Press.

Nussbaum, M. (1993) Non-relative values: an Aristotelian approach. In *The Quality of Life* (M.Nussbaum and A.Sen, eds). Oxford: University Press, pp. 242–269.

O'Brien, G. and Opie, J. (1997) Cognitive science and phenomenal consciousness: a dilemma and how to avoid it. *Philosophical Psychology* **10**(3); 269–287.

Ofshe, R.J. (1989) Coerced confessions: the logic of seemingly irrational action. *Cultic Studies Journal* **6**; 1–15.

Orbach, S. (1993) *Hunger Strike*. London: Penguin.

Parfit, D. (1971) Personal identity. *Philosophical Review* **80**(1); 3–27.

Parfit, D. (1984) *Reasons and Persons*. Oxford: Clarendon.

Parkin, A.J. (1996) *Explorations in Cognitive Neuropsychology*. Oxford: Blackwell.

Peacocke, C. (1985) Intention and akrasia. In *Essays on Davidson's Actions and Events* (M. Vermazen and M.B. Hintikka, eds). Oxford: Clarendon.

Peacocke, C. (1986) *Thoughts: An Essay on Content*. Oxford: Blackwell.

Perry, W. and Braff, D.L. (1994) Information processing deficits and thought disorder in schizophrenia. *American Journal of Psychiatry* **151**(3); 363–367.

Piaget, J. (1972) *Psychology and Epistemology* (P. Wells, tr). London: Penguin.

Pickering, N. (2006) *The Metaphor of Mental Illness*. Oxford: University Press.

Pigden, C.R. and Gillett, G. (1996) Milgram, method and morality. *Journal of Applied Philosophy* **13**(3); 233–250.

Pinker, S. (1994) *The Language Instinct*. New York: Penguin.

Pinker, S. (1997) *How the Mind Works*. New York: Penguin.

Piper, A. Jr. (1994) Multiple personality disorder: a critical review. *British Journal of Psychiatry* **164**; 600–612.

Plantinga, A. (1993) *Warrant: The Current Debate*. New York: Oxford University Press.

Plato (1961) The ion. In *Plato: The Collected Dialogues* (L. Cooper, tr; Hamilton, E. and Cairns, H. eds). New York: Pantheon.

Pope, H.G. and Hudson, J.I. (1988) Is bulimia nervosa a heterogeneous disorder: lessons from the history of medicine. *International Journal of Eating disorders* **7**; 155–166.

Potter, N. (1996) Loopholes, gaps and what is held fast: democratic epistemology and claims to recovered memories. *Philosophy, Psychiatry, and Psychology* **3**(4); 237–254.

Pressman, J. (1998) *The Last Resort: Psychosurgery and the Limits of Medicine*. Cambridge: University Press.

Putnam, F.W. (1991) Recent research on multiple personality disorder. *Psychiatric Clinics of North America* **14**(3); 489–502.

Putnam, F.W., Guroff, J.J., Silberman, E.K., Barban, L., and Post, R.M. (1986) The clinical phenomenology of multiple personality disorder: review of 100 recent cases. *Journal of Clinical Psychiatry* **47**; 285–293.

Quine, W.V.O. (1953) *From a Logical Point of View*. Cambridge (Mass.): Harvard University Press.

Quine, W.V.O. (1960) *Word and Object*. Cambridge (Mass.): Harvard University Press.

Quinton, A. (1955) The problem of perception. *Mind* **64**; 28–51.

Radio NZ (1997 Jun) Children of Lake Alice.

Raine, A. (2002) Biosocial studies of antisocial and violent behavior in children and adults: a review. *Journal of Abnormal Child Psychology* **30**(4); 311–326.

Rangihau, J. (1992) Learning and Tapu. In *Te Ao Hurihuri* (M. King, ed). Auckland: Reed.

Rapoport, J., Buchsbaum, M., and Weingartner, H. (1980) Dextroamphetamine: its cognitive and behavioral effects in normal and hyperactive boys and normal men. *Archives of General Psychiatry* **37**; 933–943.

Reich, W. (1981) Psychiatric diagnosis as an ethical problem. In *Psychiatric Ethics* (S. Bloch and P. Chodoff, eds). Oxford: University Press.

Rohrbaugh, J.B. (1981) *Women: Psychology's Puzzle*. London: Sphere.

Rosenham, D. (1973) On being sane in insane places. *Science* **179**; 250–258.

Ross, C.A. (1991) Epidemiology of multiple personality disorder and dissociation. *Psychiatric Clinics of North America* **14**; 503–517.

Rumelhart, D.E., McClelland, J.L., and the PDP Research Group (1986) *Parallel Distributed Processing Explorations in the Microstructure of Cognition*. Cambridge (Mass.): MIT Press.

Rumsey, J.M. (1992) Neuropsychological studies of high-level autism. In *High Functioning Individuals with Autism* (E. Schopler and G. Mesibov, eds). New York: Plenum.

Russell, B. (1959) *The problems of philosophy*. London: Unwin.

Russell, D. (1995) *Women, Madness, and Medicine*. Cambridge (Mass.): Polity Press.

Rutter, M., Cox, A., Tupling, C., Berger, M., and Yule, W. (1975) Attainment and adjustment in two geographical areas. I: the prevalence of psychiatric disorders. *British Journal of Psychiatry* **126**; 493–509.

Rymer, R. (1994) *Genie: A Scientific Tragedy*. London: Penguin.

Sacks, O. (1995) *An Anthropologist on Mars*. Sydney: Picador.

Salmon, W. (1993) Scientific explanation and the causal structure of the world. In *Explanation* (D. Hillel Rueben, ed). Oxford: University Press.

Sandberg, S. (1996) Hyperkinetic or attention deficit disorder. *British Journal of Psychiatry* **169**; 10–17.

Sartre, J.P. (1958) *Being and Nothingness* (H. Barnes, tr). London: Methuen & Co.

Sartre, J.P. (1972) *The Psychology of Imagination* (P. Fechtman, tr). London: Methuen.

Sass, L.A. (1992) Phenomenological aspects of 'Zerfarenheit' and incoherence. In *Phenomenology, Language, and Schizophrenia* (M.S pitzer, F. Uehlein, M. Schwartz, and C. Mundt, eds). New York: Springer-Verlag.

Sass, L. and Parnas, J. (2003) Schizophrenia, consciousness and the self. *Schizophrenia Bulletin* **29**(3); 427–444

Sass, L. and Parnas, J. (2007) Explaining schizophrenia: the relevance of phenomenology. In *Reconceiving Schizophrenia* (M.C. Chung, K.W.M. Fulford, and G. Graham, eds). Oxford: University Press, pp. 63–96.

Schechtman, M. (1994) The truth about memory. *Philosophical Psychology* **7**(1); 3–20.

Schechtman, M. (1996) *The Constitution of Selves*. Ithaca (N.Y.): Cornell University Press.

Schechtman, M. (2005) Personal identity and the past. *Philosophy, Psychiatry, and Psychology* **12**(1); 9–22.

Schore, A. (1998) The experience-dependent maturation of an evaluative system in the cortex. In *Brain and Values: Is a Biological Science of Values Possible?* (K. Pribram, ed). Mahwah N.J. Lawrence Erlbaum.

Schou, M. (1979) Artistic productivity and lithium prophylaxis in manic-depressive illness. *British Journal of Psychiatry* **135**; 97–103.

Schou, M. (1997) Forty years of lithium treatment. *Archives of General Psychiatry* **54**; 9–13.

Searle, J. (1992) *The Rediscovery of Mind*. Cambridge (Mass.): Bradford Books.

Seedhouse, D. (1994) The trouble with well-being: a response to 'Mild mania and well-being'. *Philosophy, Psychiatry, and Psychology* **3**(1); 185–192.

Servan Schreiber, D., Cohen, J.D., and Steingard, S. (1996) Schizophrenic defects in the processing of context. A test of a theoretical model. *Archives of general psychiatry* **53** (12); 1105–12.

Shaffer, D. (1994) Attention deficit disorder in adults. *American Journal of Psychiatry* **151**(5); 633–638.

Shapiro, D. (1965) *Neurotic Styles*. New York: Basic Books.

Sharfstein, S. (2005) Big pharma and American psychiatry: the good, the bad, and the ugly. *Psychiatric News* **40**(16); 3–4.

Shoemaker, S. (1963) *Self-Knowledge and Self-identity*. Ithaca (N.Y.): Cornell University Press.

Shoemaker, S. (1984) *Identity, Cause and Mind*. Cambridge: University Press.

Showalter, E. (1987) *The Female Malady: Women, Madness and English Culture 1830–1980*. London: Virago.

Sims, A. (1994) 'Psyche'—spirit as well as mind? *British Journal of Psychiatry* **165**; 441–446.

Sinclair, J. (1992) Bridging the gaps: an inside-out view of autism, or do you know what I don't know? In *High Functioning Individuals with Autism* (E. Schopler and G. Mesibov, eds). New York: Plenum.

Sinclair, J. (1993) Don't mourn for us. *Conference Proceedings: A World of Options*. Autism Network International. Toronto, Canada.

Slater, E. (1965) The diagnosis of hysteria. *British Journal of Medicine* **1**; 1395–1399.

Sleator, E.K., Ullman, R.K., and von Neumann, A. (1982) How do hyperactive children feel about taking stimulants and will they tell the doctor. *Clinical Paediatrics* **21**(6); 474–479.

Smith, M. (1994) *The Moral Problem*. Oxford: Blackwell.

Smith, S.M. and Blankenship, S.E. (1991) Incubation and the persistence of fixation in problem solving. *American Journal of Psychology* **104**; 61–87.

Smolensky, P. (1988) On the proper treatment of connectionism. *Behavioural and Brain Sciences* **11**; 1–74.

Smolensky, P. (1995) Connectionism, constituency and the language of thought. In *Debates on Psychological Explanation: Philosophy of Psychology* (C. Macdonald and G. Macdonald, eds). Oxford: Blackwell.

Snowdon, P. (1990) Persons, animals and ourselves. In *The Person and the Human Mind* (C. Gill, ed). Oxford: Clarendon.

Solomon, R. (1989) *From Hegel to Existentialism*. Oxford: University Press.

Solomon, P.R., Crider, A., Winkelman, J.W., Turi, A., Kamer, R.M. and Kaplan, L.J., (1981) Disrupted latent inhibition in the rat with chronic amphetamine or haloperidol induced supersensitivity: relationship to schizophrenic attention disorder. *Biol. Psychiat.* **16**; 519–537.

Sorenson, R.A. (1986) Self-deception and scattered events. *Mind* **XCVI**; 64–69.

Spanos, NP. (1994) Multiple Identity Enactments and Multiple Personality Disorder: a socio-cognitive perspective. *Psychological Bulletin* **116**(1); 143–65.

Spence, S. (1996) Free will in the light of neuropsychiatry. *Philosophy, Psychiatry, and Psychology* **3**(2); 75–90.

Sperry, R. (1979) Brain bisection and the mechanisms of consciousness. In *The Brain and Conscious Behaviour* (J.C. Eccles, ed). New York: Springer.

Spitzer, M. (1990a) Why philosophy. In *Philosophy and Psychopathology* (M. Spitzer and B. Maher, eds). New York: Springer-Verlag.

Spitzer, M. (1990b) On defining delusions. *Comprehensive Psychiatry* **31**; 377–397.

Spitzer, M. (1990c) Kant on schizophrenia. In *Philosophy and Psychopathology* (M. Spitzer and B. Maher, eds). New York: Springer-Verlag; pp. 44–58

Spitzer, M. (1992) Word-associations in experimental psychiatry. In *Phenomenology, Language, and Schizophrenia* (M. Spitzer, F. Uehlein, M. Schwartz, and C. Mundt, eds). New York: Springer-Verlag.

Stanghellini, G. (2004) *Disembodied Spirits and Deanimated Bodies*. Oxford: University Press.

Stein, M.B., Koverola, C., Hanna, C., *et al.* (1997) Hippocampal volume in women victimized by childhood sexual abuse. *Psychological Medicine* **27**; 951–959.

Stek, M.L., Wurff van der, F.F.B., Hoogendijk, W.J.G., Beekman, A.T.F. (2003) Electroconvulsive therapy for the depressed elderly. *Cochrane Database of Systematic Reviews* 2003, Issue 2. Art. No.: CD003593. DOI: 10.1002/14651858.CD003593.

Stephens, G.L. (1996) Commentary on 'Free will in the light of neuropsychiatry'. *Philosophy, Psychiatry, and Psychology* **3**(2); 97–98.

Stephens, G.L. and Graham, G. (2000) *When Self-consciousness Breaks*. Cambridge (Mass.): MIT Press.

Stevenson, R.L. (1886/1994) *The Strange Case of Dr. Jekyll and Mr. Hyde*. Ware (Herts; UK): Wordsworth.

Stich, S. (1990) *The Fragmentation of Reason*. Cambridge (Mass.): MIT Press.

Stone, J., Smyth, R., Carson, A. *et al.* (2005) Systematic review of misdiagnosis of conversion symptoms and 'hysteria'. *British Medical Journal* **331**; 989–993.

Storr, A. (1987) Jung's concept of personality. In *Persons and Personality* (A. Peacocke and G. Gillett, eds). Oxford: Blackwell.

Storr, A. (1989) *Churchill's Black Dog and Other Phenomena of the Human Mind*. London: Collins.

Strawson, P. (1966) *The Bounds of Sense*. London: Methuen.

Strawson, P. (1974) *Freedom and Resentment and Other Essays*. London: Methuen.

Strawson, P. (1985) Causation and explanation. In *Essays on Davidson's Actions and Events* (M. Vermazen and M.B. Hintikka, eds). Oxford: Clarendon.

Sullivan, R.C. (1992) *Rain Man and Joseph*. In *High Functioning Individuals with Autism* (E. Schopler and G. Mesibov, eds). New York: Plenum.

Szasz, T. (1962/1972) *The Myth of Mental Illness*. London: Paladin.

Szatmari, P. (1991) Asperger's syndrome: diagnosis, treatment, and outcome. *Psychiatric Clinics of North America* **14**(1); 81–93.

Szekeley, E. (1988) *Never Too thin*. Toronto: Women's Press.

Taylor, C. (1964) *The Explanation of Behaviour*. London: Routledge and Kegan Paul.

Taylor, C. (1989) *Sources of the Self*. Cambridge (Mass.): Harvard University Press.

Taylor, C. (1991) *The Malaise of Modernity*. Toronto: Anansi.

Taylor, W.S. and Martin, M.F. (1944) Multiple personality. *Journal of Abnormal and Social Psychology* **39**; 281–300.

Thigpen, C.H. and Cleckley, H. (1957) *The Three Faces of Eve*. New York: McGraw-Hill.

Tobin, B.M. (1989) An Aristotelian theory of moral development. *Journal of Philosophy of Education* **23**(2); 195–211.

Torrance, E.P. (1976) Education and creativity. In *The Creativity Question* (A. Rothenberg and C.R. Hausman, eds). Durham (N.C.): Duke University Press.

Treasure, J.L., Schmidt, U., and van Furth, E. (eds.) (2003) *Handbook of Eating Disorders*. Chichester: Wiley.

Trevarthen, C. (1979) Communication and cooperation in early infancy: as description of primary intersubjectivity. In *Before Speech* (M. Bullowa, ed). Cambridge: University Press.

Vaillant, G.E. (1975) Sociopathy as a human process: a viewpoint. *Archives of General Psychiatry* **32**; 178–183.

Vallacher, R.R. and Wegner, D.M. (1987) What do people think they're doing? Action identification and human behaviour. *Psychological Review* **94**; 3–15.

Vanderwolf, C.H. (1985) Nineteenth-century psychology and twentieth-century electrophysiology do not mix. *The Behavioural and Brain Sciences* **8**; 555.

Van t'Hof, S.E. (1994) *Anorexia Nervosa: The Historical and Cultural Specificity.* Lisse Netherlands: Swets and Zeitlinger.

Venables, P.H. (1960) The effect of auditory and visual stimulation on the skin potential responses of schizophrenics. *Brain* **83**; 77–92.

Verrier, N.N. (1992) The primal wound: legacy of the adopted child. Paper presented at the American Adoption Congress International Convention, 1991. Garden City, California.

Vygotsky, L.S. (1962/1929) *Thought and Language* (E. Hanfmann and G. Vakar, trs). Cambridge (Mass.): MIT Press.

Vygotsky, L.S. (1978) *Mind in Society.* Cambridge (Mass.): Harvard University Press.

Walker, A.F. (1988) The problem of weakness of the will. *Nous* **23**(5); 653–676.

Walker, R. (1992) The relevance of Maori myth and tradition. In *Te Ao Hurihuri* (M. King, ed). Auckland: Reed.

Wallach, M.A. and Kogan, N. (1976) Creativity and intelligence in children. In *The Creativity Question* (A. Rothenberg and C.R. Hausman, eds). Durham (N.C.): Duke University Press.

Walsh, B.T. (1991) Fluoxetine treatment of bulimia nervosa. *Journal of Psychosomatic Research* **35**(Suppl); 33–40.

Wegner, D. (2002) *The Illusion of the Conscious will.* Cambridge (Mass.): MIT Press.

Weinberg, J.R. and Yandell, K.E. (1971) *Problems in Philosophical Inquiry.* New York: Holt, Rinehart, and Winston.

Weiskrantz, L. (1986) *Blindsight: A Case Study and Its Implications.* Oxford: Clarendon.

Weiskrantz, L. (1987) Neuropsychology and the nature of consciousness. In *Mindwaves* (C. Blakemore and S. Greenfield, eds). Oxford: Blackwell.

Weiss, G. (1985) Hyperactivity overview and new directions. *Psychiatric Clinics of North America* **8**(4); 737–753.

Wexler, D.B. (1996) Therapeutic jurisprudence in clinical practice. *American Journal of Psychiatry* **153**(4); 453–455.

Whitlock, F.A. (1967) Prichard and the concept of moral insanity. *Australian and New Zealand Journal of Psychiatry* **1**; 72–79.

Whybrow, P.C. (1994) Of the muse and moods mundane. *American Journal of Psychiatry* **151**; 477–479.

Wiggins, D. (1987) The person as object of science, as subject of experience and as locus of value. In *Persons and Personality* (A. Peacocke and G. Gillett, eds). Oxford: Blackwell.

Wiggins, O., Schwartz, M.A., and Northoff, G. (1990) Toward a Husserlian phenomenology of the initial stages of schizophrenia. In *Philosophy and Psychopathology* (M. Spitzer and B. Maher, eds). New York: Springer-Verlag.

Wilbur, C.B. (1984) Multiple personality and child abuse. *Psychiatric Clinics of North America* **7**(1); 3–7.

Wilens, T.E. and Biederman, J. (1992) The stimulants. *Psychiatric Clinics of North America* **15**(1); 191–222.

Williams, B. (1981) *Moral Luck.* Cambridge: University Press.

Williams, B. (1985) *Ethics and the Limits of Philosophy.* London: Collins.

Williams, L.M. (1994) Recall of childhood trauma: a prospective study of women's memories of child sexual abuse. *Journal of Consulting and Clinical Psychology* **62**; 1167–1176.

Wilson, P. (1974) *Oscar: An Inquiry into the Nature of Sanity.* New York: Random House.

Wilson, P. (1973) *Crab Antics: The Social Anthropology of English-Speaking Negro Societies of the Caribbean.* New Haven (Conn.): Yale University Press.

Wilson, C. and Seaman, D. (1992) *The Serial Killers.* London: Virgin.

Winch, P. (1958) *The Idea of a Social Science and Its Relation to Philosophy.* London: Routledge.

Winchester, E. and Collier, D. et al. (2003) *Genetic Aetiology of Eating Disorders and Obesity in Treasure.*

Wing, J. (1978) *Reasoning about Madness.* Oxford: University Press.

Winnicott, D.W. (1964) *The Child, the Family, and the Outside World.* London: Penguin.

Wittgenstein, L. (1922) *Tractatus Logico Philosophicus* (D. Pears and B. McGuiness, eds). London: Routledge and Kegan Paul.

Wittgenstein, L. (1953) *Philosophical Investigations* (G.E.M. Anscombe, tr). Oxford: Blackwell.

Wittgenstein, L. (1967) *Zettel.* (G.E.M. Anscombe and G.H. von Wright, trs and eds). Oxford: Basil Blackwell.

Wittgenstein, L. (1969) *On Certainty* (G.E.M. Anscombe and G.H. von Wright, trs and eds). New York: Harper.

Wittgenstein, L. (1976) Cause and effect: intuitive awareness. *Philosophia* **6**(3–4); 415ff.

Wittgenstein, L. (1980a) *Remarks on the Philosophy of Psychology I and II* (G.E.M. Anscombe and G.H. von Wright, trs and eds). Oxford: Basil Blackwell.

Wittgenstein, L. (1980b) *Culture and Value* (P. Winch, tr). Oxford: Blackwell.

Worley, S. (1997) Belief and consciousness. *Philosophical Psychology* **10**(1); 41–56.

Young, J.Z. (1986) *Philosophy and the Brain.* Oxford: University Press.

Zahavi, D. (2004) *Subjectivity and Selfhood.* Cambridge (Mass): MIT Press.

Zerbe, K.J. (1996) Feminist psychodynamic psychotherapy of eating disorders. *Psychiatric Clinics of North America* **19**(4); 811–827.

Index